Hands in Health Care

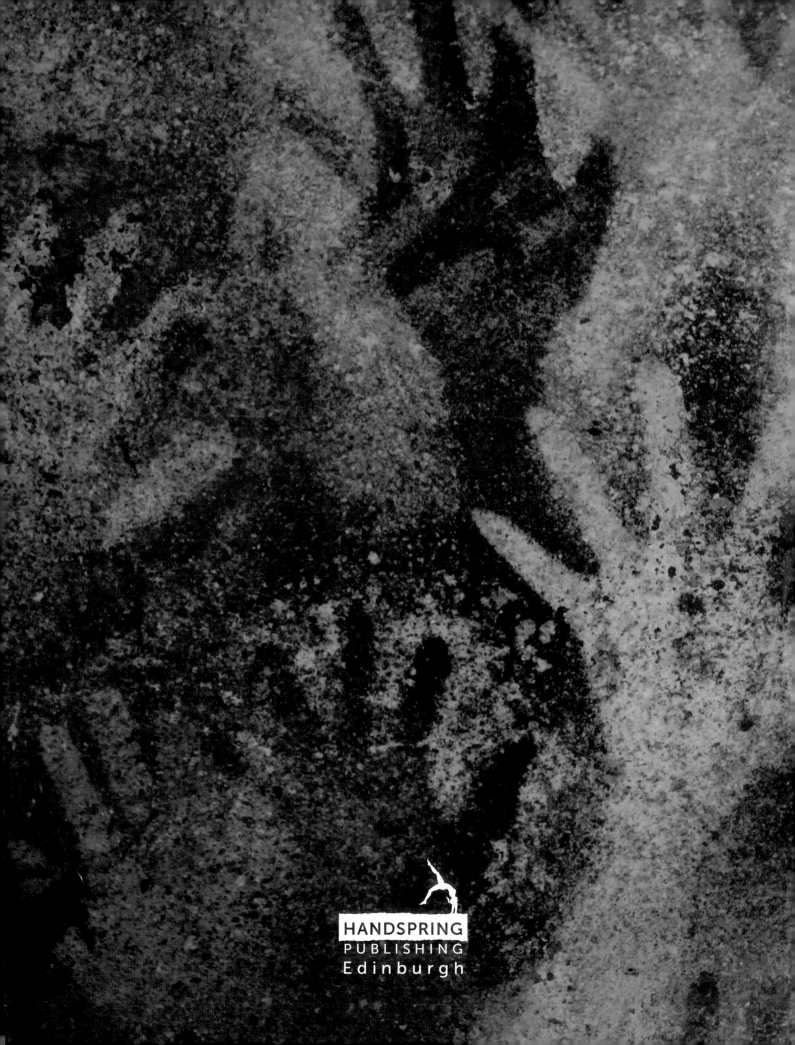

HANDSPRING
PUBLISHING
Edinburgh

Second edition

Hands in Health Care

Massage therapy for the adult hospital patient

Gayle MacDonald ◆ Carolyn Tague

Forewords

Ruth Werner ◆ Wolf E Mehling

HANDSPRING PUBLISHING LIMITED
The Old Manse, Fountainhall,
Pencaitland, East Lothian
EH34 5EY, United Kingdom
Tel: +44 1875 341 859
Website: www.handspringpublishing.com

The first edition of *Massage for the Hospital Patient and Medically Frail Client* by Gayle MacDonald was published by Lippincott Williams and Wilkins in 2004.

First published 2021 in the United Kingdom by Handspring Publishing

ISBN 978-1-912085-54-5
ISBN (Kindle eBook) 978-1-912085-55-2

British Library Cataloguing in Publication Data
A catalogue record for this book is available from the British Library

Library of Congress Cataloguing in Publication Data
A catalog record for this book is available from the Library of Congress

Notice
Neither the Publisher nor the Authors assume any responsibility for any loss or injury and/or damage to persons or property arising out of or relating to any use of the material contained in this book. It is the responsibility of the treating practitioner, relying on independent expertise and knowledge of the patient, to determine the best treatment and method of application for the patient.

All reasonable efforts have been made to obtain copyright clearance for illustrations in the book for which the authors or publishers do not own the rights. If you believe that one of your illustrations has been used without such clearance please contact the publishers and we will ensure that appropriate credit is given in the next reprint.

Commissioning Editor Mary Law
Copy Editor Susan Stuart
Project Managers Susan Stuart, Morven Dean
Designer Bruce Hogarth
Indexer Aptara, India
Typesetter DiTech Process Solutions, India
Printer Replika, India

The
Publisher's
policy is to use
paper manufactured
from sustainable forests

CONTENTS

Foreword by Ruth Werner   vii
Foreword by Wolf E Mehling   viii
About the authors   ix
Acknowledgments   x
Figure permissions   xi
Preface   xii
Glossary   xiii
Introduction   xxix

1 Holders of a legacy: The evolution of hospital-based massage therapy   1

2 A frontier of knowledge: Exploring the research   5
Gayle MacDonald with Carolyn Jauco-Trott

3 Adapting to hospital culture: Traveling in a foreign land   45

4 The spectrum of caring: Understanding the therapeutic relationship   61

5 Protecting patients and practitioners: Infection control practices   71

6 Pressure, site and position: A clinical framework   91

7 An overview of common diseases requiring health care treatment   107

8 Common symptoms and conditions: Sign posts for the massage therapist   153

9 What's that beeping? Medical devices and procedures   177

10 Pharmaceutical factors: Adjustments for medications   203

11 Gathering information: Referrals, orders and intake   227

12 One on one: The massage therapy session   243

13 Beyond touch: Aromatherapy massage sessions in health care   263
Angela Secretan

14 Sacred time: Touch at the end of life   283
Cindy Spence

15 The value of documentation: Charting protocols   305

16 Trending into the future: Possibilities and probabilities   319

Appendix   323

Test answers   331

Index   333

A legacy to be proud of

I entered the massage therapy profession in the early 1980s. At that time education programs were short and informal. We had no textbooks specifically for massage therapists. We entered the field ready to give high-quality Swedish massage to healthy people – and not much else.

Back in those days we were taught that: "Massage and cancer don't go in the same sentence" (a verbatim quote from my first pathology teacher), and we received no education whatever about working in health care settings. The thought of working with other than perfectly healthy clients was alien and terrifying. No one I knew at that time intended to build a career in working with clients with chronic or life-threatening illnesses. And the thought of working in a hospital or hospice? Inconceivable.

Fast-forward a few decades and my, how things have changed! Massage therapy in hospitals and other health care facilities is a fast-growing specialty. Scientific research demonstrates that our work offers significant benefits for patients in settings from pre-op suites to post-surgical rehabilitation, and beyond. Outstanding education for working in this environment is available now, from a variety of talented practitioners and teachers – education that can easily be based on this important text. Most importantly, the people who most need skilled massage: the sick, the frail, the medically complex, can now have access to our work.

It has been my pleasure and honor to know Gayle Mac-Donald for many years. She and I were among the first authors to write and publish texts specifically for massage therapists, and oh, we have some stories from the old days! Gayle is one of a handful of massage therapists from that era who was willing to push back on the common wisdom about who was safe to receive massage, and as such, she was a pioneer, bravely exploring new pathways for massage therapists to work with medically complex patients. It's hard to explain how courageous that was: she was challenging a deeply held tradition that kept massage therapy firmly separate from conventional health care. Ironically, she did that by reminding us of a time when compassionate, educated touch (as opposed to skilled but hurried task-related handling) was an integral part of caring for sick people.

I remember when the first edition of this book, titled *Massage for the Hospital Patient and Medically Frail Client*, came out in 2004. I read it with gratitude, and then gave it to a student who had an opportunity to create a hospital-based massage therapy program. Then I bought it again, and passed it on – again. I have used it to inform my writing and my teaching, and I have waited impatiently for a new edition.

With *Hands in Health Care*, Gayle MacDonald and Carolyn Tague have cemented a legacy in the massage therapy field. This beautifully written text is grounded in current research, but it is rich in the grace and compassion that inspire us to serve people who are in need. I love their thoughtful voices, along with their many examples of practical application of basic principles. Reader, you are in for a treat.

Thank you, Gayle and Carolyn, for helping to open this pathway for massage therapists. Thank you for reminding us where we came from, and showing us where we can go next. Our profession is better for your contribution.

Ruth Werner BCTMB

Author, *A Massage Therapist's Guide to Pathology: Critical Thinking, Practical Application*

Waldport, Oregon, USA
September, 2020

Massage has a long tradition, thousands of years, in many cultures around the world. In the late 1700s, French missionaries returned from China and brought home a variety of clearly described massage techniques. These techniques still carry their French names, although they were classified originally in China. Later in the 1800s, these became also known and taught in Sweden, from where they were imported to New York in the mid-1800s, acquiring the name "Swedish" massage. Until the early and mid-1900s these techniques were still taught to, and often practiced by, nurses or physical therapists in medical settings. Then massages became more and more relegated to "alternative medicine" or luxurious spa culture. Now, in the past two decades, massage has gained renewed interest in the healing professions and even become a topic for medical research. And with its growing support from studies published in high-impact medical journals, it is (very slowly) finding its way again, from complementary treatments reserved for those who can afford it, into major hospitals. So it is the perfect time to have here in hand a comprehensive book on the topic of massage in the hospital setting, written by experienced practitioners, who can explain these techniques to other massage practitioners and health care providers.

Beginning in 2007, I was lucky enough to author the first massage studies conducted at our academic institution. During pre-operative assessments and the recruitment for the first study, 85% of all invited potential participants immediately agreed to be in the study. Eighty-five percent wanted a massage! This was a first and big surprise for everybody in the hospital and the research team. A second surprise came when patients were discharged from the hospital after recovery from cancer surgery. On the day of discharge, patients did not want to go home early in the morning when they were expecting another study massage later in the day: another massage was worth the wait. The third surprise for the hospital leadership was that, coincidentally or not, the patients' satisfaction with in-hospital care had improved just during the time of the study, according to the regular routine surveys. In a second study, conducted on the isolation ward for children undergoing bone marrow transplantation, it was reported that a mother stood guard outside the room of her sleepless daughter to prevent the nursing staff from interrupting the one relaxing moment of the day when she received tender care. That was when her beloved daughter received the study intervention, a foot massage that made her fall asleep.

So, massage should come with a warning: if hospitals want to offer massages to their patients, they may not want to go home. And they may not want to be interrupted for temperature taking, blood draws or blood pressure checks. But patient satisfaction may go up, coincidentally or not.

Wolf E Mehling MD
Professor, Family and Community Medicine
University of California at San Francisco, USA
September, 2020

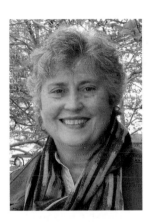

Gayle MacDonald MS, LMT began her career as a secondary school health teacher. In 1989, she became a massage therapist, which led to the blending of her experience from these two careers. After finishing massage school, she started teaching body-mind education for massage students. A serendipitous phone call in 1993 led her to develop a hospital massage program for cancer patients at Oregon Health and Science University (OHSU) in Portland, Oregon. Over time, she worked with heart transplant patients, women hospitalized because of high-risk pregnancy, orthopedic, and general medicine patients.

Gayle is a pioneer. Her book, *Medicine Hands: Massage Therapy for People with Cancer* (Findhorn Press), was pivotal in overcoming the myth that people with cancer could not have massage due to the fear of metastases. Gayle has travelled and taught in the United States, Canada, Scotland, Ireland, Australia, The Netherlands, and Belgium, sharing what she has learned since starting at OHSU over 25 years ago.

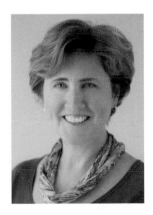

Carolyn Tague MA, CMT first studied with Gayle MacDonald in 2005 when the original version of this book was published. Since then she has worked in four hospital systems. For six years Carolyn taught in a hospital-based integrative medicine education program and then went on to establish Tague Consulting where she provides continuing education courses including Oncology Massage Therapy, Massage for People Living with Neurological Challenges, and Building Therapeutic Relationships, among others. She continues to work and teach in hospital settings including the University of California, San Francisco Medical Center and Laguna Honda Hospital. Carolyn is a frequent speaker at massage therapy and integrative medicine conferences and participates in hospital-based massage therapy research at UCSF. She serves on the Hospital-Based Massage Therapy Task Force of the Academic Collaborative for Integrative Health and on the Educator's Forum of the Society for Oncology Massage. With over 15 years teaching experience, being invited to co-author this book was a dream come true.

ACKNOWLEDGMENTS

The first big thanks go to Carolyn Jauco-Trott (KK) for the inspiration that brought this book into being. Her energy and vision compelled us forward!

There have been many wonderful contributors to this text, which we hope the reader will agree adds depth and breadth to the content presented. For sharing poems, stories and cases, much gratitude to: Sharon Brahms, Christine Douglass, Grace Dammann, Lee Daniel Erman, Christine Knapp, Yukiko Kukimoto, Kate Phelan, Meg Robsahm LMT, Irene Smith, Mary Aguilera-Titus LMT, BCTMB, Allison Young, Del Delamutt LMT, Tammy Walker LMT, BCTMB, Mary Malinski RN, LMT, Ann Marie McGrath RGN, BSc, Jacki Sellers LMT, Dayle Halverson, Cathrine Weaver MSN, RN, and Heather Stauffer LMT.

Thanks to Lauren "Cal" Cates LMT and Kerry Jordan LMT for taking time to write the ICU section in Chapter 7, to Rachel Zoffness PhD who shared her expertise regarding the study of pain, and to Karen Armstrong for her review of the Maternity section.

Appreciation goes to Carolyn Jauco-Trott for searching out, ordering, and boxing up many of the studies in Chapter 2.

For sharing documentation samples and perspectives, it wasn't always easy to get permissions, so thank you for the extra efforts to: Karen Armstrong, Beaumont Health; Lauren Cates and Kerry Jordan, Healwell; Mary Kathleen Rose; Shawnee Isaac Smith, Heart Touch Project; Estelle Smits, Massage bij Kanker; UCSF.

For reviewing Chapter 9, many thanks to Amie Mascarinas-Galleri RN and Sanjay Reddy MD; and many thanks to Cathrine Weaver from Lexington Baptist Hospital who provided cardiac expertise for the Clinical considerations section.

For their major contribution to Chapter 10 – which we could not have attempted alone – our deepest gratitude goes to Carol Baillie RN, CMT and Hannah Baillie RN, amazing nurses and mother and daughter team.

Deep gratitude to Angela Secretan for overcoming her fear of writing in order to take on Chapter 13, and to Cindy Spence for writing Chapter 14. Cindy would like to thank Susan Gee for assisting; Nurse Practitioner Deb Rice of Faith Presbyterian Hospice, Dallas, Texas; Valerie Hartman for her encouragement and inspiration; and Tracy Walton for positioning training.

One idea that we and the publishers committed to early was to feature full color, quality photographs that could help guide readers as only pictures can. Thank you to the teams of photographers, practitioners and volunteer patients in sourcing these. Sincerest gratitude for vital contributions goes to:

Photographers: John Welander (Portland, Oregon) and Andrew Secretan (St. Boswells, Scotland).

Baptist Health Lexington Team: Cathrine Weaver, Lee Ball, Jill Cole, Carolyn Jauco-Trott, Jessica Newton, Rebecca Roark, Erin Mills and Tracy Baker. With a special thanks to their nurse champion, Cathrine Weaver. Thank you for making it all happen!

Oregon Health and Sciences University team: Annette Lovett and Gayle MacDonald.

University of California, San Francisco team: Alexa Ehlen, Mary Destri, Barbara Gideon, Rachael Newsom, Kate Phelan, and Carolyn Tague.

Many volunteer hours go into the various bits and pieces of a book. There are numerous people whose names don't appear anywhere but who made a vital contribution: Karen Casciato, massage therapist in Portland, Oregon; Kaman Cheung, aroma massage therapist, Hong Kong; Marcella MacDonald, retired nurse; and Gillian Jackson, palliative care specialist from Melbourne, Australia.

And finally, big thanks go to Handspring, and specifically Mary Law and Andrew Stevenson, for the opportunity to advance this aspect of massage therapy. Working with them has been the best of all worlds; they are heart-centered professionals.

ACKNOWLEDGMENTS *continued*

Gayle's acknowledgments

Writing a book is an arduous process. I knew from the beginning I couldn't do this on my own. I am eternally grateful to Carolyn Tague for saying, "Yes." Her tenacity, responsibility, good humor in the face of stress, and love of the subject carried me through.

Thank you to Sharon Fisher for being my IT angel and for always being there when I needed her.

I am so grateful for the opportunity to work with such a generous, loving, and devoted group of people. You are my inspiration.

Carolyn's acknowledgments

I want to take this opportunity to not only acknowledge, but to publicly express my most heart-felt gratitude to Gayle MacDonald. Not only was it an honor to be invited to co-author her second edition of this textbook, it has been a truly fulfilling experience. Gayle's gentle guidance and openness, without ever a tinge of pressure has in itself been an amazing learning experience. Gayle stayed open, encouraging and always kind. This was an unexpected but most appreciated gift to my soul. Along the way, my associate Barbara Gideon offered to help with the time-consuming and stress-producing reference and citation clean up. That offer and her subsequent detailed work allowed me to sleep for the first time in months. Thank you Barbara for saving my health!

In addition to my gratitude to my co-author and all our colleagues, I wish to state here my mind-body-spirit gratefulness to my spouse Nancy, whose support and patience has been beyond what one could hope for. Thank you, my Nancy.

And finally, the students whom I have spoken to in my head over the course of this project: You are the vision of the future, thank you for showing up and finding this text! You will be relatively few in number, but you will be great on the path of keeping the "care" in health care.

Figure permissions

Figure 1.2
From the *Otago Witness*, Issue 3403, June 4, 1919. Courtesy of the National Library of New Zealand.

Table 6.1
The Pressure Scale was developed by and is used by the gracious permission of Tracy Walton, Tracy Walton and Associates, Cambridge, Massachusetts, USA.

Figures 9.3, 9.6, 9.8
Photos courtesy of Baptist Health, Lexington, Kentucky, USA.

Figure 11.3
Courtesy of University of California, San Francisco, USA.

Figure 11.5
Courtesy of Karen Armstrong, Beaumont Hospital, Royal Oak, Michigan, USA.

Figure 11.6
Courtesy of Shawnee Isaac Smith, Founder, Heart Touch Project, Santa Monica, California, USA.

Figure 15.1
Courtesy of Beaumont Hospital, Royal Oak, Michigan, USA.

PREFACE

Massage therapy has a place in restoring well-being to people who are affected by illness, accident, aging, or medical treatment. *Hands in Health Care: Massage Therapy for the Adult Hospital Patient* is a resource for manual therapists whose practice is to care for patients who are within the health care establishment. Although the title might lead one to believe that the focus is just on hospital care, and that the book is just for massage therapists, it is far from that. This book is for the therapist who works in the rehabilitation setting, palliative care and hospice, skilled nursing facility, outpatient clinic, or doctor's office. This is a text for all bodyworkers, whether employees, contractors, or volunteers. It is for nursing staff or others who provide touch therapies, such as Reiki, Craniosacral Therapy, or Healing Touch, for medically complex people.

Hands in Health Care is the second edition of a text originally titled *Massage for the Hospital Patient and Medically Frail Client*, a publication of Lippincott Williams and Wilkins (Wolters Kluwer). Nearly a full generation has passed since the first edition, which was published in 2004. That is eons in the health care field as well as in the global domain. The changes that have occurred in that amount of time are astonishing. Technological developments, political pressures, and limited resources have changed many aspects of life, and without a doubt have altered the delivery of health care, in some ways for better and in some for worse.

Despite the mind-boggling changes over the past 16 years, massage, at its core, remains much the same. It is a timeless art that still brings comfort, relaxation, and a feeling of acceptance. The types of strokes, the adjustments due to procedures or disease, and the reverence practiced in a hospital, are unchanged. The basic question behind this book also remains the same: how do we adapt our massage skills to a specialty setting like a hospital, nursing facility, or rehabilitation center?

The obvious justification for a second edition was the need to update the research, new medications, clinical information, and current infection control practices. Additionally, we wanted to provide instruction in new topics, such as massage for people with neurological disorders, substance abuse, end of life care, aromatherapy, and the therapeutic relationship between patient and practitioner.

As massage educators, we want to lend support to the creation of new hospital massage programs. A textbook lends validity to such an endeavor. A book is also an important contributor in setting standards and creating a framework. It can become a hub around which a community can gather, especially in this day and age of advanced technology.

The meat and potatoes of *Hands in Health Care* are the clinical recommendations for specific circumstances, such as cardiac conditions, kidney disease, or diabetes-related problems. The act of massaging these patients is simple, even though they may have complex conditions and needs. The medical milieu in which we work is also complex, involving as it does the dynamics of working with hospital staff, strict infection control practices, dress and grooming standards, the psychology of the patient-therapist relationship, and the influence of medications, medical devices and procedures. There are also legal considerations, such as rules of confidentiality, liability, and documentation. To be sure, the institutional environment requires skills and knowledge outside the normal experience of most massage therapists.

Our hope is that therapists, administrators, and medical and nursing staff see the benefit of massage for their patients. Equally important is an understanding that therapists need to receive specialized training in order to deliver outstanding care in the health care domain. This education can come in a variety of ways: via a nurse mentor, through a formal training program, or a self-prescribed slate of professional development courses. It is our wish that no matter how a person trains for this rewarding work, *Hands in Health Care* will be a valuable teacher, guide, inspiration, support, and resource.

Gayle MacDonald MS, LMT
Portland, Oregon, USA
Carolyn Tague MA, CMT
San Francisco, California, USA
September 2020

GLOSSARY

The first use of a word in the text is highlighted in orange

Ablation
To remove or destroy part of the body or its function. Common methods include surgery or electrode catheter.

Abscess
Localized collection of pus in any part of the body.

Abstract
Summary of a research article.

ACE inhibitors
A group of medications that cause vasodilation.

Acidosis
The build-up of acid in the blood from kidney disease.

Acquired
Characteristic, disease, or abnormality that is not inherited.

Activities of daily living
Self-care, communication, and mobility skills needed to live independently. Includes the unaided ability to perform six basic personal care activities: eating, toileting, dressing, bathing, transferring, and continence.

Acute care
Health care that is given for a brief but severe episode of illness, usually in a hospital by specialized personnel.

Adverse event
An incident that results in harm to the patient. These events commonly include falls, medication errors, incontinence, hospital-acquired infections, and pressure injuries.

Afferent
Carrying impulses to a center, such as a nerve carrying an impulse to the brain.

Airborne transmission
Transfer of a disease-causing organism through the air. Chickenpox is an example.

Alkylating
Therapy that introduces an alkyl radical into a compound in place of a hydrogen atom, interfering with cell metabolism and growth. These drugs are used in cancer treatment.

Allogeneic transplant
Stem cells donated by someone other than the patient.

Ambulatory
The ability to walk.

Amyotrophic lateral sclerosis (ALS)
A progressive disease of motor neurones that causes degeneration of muscles.

Analgesics
Medications that relieve the normal sense of pain.

Anastomosis
Connection of two tubular structures such as an artery and a vein by which the capillary bed is bypassed.

Anecdotal
Information based on testimony.

Anesthesia
Partial or complete loss of sensation due to disease, injury, or the administration of an agent usually by injection or inhalation.

Aneurysm
An abnormal enlargement of a blood vessel, usually an artery, which causes weakening of the vessel wall.

Angina
Severe pain around the heart caused by oxygen deficiency to the heart muscle.

Angiogenesis
Creation of new blood vessels.

Angiogram
A radiographic record of the size, shape, and location of the heart and blood vessels.

Angiography
The use of a contrasting dye and x-ray to examine the functioning of blood vessels.

Angioplasty
Dilation of blood vessels by surgery or through the use of a balloon inside the lumen.

Antecubital
In front of the elbow.

Antenatal, antepartum
The time before birth, prenatal.

Antiangiogenic
A substance that reduces the growth of new blood vessels.

Anticholinergic
An agent that blocks parasympathetic nerve impulses, such as an antidepressant.

Anticoagulant
An agent that prevents or delays blood from clotting.

Antiemetic
Medications to relieve nausea and vomiting.

Antihypertensives
A group of drugs that lower blood pressure.

Antimetabolites
Drugs used against rapidly growing tumors.

Anxiolytics
A group of drugs that relieve anxiety.

Apheresis
A hemodialysis-type of procedure that separates and removes specific blood components.

Aplastic anemia
Anemia caused by decreased red blood cell production as a result of a bone marrow disorder.

Arrhythmia
Irregular heart rhythm.

Arteriograph
A procedure using x-rays and a contrasting dye to study arteries.

Arteriosclerosis
Hardening of the arteries.

Arteriovenous malformation
An abnormal tangle of blood vessels that connect arteries and veins, which disrupts normal blood flow.

Arthrectomy
Removal of a joint.

Arthrograph
Machine used to examine a joint by radiography.

Arthrography
A radiographic report of a synovial joint after injecting a dye.

Arthroscope
An endoscope for examining the inside of a joint.

Ascites
A collection of fluid in the abdominal area often related to liver disease.

Aspiration
The drawing in or out by suction, such as foreign bodies breathed into the lungs, or the withdrawing of fluid from the body.

Asthma
Breathing difficulty caused by bronchial spasm or swelling of the mucous membrane.

Ataxia
The inability to coordinate voluntary muscle activity.

Atelectasis
Collapse or airless condition of the lung.

Atherectomy
Removal of fatty deposits from the inside of arterial walls.

Atherosclerosis
Fatty deposits on the interior of arteries causing narrowing and fibrosis.

Atrial fibrillation
Irregular heartbeat. Cardiac arrhythmia.

Autologous transplant
Stem cells donated by the patient.

Axillary/axilla
Pertaining to the armpit.

Benzodiazepines
A group of drugs given to reduce anxiety or induce sleep.

Beta-blockers
A group of drugs that relieve cardiac stress by slowing heart contractions, improving rhythm, and reducing blood vessel constriction.

Beta-cells
Cells in the islets of Langerhans in the pancreas that secrete insulin.

Biofield therapies
Noninvasive therapies in which the therapist works with the patient's interacting fields of energy and information that surround living systems. Reiki, Healing Touch, and Therapeutic Touch are common examples.

Biopsy
Excision of a small piece of tissue for microscopic study.

Brace
Device used in orthopedics for holding joints or limbs in place.

Brachytherapy
A type of radiotherapy in which the radioactive material is placed inside the body.

Bradycardia
Slow heartbeat, usually below 60 beats per minute.

Cachexia
A state of health resulting in malnutrition and wasting noted in chronic disease such as cancer or AIDS.

Calcium channel blocker
A group of vasodilating drugs that block the influx of calcium into smooth muscle cells. This causes the muscle tone in the vessel wall to relax.

Candida
A yeast-like fungus that is naturally occurring in the human body but that can become pathogenic if the balance is disturbed.

Candida auris
A type of fungal infection that can infect the bloodstream and is often resistant to fungal drugs.

Cardiac
Pertaining to the heart.

Cardiac ablation
A procedure used to remove or terminate a faulty electrical pathway from sections of the heart. It is used for people with cardiac arrhythmias such as atrial fibrillation, atrial flutter, and supraventricular tachycardia.

Cardiac output
The amount of blood the heart pumps through the circulatory system in one minute.

Cardiomyopathy
Disease of the heart muscle.

Catheter
A tube passed through the body for the purpose of removing or injecting fluids into body cavities.

Catheterization
The act of passing a tube through the body for the purpose of removing or injecting fluids into body cavities.

Cellulitis
Bacterial skin infection that can become invasive.

Central IV catheter, central line, central venous catheter
A tube which is inserted into and kept in the vein for a lengthy period of time in order to inject drugs or extract fluids. Types are Groshong, Hickman, Quinton, and Portacath.

Cerebrospinal
Referring to the brain and spinal cord.

Cerebrovascular accident (CVA)
Caused by disruption of the brain's blood supply and commonly referred to as a stroke.

Cesarean section
Surgical delivery of a baby in which an incision is made into the uterus through the abdominal wall.

Chronic bronchitis
Long-term inflammation of the bronchial tubes.

Chronic obstructive pulmonary disease (COPD)
A group of lung diseases that cause decreased lung functioning, such as asthma, emphysema, and chronic bronchitis.

***Clostridioides difficile* (C. diff)**
Common spore-forming bacteria of the intestine. An overgrowth, which leads to infection, can be caused by antibiotics and immunosuppression.

Coagulation
Clotting, usually in reference to blood.

Coagulopathy
Defect in the clotting ability of the blood.

Colitis
Inflammation of the large intestine.

Colostomy
The opening of some part of the colon onto the abdominal surface.

Colposcopy
An instrument used to examine the tissues of the vagina and cervix through a magnifying lens.

Commode
A bedside toilet that can be used instead of a bedpan when the patient is able.

Comorbidity
Presence of multiple diseases simultaneously.

Computed tomography (CT)
A diagnostic scan that images cross-sections of the body with x-rays.

Congenital
A condition present since birth.

Congestive heart failure (CHF)
The progressive deterioration of the heart muscle, causing it to pump insufficiently. Fluid build-up around the heart is the specific cause of inefficient contraction.

Conjunctivitis
Inflammation of the membrane that lines the eyelids and covers the eyeball.

Contact Precautions
Practices employed to protect health care workers, families, and other patients from infections that are transmitted by direct contact, such as VRE (see entry below), herpes, or conjunctivitis. These precautions involve handwashing, gloving, and gowning.

Continuous passive motion device
A mechanical device used to provide continuous movement through specific ranges of motion at selected joints. Used following surgery to reduce complications and promote recovery.

Continuous positive airway pressure (CPAP)
The provision of positive airway pressure during both inhalation and exhalation.

Contracture
Shortening and hardening of muscles and connective tissue.

Control group
A group involved in a research project that does not receive the treatment being tested.

Co-occurring conditions
The occurrence of two or more disorders or illnesses in the same patient.

Coronary
Referring to the heart, specifically the vessels that feed the heart.

Coronary artery bypass graft (CABG)
A surgical procedure routing blood from the aorta to a part of the coronary artery past the site of the blockage.

Corticosteroids
Hormonal steroid substances produced in the cortex of the adrenal glands.

Crossover design
Two groups are used. Each receives the experimental intervention and each serves as the control, but in opposite order from the other. Halfway through, the groups switch.

Cutaneous
Relating to the skin.

Cutaneous diphtheria
An acute, infectious disease characterized by the development of a false membrane lesion on the skin.

Cyanosis
Blue discoloration of the skin due to lack of oxygen and excess carbon dioxide in the blood.

Cystoscope
Instrument used to examine the interior bladder and ureter.

Cytokines
A category of small proteins important in cell signaling.

Cytomegalovirus
A herpes virus found in human salivary glands. The virus may produce infection during periods of immunosuppression.

Cytotoxic
Toxic to cells.

Decompensation
Functional deterioration of a system or structure.

Deep vein thrombosis
A blood clot in the deep venous system of the upper or lower extremities.

Dermatitis
Skin irritation.

Dialysis
See Hemodialysis.

Diastolic
The period of relaxation after the heart contracts, during which time the chambers fill with blood. The pressure in arteries is at its lowest during this time.

Diphtheria
A bacterial infection that most often affects children. Inflammation is caused in the nose, throat, and bronchial tubes. The toxins can damage peripheral nerves, heart muscle, and other tissue.

Dissociation
Disconnecting from thoughts, feelings, memories.

Diuretic
An agent that increases the output of urine.

Double blind
A method of scientific study in which neither the subject nor the investigator knows what treatment, if any, the subject is receiving.

Doula
A person trained to give nonmedical support to women who are preparing for birth and to assist during and after the event.

Draw sheet
A sheet placed under the patient to assist in repositioning.

Droplet infection
Infection transferred by means of spray from the mouth or nose. An example is the common cold.

Dyskinesia
Difficulty in performing voluntary movements.

Dyspnea
Shortness of breath.

Dysrhythmias
Abnormal, disordered, or disturbed rhythm, such as cardiac dysrhythmia.

Eclampsia
Coma and convulsive seizures occurring between the 20th week of pregnancy and the first week after the birth. The cause is still unknown. It occurs more often during first pregnancies. Preexisting high blood pressure and infections that damage the kidney contribute to the condition.

Edema
A local or generalized swelling.

Electrocardiograph
Device for recording changes in the electrical energy produced by the action of heart muscles.

Electrode
A device placed on the skin to measure electrical current.

Electroencephalograph
Device for recording changes in the electrical energy produced by the brain.

Electrolyte
Minerals that conduct an electrical current in the body.

Embolism
Obstruction of a blood vessel, usually by a blood clot or other foreign substance.

Emesis
Material ejected from the stomach.

Emetic
Nausea-producing.

Emphysema
A disease process of the lungs in which the air sacs increase in size.

Encephalitis
Inflammation of the brain.

Endoscope
Device for examining the inside of a hollow organ or cavity.

Endoscopic
Pertains to an examination of the internal organs or cavity by use of an endoscope.

Endotracheal
Inside the trachea. Usually referring to a tube inserted into the trachea, which is then inflated to provide an airway. It also prevents aspiration of foreign material into the bronchus.

Engraft
The process of stem cells traveling to the bone marrow and producing new blood cells.

Enteric
Pertaining to the small intestine.

Enterococcus
Any species of streptococcus found in the intestine.

Epidural
Located over or on the outer layer of the spinal cord or the brain, also known as the dura. Also refers to anesthesia placed in the epidural space.

***Escherichia coli* (*E. coli*)**
Usually a nonpathogenic bacterium present in the digestive tract of all humans. It will cause infection if it enters the urinary tract. If found in milk or water, it is an indication of fecal contamination. It is the chief cause of "traveler's diarrhea."

Evidence-informed practice
The use of interventions that are scientifically proven.

Experimental
A scientific procedure to gain further knowledge. Also refers to the group in an experiment that is receiving the trial intervention.

External beam therapy
Radiotherapy beams delivered externally to a patient's tumor site.

Extubation
Removal of a tube, such as an endotracheal tube.

Exudate
Body fluid, cells, or cellular debris, which has escaped from blood vessels and been deposited in tissues or on tissue surfaces, usually as a result of inflammation.

Feasibility study
One that examines whether it is possible, under certain circumstances, to study a specific intervention.

Febrile
Relating to fever.

Feces
Bodily waste.

Fetal
Pertaining to the unborn child in the uterus from the third month of pregnancy until birth.

Fiberoptic instruments
Highly flexible instruments that allow access to channels in the body, such as the colon. They are composed of bundles of hairlike glass rods that transmit intense light allowing the physician see the walls of an organ during an endoscopic exam.

Fibrillation
Quivering, spontaneous, or incomplete contractions of individual muscle fibers, such as in the heart. Often seen in sudden cardiac arrest.

Fistula
Abnormal tube-like passage from a normal cavity or tube to another surface opening or cavity, such as an arteriovenous fistula, which is created by connecting an artery and a vein.

Fixator
Orthotic device that can be internal or external. It uses a combination of pins, nails, screws, and plates to hold bones together.

Foley catheter
A tube that is placed in the bladder to provide continuous urinary drainage.

Formulary
A book that provides standards and specifications for drugs.

Fowler's position
Semi-reclining position.

Gamma-aminobutyric acid (GABA)
An amino acid that is the principal inhibitory neurotransmitter in the central nervous system.

Gangrene
The death of tissue due to a lack of blood supply.

Gastroenterologist
A specialist in the study of the stomach, intestines, and other digestive organs.

Gastrostomy
Surgical creation of a gastric fistula (opening) through the abdominal wall.

Glycoprotein
A compound consisting of a carbohydrate and protein.

Graft-versus-host disease (GVHD)
A group of side effects of an allogeneic bone marrow transplant in which the donor's cells see the host's tissues

as foreign and attack them. Often affected are the skin, nails, hair, GI tract, liver, lungs, muscles, and joints.

Groshong
A type of central IV catheter.

Guillain-Barré syndrome
Acute, inflammatory destruction of the peripheral nerves' myelin sheaths. Causes rapid and progressive loss of motor function. Believed to be an autoimmune response.

Handrub
Waterless antibacterial hand cleanser.

Head lice
A type of parasitic insect that resides in the human scalp.

Health care-acquired infections (HAIs)
Infections acquired while receiving care in the health care setting.

HELLP syndrome
A complication of pregnancy-induced hypertension that causes low platelets and destruction of red blood cells.

Hematocrit
Percentage of the blood volume occupied by cells.

Hematoma
A collection of clotted blood in an organ, tissue, or space caused by a broken blood vessel.

Hematopoietic stem cell transplantation (HSCT)
The transplantation of stem cells usually derived from bone marrow, peripheral blood, or umbilical cord blood.

Hemiparesis
Partial paralysis.

Hemodialysis
A method for providing the function of the kidneys by circulating blood through tubes made of semipermeable membranes. These dialyzing tubes are continually bathed by solutions that selectively remove unwanted material.

Hemorrhagic
Pertaining to bleeding.

Hepatitis
Inflammation of the liver.

Herpes
The common term for two different viruses known as herpes simplex virus 1 (HSV1) and herpes simplex virus 2 (HSV2). HSV1 cause vesicles to erupt most commonly on the mouth, frequently referred to as cold sores. HSV2 causes vesicles on the genitalia, thighs, or buttocks.

Hickman
A type of central IV catheter.

Histamine
A substance produced from the amino acid histidine. It causes a reaction, such as swelling, redness, and rash, when released from injured cells. If injected, histamine stimulates gastric secretion and causes flushing of the skin, lowered blood pressure, and headache.

Homeostatic
A state of equilibrium.

Hormone
Chemical substances formed in organs or glands. They travel through the blood to other parts of the body, stimulating their function or the secretion of more hormones.

Hospitalist
A physician that specializes in hospital care.

Hydrocephalus
A condition in which an excessive amount of cerebrospinal fluid accumulates in the brain.

Hypercholesterolemia
Excess cholesterol in the blood.

Hypercoagulable
Increased tendency for blood to clot.

Hypertension
High blood pressure.

Hypotension
Low blood pressure.

Hypothalamus
A part of the brain located in the middle of the base of the brain. It is involved with the autonomic nervous system, endocrine mechanisms, and mood states.

Hypothermia
Insufficient body heat.

Hypoxia
Deficiency of oxygen in the blood.

Ileostomy
An opening into the ileum (lower intestine) by way of the abdominal surface. Fecal material drains into a bag worn on the abdomen.

Ileum
The longest and final part of the small intestine before it leads into the colon.

Immunosuppressed (immunocompromised)
An immune system that is incapable of reacting to pathogens. The cause can be drug-induced, genetic, or disease-related.

Immunotherapy
Therapy that boosts the body's natural defenses to restore immune function in order to fight cancer.

Impetigo
A contagious condition caused by streptococci or staphylococci bacteria in which the skin becomes inflamed and isolated pustules form. They eventually rupture and become crusted. The skin of the nose and mouth is the most often affected area.

Incontinence
Inability to retain urine, semen, or feces due to loss of sphincter control, or brain or spinal lesions.

Infarct
Part of an organ in which the tissue has died due to lack of blood supply.

Inguinal
Related to the groin.

Inherited
Characteristics or conditions with a genetic connection.

In situ
Positioned, undisturbed, in place.

Interstitial
Refers to spaces within a tissue or organ.

Intervention
Taking action so as to modify the result. Examples are the use of medication, massage, physical therapy, or chiropractic treatments.

Intravenous (IV) catheter
A catheter inserted into a vein to administer fluids or medications or to measure pressure.

Intubation
Insertion of a tube into any hollow organ for entrance of air or to dilate a structure.

Ischemia
Obstructed blood supply to a localized area.

IV pole
Equipment that supports a hanging IV bag.

Jejunostomy
A surgical opening into the jejunum by way of the abdominal surface.

Jejunum
The middle portion of the small intestine.

J-Pouch
A bag attached at the site of a jejunostomy for the purpose of collecting intestinal contents.

Jugular vein
Main vein in the neck.

Kinins
General term for a group of polypeptides that have considerable biological activity. They influence smooth muscle contraction, induce hypotension, increase blood flow and permeability of small blood capillaries, and incite pain.

Laparoscope
Instrument used to examine the inside of the abdominal cavity.

Lesion
A pathological change in tissue from an injury, infected patch, cyst, or cancer.

Leukemia
Cancer in which the bone marrow produces too many white blood cells, which don't function normally.

Leukopenia
Less than the normal number of leukocytes.

Lewy body dementia
Characterized by abnormal deposits of a protein called alpha synuclein. The deposits are called Lewy bodies.

Liability
Obliged by law.

Likert scale
A written research tool that measures patient feedback on a scale of 1 to 5.

Lupus
A chronic autoimmune disease in which the immune system attacks normal healthy tissue.

Lymphangitis
Inflammation of the lymphatic system.

Lymphedema
A collection of lymphatic fluid due to a congenital defect, obstruction of the lymph vessels, or removal of lymph nodes.

Lymphoma
Cancer that begins in the lymphocytes, one of the five types of white blood cells.

Magnetic resonance imaging (MRI)
Use of magnetic fields and radio-frequency waves in combination with computer technology to view images of soft tissue in the body.

Malignant ascites
Ascites resulting from a disease process, such as cancer.

Mechanical ventilator
Mechanical device for artificially oxygenating the lungs as well as monitoring the flow of air to the lungs.

Medical
Related to the term "medicine," the art and science of diagnosing, treating, and preventing disease. Also, the treatment of disease through the use of drugs or other remedies that are nonsurgical. Physicians and nurse practitioners are involved in the medical side of health care.

Meningitis
Inflammation of the membranes of the spinal cord and brain, the meninges.

Meta-analysis
A way to statistically analyze a group of studies that meet certain criteria.

Metabolite
A by-product of the body breaking down food, drugs, or its own tissue, as with cachexia.

Metastases
Secondary cancerous tumors that form distant to the site of the primary tumor.

Metastasis
The movement of bacteria or body cells, such as cancer cells, from one part of the body to another.

Motor neurone disease (MND)
See Amyotrophic lateral sclerosis.

MRSA (methicillin-resistant *Staphylococcus aureus*)
A bacteria that is resistant to the antibiotic methicillin.

Mucositis
Inflammation of the mucosal lining, generally occurring in the mouth and esophagus as a side effect of some chemotherapies.

MUGA (multiple gated acquisition) scan
A diagnostic scan that employs nuclear technology to assess heart function.

Multiple myeloma
Cancer of the plasma cells, a type of white blood cell found in the bone marrow. Plasma cells normally produce antibodies, which are used to attack viruses and bacteria, for the body's immune system.

Multiple sclerosis
A disorder of the central nervous system caused by loss of the myelin sheath around nerve fibers.

Myalgia
Muscle pain.

Myelodysplastic syndrome
A group of cancers in which blood cells in the bone marrow don't mature into healthy blood cells.

Myelofibrosis
Extensive scarring in the bone marrow that disrupts the body's ability to produce healthy blood cells.

Myocardial infarction
A condition caused by a partial or complete occlusion of one or more coronary arteries, which carry blood necessary to keep heart muscle alive. It is commonly referred to as a heart attack.

Narcotics
Opiate-based drugs that depress the central nervous system, thereby relieving pain and inducing sleep.

Nasal cannula
Tubing used to deliver oxygen. It extends approximately 1 cm into each nostril and is connected to a common tube, which is then connected to the oxygen source. It is used in situations such as cardiac disease in which a low flow of oxygen is desired.

Nasogastric
Relating to the nose and stomach. Usually pertains to intubation of the stomach via the nasal passage.

Nephrostomy
The formation of an artificial fistula into the renal pelvis.

Neuropathy
A pathological condition of the nervous system that results in tingling, loss of feeling, and pins and needles in a body part.

Neurotransmitter
A chemical substance that is released by a presynaptic neurone, which then travels across the synapse to act on the target cell to either inhibit or excite it. Norepinephrine and dopamine are examples.

Neutropenia
Lower than normal numbers of neutrophils, a type of white blood cell. These cells are responsible for much of the body's defense against disease. Low levels increase the chance of infection.

Norovirus
A highly contagious virus that causes vomiting and diarrhea, often mistaken for influenza.

Nosocomial
Pertaining to the hospital or infirmary.

Nurse
A health care provider who manages the patient's plan of care and assists the patient to perform activities that contribute to health or their recovery (or to a peaceful death). Nurses do not diagnose or prescribe treatment but act under the orders of the doctor.

Nystagmus
An involuntary condition that causes the eye to rapidly move up and down or right and left.

Obstetrics
The branch of medicine that cares for pregnant women before, during, and after birth.

Occlusion
A blockage.

Oncology
The branch of medicine dealing with cancer.

Orogastric
Refers to the mouth and stomach.

Orthopedic
The branch of medicine that treats problems of the muscular and skeletal systems of the body.

Orthopedic fixation devices
These can include items such as pins, plates, screws, and wires.

Orthostatic hypotension
Low blood pressure that occurs when a person rises from a lying or seated to a standing position.

Osteoarthritis
A chronic disease of the joints resulting in the destruction of the cartilage intended to cushion the joints. It is often found in the aged population and is disabling.

Osteoporosis
A disease process that results in the reduction of bone mass. Fractures often occur where they would not normally. Vertebrae are most commonly affected.

Outcomes
Variables measured during a study.

Pacemaker
An electrical device implanted in the chest to regulate heart rhythm.

Palliative care
A supportive type of care that is provided alongside ongoing treatment to optimize the quality of life for the person with a life-limiting illness.

Paracentesis
A procedure that removes fluid from the peritoneal cavity using a hollow needle or tube.

Parasympathetic nervous system
Part of the autonomic nervous system that slows the heart, encourages digestion, and supports rest.

Pathogen
A micro-organism or substance that is capable of causing a disease.

Patient-controlled analgesia
Pain medications that can be administered in measured doses by the patient.

Percutaneous
Application of medication through the skin, such as an ointment or by injection.

Pericardial
Pertaining to the double walled sac surrounding the heart and the origin of the main vessels, such as the aorta and superior and inferior vena cava.

Pericardial effusion
Excess fluid between the heart and the sac surrounding the heart, known as the pericardium. Most are not harmful, but they sometimes can make the heart work poorly.

Peripheral artery disease
A circulatory condition in which the arteries of the extremities are narrowed.

Peripheral IV catheter
An IV catheter usually placed in the lower arm for temporary use. Also called a peripheral line.

Peripheral neuropathy
Neuropathy that generally affects the hands, feet, or lower legs.

Peripherally inserted central catheter (PICC)
A catheter that is placed into a central vein either in the antecubital space or the upper arm. It is for patients needing long-term care.

Peristaltic
The wave-like contraction and relaxation movements of the intestines that propels waste.

Peritoneal (peritoneum)
Pertaining to the membrane over the abdominal organs and the lining of the abdominal cavity.

Peritoneal dialysis
Treatment that filters the blood and rids the body of extra fluids by using the peritoneum, the lining of the abdomen.

Permacath
A large-bore catheter that remains in place on a long-term basis. Often used for hemodialysis.

Personal protective equipment (PPE)
Items such as mask, gown, and gloves used as part of Standard Precautions to protect both patients and health care workers.

Personalized medicine
Treatments customized to a patient's particular genetic and molecular make-up.

Petechiae
Small purplish, hemorrhagic spots that appear on the skin or mucous membranes with certain severe fevers or as a side effect of drugs.

Pharmaceutical
Pertaining to drugs or pharmacy.

Pharyngitis
Inflammation of the throat.

Phlebitis
Inflammation of a vein.

Placenta previa
A condition in which the placenta implants in the lower part of the uterus.

Plaque
Deposits on tissue. An example is deposits of fatty substance inside blood vessels.

Plasma
The somewhat clear fluid of the blood that caries corpuscles and platelets. It consists of serum, protein, and chemical substances in aqueous solution. The chemical substances include electrolytes, glucose, proteins, enzymes, hormones, and fats.

Platelet
A blood component necessary for coagulation.

Pleural
Pertaining to the membrane that enfolds both lungs, lines the chest cavity, and covers the diaphragm.

Pneumonia
Inflammation of the lung caused by bacteria or chemical irritants.

Portacath
Type of long-term central venous catheter that is surgically placed under the skin. Also known as a "port."

Positrons
A particle having the same mass as a negative electron but possessing a positive charge.

Postpartum
The period after childbirth.

Post-traumatic stress disorder (PTSD)
Psychological damage caused by a traumatic event.

Precision medicine
See Personalized medicine.

Pre-eclampsia
A condition associated with pregnancy that causes hypertension with proteinuria or edema.

Preterm labor
Premature start of pregnancy contractions.

Pre-/post-test design
A design that compares the data collected before the intervention to the data following the intervention between groups.

Prophylactic
Any agent or regimen that contributes to the prevention of infection or disease.

Prostaglandin
Any of a group of fatty acid derivatives that are biologically very active. They affect a number of systems, such as the cardiovascular, gastrointestinal, and respiratory systems.

Protective isolation
Infection control practices that protect the patient from infections that might be transferred to them from health care staff and family. Also known as reverse isolation.

Prothrombin
A coagulation factor synthesized by the liver that is converted to thrombin.

Pruritus
Itching.

Psychosocial
Pertaining to the emotional and social component of patient care.

Pulmonary
Concerning the lungs.

Qualitative
Study design that uses the client's subjective experience rather than statistical data to measure the effect of the intervention.

Quantitative
Study design that uses statistical data to measure the effect of the intervention.

Quasi-experimental
Study design that is similar to a randomized controlled trial but lacks the element of randomly assigning people to experimental or control groups.

Radioactive isotope
One of a series of chemical elements that have nearly identical chemical properties but different atomic weights and electric charges. An isotope in which the nuclear composition is unstable.

Radiopharmaceutical
A radioactive chemical used in testing the location, size, outline, or function of tissues, organs, vessels, or body fluids. The presence and location of radiopharmaceuticals in the body are detected by special methods or devices that record the radioactivity being emitted. They may also be used in the treatment of diseases such as prostate cancer.

Randomized
A research method in which individuals are arbitrarily assigned to one of two groups, experimental or control.

Renal
Pertaining to the kidneys.

Retroperitoneal
Behind the peritoneum and outside the peritoneal cavity, such as the kidneys.

Retrospective study
Measuring data collected via medical records or health intake charts. The data could have been collected expressly for research or to evaluate patient care.

Reverse isolation
See Protective isolation.

Reye's syndrome
A rare illness affecting children who have taken aspirin. Causes acute encephalopathy and fatty infiltration of the

liver and possibly of the pancreas, heart, kidney, spleen, and lymph nodes. May involve the central nervous system to varying degrees.

Rheumatoid arthritis
Inflammatory changes of joints and surrounding tissues resulting in crippling deformities.

Rubella
Commonly known as German measles, an acute, short-lasting, infectious disease resembling both scarlet fever and measles but differing in the short course. The rash begins on the face and quickly spreads over the whole body but fades very rapidly. Serious fetal anomalies may result if the mother contracts the disease in the first trimester of pregnancy.

Rubeola
Commonly known as measles, an acute contagious disease with fever, non-elevated rash found in patches, and a runny nose.

Scarlet fever
A bacterial infection that is highly contagious. Characterized by a sore throat, red tongue, fever, and scarlet rash.

Sedative
A substance that produces a calming, soothing, or tranquilizing effect.

Self-limiting
Limitations controlled by the patient.

Semi-reclining
Supine lying position, typically at a 45-degree angle. Also known as Fowler's position.

Sepsis
A life-threatening condition that arises when the body's response to infection causes injury to its tissues and organs.

Septicemia
An infection caused by the presence of bacteria in the bloodstream.

Shingles (herpes zoster)
Eruption of acute inflammatory herpes vesicles usually on the trunk of the body along the course of a peripheral nerve.

Shunt
An artificially constructed passage, akin to a miniature garden hose, to divert flow from one main route to another.

Sickle cell anemia
A condition in which the red blood cells are sickle shaped rather than round, which disrupts the smooth flow of blood through the circulatory system. These cells also die early, causing a shortage of red blood cells.

Spasticity
Abnormal muscle tightness due to prolonged muscle contraction.

Splint
An apparatus used for the fixation, union, or protection of an injured part of the body. Construction may be of wood, plastic, plaster, or metal.

Sputum
Substance discharged by coughing or clearing the throat.

Standard Precautions
The practices used to protect against infection from all body fluids regardless of a person's diagnosis or presumed infectious status.

Staphylococcus
A term used loosely for any disease-causing bacteria that appear in "grape-like" clusters microscopically.

Statins
A group of drugs that block the liver enzyme responsible for making cholesterol.

Statistical significance
After appropriate analysis of numerical data, it is decided that the results are not happening by chance.

Stem cell
Primordial, all-purpose cells that can develop into any tissue in the body.

Stem cell therapy
Often refers to the use of stem cells to regenerate joints.

Stenosis
The constriction or narrowing of a passage or orifice.

Stent
Any material or device used to hold tissue in place or to provide a support for a graft or anastomosis while healing is taking place.

Sternal
Related to the breastbone.

Sternotomy
A procedure in which the sternum is cut through.

Sterol
One of a group of substances, such as cholesterol, belonging to the lipids.

Stoma
An artificial opening between two passages or body cavities or between the body's surface and a cavity or passage. The opening created by a colostomy is an example.

Streptococcus
Spherically shaped bacteria that usually grow in chains.

Subcutaneous
Beneath the skin.

Subjective
Information arising from individual opinion not from research.

Supine
Lying on the back with the face upward.

Supine hypotensive syndrome
Low blood pressure when in a supine position.

Swan-Ganz catheter
A flexible catheter with a balloon near the tip that is used in testing or monitoring pressures in the lung and heart.

Sympathetic nervous system
Part of the autonomic nervous system that is activated during conditions of stress.

Synovial
Pertaining to the lubricating fluids of the joints.

Systolic
The period of cardiac contraction. Blood pressure is highest during this action.

Tachycardia
An abnormally fast heartbeat, usually defined as a heart rate greater than 100 beats per minute in adults.

Telemetry
The transmission of data electronically to a distant location.

Thalassemia
A group of inherited hemoglobin disorders.

Therapeutic
A healing agent having medicinal or healing properties or results obtained from treatment.

Thoracic
Related to the chest.

Thrombin
A plasma protein substance used topically to control capillary bleeding during surgical procedures. A blood-clotting agent.

Thrombocytopenia
An abnormal reduction in the blood platelets.

Thrombolytic
The breaking up of a blood clot.

Thrombophlebitis
Occurrence of a blood clot in conjunction with an inflamed vein.

Thrombosis
Formulation or presence of a thrombus.

Thrombus
A blood clot that obstructs a blood vessel or cavity of the heart.

Tracheotomy
Incision into the trachea through the skin and muscles of the neck.

Tracheostomy tube
Tube inserted into the trachea following a tracheotomy to maintain the opening.

Traction
Usually used to pull and align structures such as the vertebrae or a structure that has been fractured.

Transdermal patch
A method of delivering medicine by placing it in a special gel-like matrix that is applied to the skin like a Band-Aid. The medicine is absorbed into the skin at a fixed rate.

Transfer
The act of moving a person with limited function from one location to another.

Transient ischemic attack (TIA)
A stroke lasting only a few minutes when the blood supply to part of the brain is briefly blocked.

Transmission-Based Precautions
The protective practices employed when caring for patients known or suspected to be infected by specific pathogens.

Transmural
Extending through or across the entire wall of an organ or structure.

Trend
With regard to research, data that lean toward a certain outcome but are not statistically significant.

Trigeminal
Pertaining to the trigeminus or fifth cranial nerve.

T-tube
A T shaped tube that is placed within another tube, such as for the patient on a vent.

Tuberculosis
Bacterial infection that most commonly affects the lungs.

Ulcer
An open sore on the skin or mucous membrane accompanied by sloughing of inflamed dead tissue.

Ulceration
Formation of an open sore or lesion of the skin or mucosal lining.

Ultrasound
A test that bounces sound waves off various tissues to detect density and elasticity. The echoes are processed into images.

Universal Precautions
The practices employed to protect against blood-borne pathogens, such as hand washing, gloving, and gowning.

Urinal
A container into which one urinates.

Urostomy
Redirection of urine outside the body after the bladder has been repaired or removed.

Urticaria
A vascular reaction of the skin characterized by a sudden general eruption of pale evanescent wheals or papules, which are associated with severe itching. May be caused by contact with an irritant such as nettles, chemicals, insect bites, or allergens.

Vaccine
Used primarily to prevent a disease, but also used as treatment in personalized medicine to train the immune system to fight a disease, such as cancer.

Vagus nerve
The longest nerve of the autonomic nervous system. It provides the parasympathetic nervous system with control of the heart, lungs, and digestive tract.

Vancomycin-resistant *Enterococcus* (VRE)
Bacteria resistant to the antibiotic vancomycin.

Variables
Measurable attributes that change or vary across the experiment, such as age, gender, type of disease, or massage pressure.

Varicella
Commonly known as chickenpox, an acute, contagious disease with fever and vesicular eruption initially on the back and face.

Varicose veins (varicosity)
Distended, swollen veins.

Vasculitis
Inflammation of a blood or lymph vessel.

Vasoconstriction
Narrowing of the blood vessels.

Vasodilation
Widening of the blood vessels.

Vasodilator
Any substance that widens blood vessels.

Vital signs
Body temperature, heart rate, respiration, and blood pressure.

INTRODUCTION

Parameters

One would think that hundreds of pages should be enough to cover every aspect of massage in the health care setting. They are not. We have had to narrow our focus and prioritize the usage of space, otherwise the book would be 500 pages long, or more!

Hands in Health Care focuses on adult patients and the practitioners who massage them. All people are able to receive some sort of touch therapy – those for whom it is a contraindication are rare. However, because of limited page count, we have had to focus on the patient populations for which massage is most common. Please forgive us if we left out a group of patients who are special to your heart. Also, we have not addressed training or curriculum specifics, which could require another book. Funding and placement within the hospital hierarchy are not discussed, nor are the how-tos of research projects. The focus is on helping practitioners adapt to the health care environment and on how to give massage to people receiving medical treatment and/or nursing care.

Definitions

It is necessary to bring clarity to words that are in common usage, such as massage, hospital, and patient. We very much hope that you will take the time to read the remainder of this introduction because it will influence your understanding moving forward into the book. Most important to the tenets of this text is the definition of massage.

Massage

Massage has become an umbrella term for many types of touch therapies. The following definition of hospital-based massage therapy is taken from Karen Gibson's manual, *Developing a Hospital-Based Massage Therapy Program*. "Massage is any skilled, systematic form of touch applied with sensitivity and compassion by professionally trained massage therapists with the specific intent of increasing comfort, complementing medical treatment, improving clinical outcomes, and promoting wholeness." This was written in 1992 and is still true today.

The words massage, touch therapy, and bodywork are used synonymously. Within this context, systematic touch modalities such as Reiki, Healing Touch, and acupressure would also be nested under this definition of massage.

CAM therapies/integrative medicine/holistic care

The acronym CAM stands for complementary and alternative medicine. Complementary therapies are those that are used alongside mainstream medicine. The term is an umbrella under which rests such modalities as massage, aromatherapy, art therapy, counseling, and yoga. Alternative medicine is that which is used instead of mainstream medicine. In this textbook, massage is viewed as a complementary therapy, NOT as an alternative treatment.

Some institutions use the term "integrative medicine", which is a combination of mainstream and complementary practices. The words are used interchangeably at times throughout the book.

Holistic care is the philosophy that forms the bedrock of complementary therapy or integrative medicine. This is care that attends to all parts of a patient: physical, emotional, mental, and spiritual.

Hospital

The term hospital has morphed into a variety of titles – medical center is common. However, in Australia, a medical center only provides care during the day. In the US, a medical center is usually a 24-hour hospital combined with day care services. In the UK, other terms are synonymous with hospital, such as infirmary, as in the Glasgow Royal Infirmary. Some care facilities go by the term institute, such as the Institut Jules Bordet, or clinic, such as the Clinique Saint-Jean. But hospital remains the term in common usage. In this book we have used the term "hospital" broadly to also mean a medical center, day clinic, doctor's surgery, extended care facility (nursing home), rehabilitation center, and hospice. At times we do want to speak directly about specific health care settings, in which case we will use specific terminology.

Patients

People who are receiving medical treatment have long been called patients. The word originally meant "one who suffers", from the Latin word *patiens*. Discussions about use of the term have occurred for decades. On one side of the argument, the word patient encapsulates a feeling of unequal relationship, a sense of passivity. There is a hierarchical positioning; the professional is the expert who knows what to do and the user of health care does as instructed.

Certainly, the traditional designation of patient created a picture of a person who would sit meekly for hours in a clinic waiting their turn, suffering in silence. This is at odds with the modern idea of the patient who is encouraged to be an equal partner, actively participating with the physician, nurse, or therapist. Professor Raymond Tallis writes in the *British Medical Journal* that: "Words acquire new meanings through custom and usage... In short, words, like their speakers, move on". He suggests continuation of this long-standing term because we have all moved on, acquiring a newer sense of patient. He also points out that there is no obvious alternative. "Health-seeker" and "service-user" are clunky substitutes. Client and consumer have also been tried, but both lack the unspoken agreement that lies at the heart of health care: compassion for someone who is often vulnerable, worried, and in need of a deep trust.[1]

We have, therefore, opted to continue with the word patient throughout the text.

Treatment

The use of the term treatment within a massage context can be controversial. In some parts of the world, the argument is that only doctors can give treatments, and so therapists avoid conflict by using the term session. Other areas of the world commonly use treatment when referencing bodywork or aromatherapy. In this book, the two words are used synonymously.

Reference

1. Tallis R. Do we need a new word for patients? Commentary: Leave well enough alone. BMJ. 1999;318(7200):1756–58.

In the early stages of their evolution, in Byzantium [eastern Roman territory], Christian hospitals demanded great sacrifices from those who committed themselves to aiding the sick. Hospital service was a form of penance.

Guenter B. Risse[1]

Much like today, the evolution of health care during ancient times was a story of cross-pollination. Asclepius, the Greek mythological god of medicine, and the writings of influential Greek figures such as Hippocrates and Galen, were known in the Arabic-speaking world. Many centuries later, Arabic medical literature was translated into Latin, providing medieval Europe with updated ideas and practices. Through those earlier times, medical theory and practice also co-mingled with ideas from Egypt, Mesopotamia, and India.[2,3]

According to the United States National Library of Medicine, the hospital is credited as being one of the greatest achievements of Islamic society.[4] It is not known for sure whether massage was given in these hospitals, but there is evidence of massage being administered in the ancient health halls and temples of India, China, Egypt, Greece, and Rome.[5]

The Latin word *hospes* means host, guest, visitor, or stranger, and forms the basis for words such as hospital, hospice, and hospitality. By the 4th century AD, Christians had created houses of refuge where religious orders of both men and women tended to the sick and dying. Much of the emphasis in these early Christian shelters was on providing spiritual solace rather than physical comfort. Their purpose was to save the soul, not the body. However, reference is made to massage in accounts of the era.[5]

Little is known about massage during the Middle Ages (roughly designated as between the 5th and 15th centuries). In *The History of Massage*, Robert Calvert reports that despite its negative attitude toward the body: "the Church … helped preserve massage within the Western world during the Middle Ages."[5] Touch, in the form

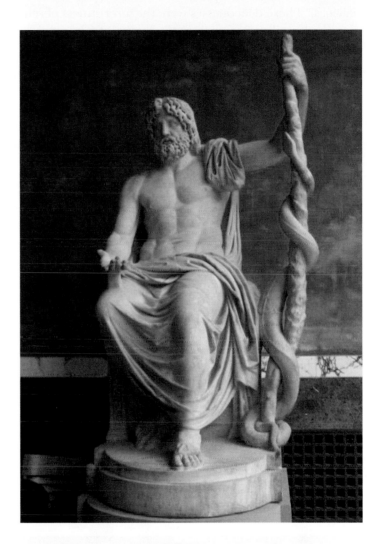

FIGURE 1.1
Asclepius, the ancient Greek god of medicine, is the representation of healing in the medical arts. The rod of Asclepius was a snake-entwined staff that is still used today as a medical symbol. The snake is an ancient symbol of fertility and vital life force.

(Photo by Nina Aldin Thune.)

of laying on of hands, became part of Christian ritual and care of the sick and dying.[5] During this period, it was church women who cared for those struck down by the plague and other epidemics, many physicians being unwilling to serve people who could not pay for their services.[6] These deaconesses were the forerunners of religious orders of sisters, such as the Sisters of Charity, Sisters of Providence, and the Augustinian nuns, founders of the Hotel-Dieu de Quebec in 1644, who established care facilities for the sick and the poor. Today a number of hospitals can trace their roots to these pioneering groups of women.

Care for the sick and dying in the Christian world was connected to monasteries. However, the Islamic hospital was largely a secular institution with a wider range of functions. It served as a center for medical treatment, a place to recover from illness or accidents, an insane asylum, and retirement home for the aged and infirm. The first recorded hospital in the Islamic world was in Baghdad in 805 AD.[2]

In European chronology, the period of transition from the Middle Ages to modern times is referred to as the Renaissance. This was a time of revival for the arts and literature that occurred between the 15th and 17th centuries. Health care practitioners of the day came to a new understanding of anatomy and physiology, which impacted the application of hands-on modalities. During the Renaissance, Christian hospitals evolved from houses of refuge, dying, and spiritual sustenance to places of rehabilitation and cure.[5,6] This idea that one could recover from illness was new. Cure, using medical knowledge and surgical techniques, became the aim of the 18th-century hospital. The transformation of health care continued through into the present day where it is based on a science, research, and technology.[6]

Massage endured highs and lows during these periods. Some health care providers embraced the science and mechanization of the era, turning away from hands-on practices. Others enthusiastically prescribed it for a plethora of medical conditions.

Massage and nursing

Massage has, at various times, been part of the physician's repertoire. The Greek physician Hippocrates is credited with saying that: "the physician must be experienced in many things, but assuredly also in rubbing."[5] However, for the past century and a half, hospital massage has been clearly associated with nursing. The creation of modern nursing practice is credited to Florence Nightingale, an English woman who took it upon herself to nurse the wounded soldiers of the Crimean War (1853–56). Although she does not specifically mention massage in her *Notes on Nursing*, it was part of her training program.[6] Nightingale's trainings became the model for early nursing training around the world.

During and following World War 1, massage was an important part of rehabilitation for British and Commonwealth troops. Begun in 1914, the Military Massage Corps, mostly made up of nurses, served in military

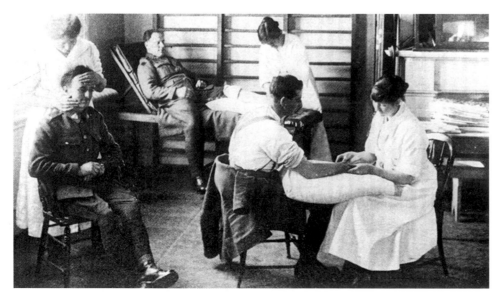

FIGURE 1.2
Soldiers in New Zealand receive massage treatments at Dunedin Hospital's orthopedic department in 1919. Trained massage therapists treated soldiers wounded in World War 1.

(From the *Otago Witness*, Issue 3403, June 4, 1919. Courtesy of the National Library of New Zealand.)

hospitals in the UK. The masseuses, as they were known at the time, saw 30–40 patients a day for the mighty sum of £3 a week. Their work established the foundation for what later became physiotherapy.[7]

Training in hands-on modalities continued to be an integral part of nurses' training and care through the mid-1950s, after which is declined to almost nothing. At various times during the 20th century, both nurses and physical therapists administered massage. While physical therapists used massage as a treatment for various medical conditions, nurses gave massage as a comfort measure. The nightly backrub is still remembered by many older patients as a standard part of the hospital experience from the 1940s up until the 1960s.

Decades ago, nurses were primarily caregivers. They straightened bedding, tidied patients' rooms, emptied the garbage, dusted the furniture, mopped the floor, gave massage, assisted the patient with exercises, and much more. Nurses were part housekeeper, physical therapist, occupational therapist, social worker, respiratory therapist, and massage therapist. They were the ultimate holistic practitioners. Today, nurses and physical therapists rarely include massage in their care or treatment. The modern-day hospital nurse not only gives direct patient care but also coordinates an array of practitioners from other disciplines, such as respiratory care, phlebotomists, and occupational therapy. This leaves little time for "luxuries" such as massage. And physical therapy, like other branches of health care, has shifted toward higher-tech treatments, such as ultrasound and electrical stimulation.

From a variety of circumstances, three main factors resulted in massage, as well as other types of personal care, being largely discontinued: 1) an increase in the patient load due to a shortage of nurses; 2) the requirement for additional documentation to be completed for governmental and insurance regulators, thereby reducing time spent with patients; and 3) the growth of medical technology, which favored drugs and machinery over hands-on methods of care.

Revolution, technology, and touch

Two global forces, both of which began in the mid-20th century, affected the present-day practice of hospital massage therapy. The first influence was the world-wide upheaval and revolution that occurred in the mid- to late-1960s. It was a decade of rebellion toward authority, a time of awakening, experimentation, and a changing consciousness toward the earth. Westerners were introduced to Eastern cosmology, James Lovelock coined the Gaia Principle, and young people revived a back-to-the-land movement. The spirit of the times was one of interrelationship between spirit and matter and was the predecessor of today's ecopsychology movement, the interrelationship between humans and nature.

The seeds of these ideas that were sown in the 1960s and early 1970s grew in popularity in the early 1990s, and have now matured into therapies that are integrated into mainstream medicine. For instance, mindfulness-based stress reduction, which has its roots in Eastern cosmology, is now a common offering in hospital settings. The terms mindbody, integrative medicine, multidisciplinary care, and holistic health, all can be traced back to that era, as can the present form of hospital massage. Now, instead of being part of nursing or rehabilitation services, massage has become incorporated into such departments as Integrative Medicine, Complementary Therapies, or Holistic Health. Massage has, once again, become part of an approach that addresses the whole person: physical, emotional, mental, social, environmental, and spiritual.

The second societal transformation from the 1960s and 1970s that influenced today's practice of massage, was the increasingly technological nature of medicine. High-tech medicine led to patients being cared for by a team of specialists. There are many advantages of being cared for by experts, but there are drawbacks to having a dozen different staff members tending to their piece of the puzzle. A patient's day in the hospital can consist of a steady stream of hospital staff, each treating only one specific part of the patient's health needs, leaving the patient feeling fragmented. The respiratory therapist cares for the lungs; the physical therapist sees to the legs; the nurse manages the plan of care; the pharmacist is responsible for managing pain; the nursing assistant sees to the personal care needs; the nutritionist oversees the food; the intravenous nurse attends to catheters; the social worker cares for the psychosocial needs; and the pastoral counselor attends to the soul.

Chapter ONE

John Naisbitt foretold of this scenario in his 1982 book, *Megatrends*. Advances in technology, he predicted, would be accompanied by a need for more touch. High-tech/high touch was one of his lead prognostications.[8] It is easy to rail against medical technology and specialization, to long for the good old days when the town doctor treated patients from childhood through adulthood. Paradoxically, however, the rise of technology is now partly responsible for the growth of hospital massage as a specialty. As health care has become more fragmented, the need for modalities that can provide a sense of wholeness, such as massage therapy, is greater. Fragmentation and wholeness, two seemingly opposite characteristics, are inextricably linked.

The nursing profession, despite being an increasingly high-tech endeavor, still leans toward creating wholeness for patients. Therefore, it is not surprising that the creation of the modern-day hospital massage therapist was pioneered in the late 1980s by nurses and is, even now, strongly influenced by many nurses. There is definitely a place for touch therapy given by nurses, respiratory therapists, social workers, and all health care staff – indeed, everyone caring for patients should see touch as part of their therapeutic mandate. However, the development of a specialist devoted to touch therapy has many advantages.

Just as medical specialists are able to provide more knowledgeable care, so too are massage specialists. Professional touch therapists have a broader and deeper level of skill. Patients who previously might have been passed by as inappropriate massage candidates, such as those with congestive heart failure or low platelet levels, can now enjoy the benefits of low-impact touch modalities that specialists are trained to administer. A bodyworker also has the luxury of unhurried time with the patient that was not available to nurses even 50 years ago. Whereas a nurse may have time to rub the back or feet, a massage practitioner has time to attend to the entire person. The sense of wholeness created by this kind of attention is an important contribution to patient care. Additionally, it is the professional massage therapist who has the knowledge and time to spend teaching family how to massage their loved one.

Summary

Today's hospital massage therapists are not unlike the attendants in the healing temples of Greece, the *hospes* workers from the Middle Ages, or the nurses who tended soldiers injured in battle. Their careers are and were ones of service and sacrifice. Guenter Risse's quote at the start of this chapter is as true today as 600 years ago: "…hospitals demanded great sacrifices from those who committed themselves to aiding the sick."[1]

Historians will look back on the present era as a time when the arc of the pendulum widened to include science and art, when West met East, modernity reached back to join with the ancient, and technology spawned a renewed need for touch. The present period is only a single chapter in a continuously evolving story: ultimately, the story will always return to the same place – hands contain medicine. No matter what the techniques of the day are or who is designated to administer them, touch is a vital component in caring for people.

References

1. Risse GB. Mending Bodies, Saving Souls: The History of Hospitals. New York: Oxford University Press; 1999.

2. US National Library of Medicine. Medieval Islamic Medicine. 2011. Available from: https://www.nlm.nih.gov/exhibition/islamic_medical/islamic_02.html

3. Das A. Greek Philosophy and Medicine. British Library. Available from: https://www.bl.uk/greek-manuscripts/articles/the-transmission-of-greek-philosophy-and-medicine

4. US National Library of Medicine. Hospitals. 2011. Available from: https://www.nlm.nih.gov/exhibition/islamic_medical/islamic_12.html

5. Calvert RN. The History of Massage. Rochester: Healing Arts Press; 2002.

6. Calvert RN. Pages from History: Massage in Nursing. Massage Magazine. 2003 May/June; pp. 158–160.

7. UK National Archives. Women in Uniform: The Almeric Paget Military Massage Corps – Introduction. Available from: http://www.nationalarchives.gov.uk/womeninuniform/almeric_paget_intro.html

8. Naisbitt J. Megatrends. New York: Warner Books; 1982.

It is important to become familiar with research results and use them to educate others and to shape our practice. If we are truly health professionals, this is our duty to our clients. It is also our professional and ethical responsibility to make responsible claims about the outcomes of our work.

Tracy Walton, Massage Therapy Educator

When back rubs were part of standard evening nursing care, it was enough that they just felt good. There was no need to analyze or dissect the experience. Patients and hospital staff knew firsthand that massage was relaxing, good preparation for sleep, and mood enhancing. However, in today's science-oriented, cost containment-driven society, many people want beneficial claims to be backed by proof. Time and financial resources are precious; health care organizations, government agencies, insurance companies, and even philanthropic organizations want to know that interventions are truly providing beneficial outcomes, rather than administering care based on assumption, hope, or myth. There is, however, no clear pathway to this goal as yet for complementary therapies such as massage.

One way of evaluating care is through the use of evidence-informed practice (EIP). This model seeks to make clinical decisions that incorporate a variety of factors. The best available research is coupled with the client's needs, values, and preferences, the wisdom of the practitioner, and prevailing theory, all within the culture of the institution and community.[1]

The EIP model is ideal for integrative health care, however, the research part of the equation is not yet well defined. Despite an increase in studies containing larger sample sizes and more randomized controlled trials, there are still too few studies for the most part, and those that have been conducted are often considered to have lower value on the levels of evidence ladder because they don't measure up to the norms traditionally used in medicine (see Info Box 2.1).

The gold standard in research is the double-blinded, randomized controlled trial (RCT) protocol, which was designed for pharmaceutical research, not holistic medicine; and yet, it is this framework that is expected of investigations, even though it has severe limitations when it comes to evaluating complementary therapies. The RCT model asks narrow, isolated questions, which is not reflective of therapies such as massage – integrative medicine is complex and patient-centered.[2]

Info Box 2.1 Levels of evidence

Level	Type of evidence
1	Meta-analysis/systematic review
2	RCTs (the larger the sample size the better)
3	Non-RCTs
4	Observational studies with a comparison group
5	Case report or case series
6	Expert opinion

There are various *levels of evidence* models such as this one. Each is based on a similar idea, which is that some types of studies have greater strength due to methodology, quality of data, or sample size. These models are designed to help weigh the evidence. Other similar versions can be found by doing an internet search of "levels of evidence."

Holistic care can be evaluated by using *whole systems research* (WSR). As of yet, WSR has not evaluated hospitalized patients, which would require more qualitative investigations. Qualitative studies explore a patient's whole experience: one example of this is the study by Arnon et al. of reflexology for women in labor.[3] These researchers set out to explore the physical and psychological components of this experience through in-depth, open interviews. Nearly all of the 36 laboring mothers felt empowered, had increased self-confidence, and a greater ability to self-manage pain during labor and delivery. They described the reflexology treatments as a holistic experience that allowed them to relax even after the therapist left the room. This is the type of feedback that is not captured with quantitative data.

Despite the lack of ideal research, it is the goal of this chapter to present the research as it does exist, which tends toward the classic RCT or quasi-experimental design. These studies have merit, but they do not yet provide crystal clear answers that clinicians and funders might wish for. Very little cost analysis has been performed through these investigations. Most lean toward how massage therapy might be used in symptom management.

Examining research may not be natural territory for massage therapists. However, it doesn't take a doctoral degree or expertise in statistical analysis to understand the basics of research. It is the aim of this chapter to distill the existing research and present it in a comprehensible way, warts and all.

Inclusion criteria

Inclusion criteria are the characteristics that prospective subjects must meet to qualify for a study. This chapter, too, used inclusion criteria to discern which studies would be reported. Only published investigations of people who were receiving care in hospitals, hospices, long-term care facilities, and rehabilitation centers were incorporated. Excluded were massage studies of healthy subjects, animals, case studies, anecdotal reports, doctoral dissertations, and massage given by family or companions. The goal was to present the most recent research that could be accessed. In a few cases, older research was included because it contained clinical information not found in newer articles.

Studies written in English that examine manual techniques in which the hands are used to touch or manipulate tissue, such as Swedish massage, acupressure, and reflex-

ology, are reported. Biofield modalities, such as Reiki or Therapeutic Touch, are often used with positive results in hospitals and other health care settings and are included in this chapter. Mechanical forms of massage, such as the use of wristbands to stimulate acupressure points or pneumatic cuffs, are not included. Most older studies and those with small sample sizes or weak methodologies were not included. However, a few of these are part of the presentation in this chapter because they instruct the therapist in clinical information that may be important.

Technology can be blamed for creating a sense of disconnection from the world, but it has also created connections and global cross-pollination in unimaginable ways. This is evident in the research that now exists from around the world. The tables in this chapter present studies from Australia, Canada, Egypt, Germany, India, Iran, Ireland, Israel, Japan, South Korea, Sweden, Turkey, Taiwan, the UK, USA, and more. The exploration in this chapter brings together studies that have examined the effects of massage in a variety of health care settings. The aim is to paint a broad picture that is inclusive rather than exclusive. While it is true that many of these studies have limitations due to sample size, methodology, or research design and would not qualify for a meta-analysis or be at the top of the levels of evidence ladder, they still have a story to tell. They show what is feasible and may inspire massage therapists with new ideas. Massage researcher Janet Kahn states: "Research is any systematic inquiry."[4] This then is the overriding criterion for inclusion: does the study show evidence of a consistent and methodical inspection?

To start with, the studies are grouped by variables, such as pain, anxiety, vital signs, and sleep. The same studies are then presented in chart form by patient population, such as surgery, intensive care, oncology, or cardiology.

Examining the variables

Variables refer to *what* is being measured, such as blood pressure, nausea, or fatigue. This section looks across the patient populations at the studies according to these measurements. Many of the results are what practitioners would expect, such as the positive effect on anxiety, pain, and sleep. At other times, the research produces surprising outcomes, such as the mixed effects on vital signs or the lack of examination of patient satisfaction.

Anxiety and pain are a good starting place for the review because they are the two most studied variables.

Anxiety

Anxiety is specific to the circumstances. It is not a "one size fits all" emotion. For example, a patient undergoing cataract surgery may be apprehensive about being awake during the procedure or they may be worried about having a claustrophobic reaction while under the drape. People who have just had open-heart surgery may fear for many things, including their survival. To be moved into a nursing facility may provoke intense uncertainty and anxiety. Many first-time mothers-to-be are anxious about the intense, almost unbearable pain of childbirth, which is one of the reasons cesarean sections are popular.

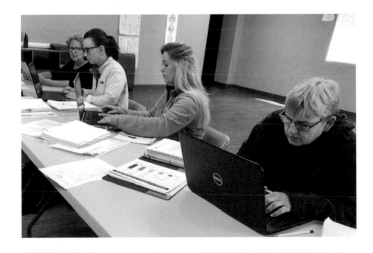

FIGURE 2.1
Lexington Healing Arts Academy (Kentucky), Hospital-based massage therapy practitioners studying the research.

(Photo by Carolyn Jauco-Trott)

No matter the source of anxiety, massage techniques have a high success rate in alleviating short-term anxiety. This finding holds true across a broad spectrum of patient groups: cardiac[5–14] and geriatric patients,[15–18] people in the intensive care unit (ICU),[19] maternity patients,[20–23] people with cancer,[24–31] and those undergoing procedures[32–34] and surgery.[35–42]

Researchers looked at a variety of massage interventions, such as a 5-minute hand massage before cataract surgery,[10] a 20–30-minute reflexology session on open-heart surgery patients on mechanical ventilation,[69] 10-minute back massage for ICU patients,[19] and a 20-minute Swedish massage combined with music prior to wound care for burn patients.[34] With a few exceptions,[43–47] each of the unique interventions reduced short-term anxiety.

In and of itself, reducing anxiety is a laudable goal. A person is more comfortable when they are at peace. However, less anxiety translates into more than just comfort – anxious energy can be put to better use. The patient often softens internally, becoming more receptive, and maybe, just for a moment, is able to interact more openly with visitors and staff, or to smile more easily. They might be receptive to the art or music therapist or walking in the halls with the PT. It's even been suggested that wounds heal faster, pain is lessened, and sleep improved.

Pain

Pain is a simple, tidy-looking word, and yet is a complex and difficult condition. It has physical and emotional components that are rooted in complicated forces: this is one of the reasons that pain is so difficult to manage. When researchers ask patients to rate their pain, the rich background that is influencing pain is not parsed out. This is one of the limitations of quantitative research.

Pain and its associated treatments are increasingly being scrutinized. In the USA, there is an urgency to the attention because of the abuse of opioids and the high number of deaths by overdose. While other countries have not had the same scale of dire outcomes, they too have renewed focus on pain. Pain, especially chronic pain, is a crisis that affects public health as well as social and economic welfare, and globally, is estimated to affect 20% of the adult population.[48]

Not all pain can be managed through drugs alone. The ideal pain management program consists of a combination of drug and nondrug interventions, such as massage. Bodywork techniques consistently reduced short-term pain in the majority of studies reviewed of patients receiving care in hospitals and nursing homes.

A study done by the Mayo Clinic of 1220 integrative service sessions found that massage therapy was the most requested service by inpatients and was highly effective in reducing short-term pain.[49] Most of the examinations of heart patients, many of who were either in the critical care unit, ICU, or recovering from open-heart surgery, showed reduced pain.[5,6,9,50–52] Only two studies showed no difference between the massage group and the control group.[46,53] These studies not only demonstrate an effectiveness on short-term pain, but they show that it is feasible for massage therapists to work in critical and intensive care arenas with patients who have had major surgery.

Pain studies for elders and ICU patients are limited. The two studies found of geriatric patients do show an improvement in pain.[18,54] One study in particular focused on restless leg syndrome pain, with good results.[54]

The study of maternity-related pain showed that touch therapy techniques were almost universally effective.[20,22,23,55–61] A variety of methods were found to be useful during labor: 30 minutes of massage to the abdomen, shoulders and back, and sacral pressure at the start of each of the three phases of labor,[55] 30 minutes of massage to the sacrum,[22] and massage with frangipani aromatherapy oil versus virgin coconut oil.[58] Postpartum pain was reduced with foot reflexology to the pituitary, solar plexus, and uterine points.[59] Following a C-section, a 5-minute foot massage using acupressure points CV7 and LV3[56] and 20 minutes of plain massage both reduced pain.[57]

People hospitalized for cancer treatment had reduced pain from massage.[25,29–31,45,62–64] Protocols ranged from a 10–15-minute Swedish massage,[29,62] 45-minute Healing

A therapist's journal 2.1
Show-and-tell

For nurses who have not witnessed the positive effects of massage on patients, all it takes is seeing someone who has struggled with pain management become relaxed, sleep more comfortably, or willingly participate in activities and engage with others to convince the nurse that this is a worthwhile intervention. This "show-and-tell" effect has proven, time and again, to be the most impactful method of promoting massage at the bedside.

Cathrine Weaver MSN, HN-BC, INFF, RN
Integrative C.A.R.E. Services Coordinator
Baptist Health Lexington, Lexington, Kentucky

Touch versus customized massage,[64] to a combination of acupuncture, Swedish massage, and foot acupressure.[45] It is akin to comparing apples and oranges to compare such a heterogeneous group of studies, and not a level of evidence that is comparative to a systematic review or meta-analysis; and yet, there is a benefit in being aware of the various protocols.

Patients who received massage for pain during medical procedures had mixed outcomes,[32,33,47,65,66] but a variety of surgical patients benefited from massage.[35,36,42,67,68] Only Miller et al. found a 5-minute hand/arm massage protocol did not improve pain ratings.[37]

Vital signs

Vital signs are a group of physiological assessments used to monitor a patient's status and include blood pressure, pulse, temperature, and respiration rate. Massage researchers use them as a measure of relaxation. Asked to hypothesize about the effect of massage on vital signs, a person might guess that massage decreases these variables. However, the pattern is inconclusive at best.

The vital signs of cardiac patients received the most scrutiny. One study[10] found reduced heart rate, respiration rate, and diastolic blood pressure; two others found decreased blood pressure only[8,46]; and one resulted in lowered heart rate only.[9] The other cardiac studies found no other improvement in vital signs.[9,50,69] Two geriatric studies measured vital signs and were also inconclusive.[15,16] Studies of surgical patients and those having procedural interventions are equally as indeterminate. Two groups of patients who had massage prior to a heart catheterization procedure showed no improvement in vital signs,[47,66] which was also true of a group of patients having cataract surgery.[40] However, another study of cataract surgery patients[41] and one of liver transplant patients[68] showed a decrease in respiration rate, heart rate, and blood pressure. The laparoscopic surgery patients studied by Çankaya et al. only had reduced systolic blood pressure.[67]

It is abundantly clear that touch therapy sessions have an inconsistent effect on vital signs. One must question the use of them as an indicator of relaxation or rest in hospital settings and nursing facilities. This doesn't mean that massage interventions are not relaxing, it might just mean that the researchers are not asking the right questions or using the best methods of measuring relaxation.

Sleep

Sleep is important in promoting recovery from illness and yet, is often lacking in health care settings. Despite receiving medications to promote sleep, patients often report insomnia.

All of the cardiac studies reviewed showed improvement in sleep or sleep quality from a variety of interventions.[7,53,71–73] One geriatric study showed improvement,[54] as did the three available studies of people in ICU,[19,74,75] two oncology studies,[29,76] and an investigation of acupressure for end-stage renal patients on hemodialysis.[77]

The successful protocols included a 5-minute acupressure treatment to the Heart 7 point for three days,[72] while another acupressure study examined Heart 7, Pericardium 6, Gallbadder 20, and Stomach 36, also for three days.[7] Other interventions ranged from a 20-minute hand/foot massage for seven days,[73] a neck/shoulder/back massage over three consecutive days,[53] and a 20-minute foot massage.[71]

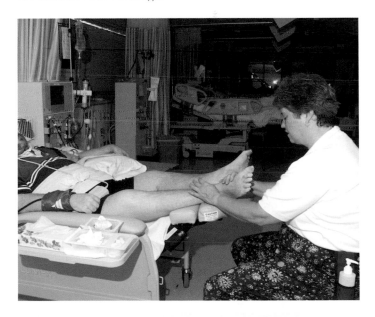

FIGURE 2.2
Hemodialysis patient receives massage during his procedure.

(Photo by Don Hamilton.)

On the other hand, three studies showed no difference between the intervention group and control.[17,63,78] It bears looking at the circumstances of these three studies. One employed a 3-minute back massage before bed,[78] another used a 5-minute hand massage,[17] both of which may not have been a large enough dose, so to speak. The third of these examinations was of people with bone metastases, a difficult symptom to ameliorate.[63]

A search of the Cochrane Library of massage-related sleep studies revealed one systematic review of non-pharmacological interventions with ICU patients. Very few massage studies met their inclusion criteria for analysis. The authors state that there was some evidence that relaxation techniques, such as foot massage and acupressure provided small improvements in various subjective measures of sleep quality, but in their opinion the quality of evidence was low.[79]

Nausea

Nausea can be a side effect of anesthesia, chemotherapy, labor, or medications. It is more than an annoyance – nausea causes serious complications, such as aspiration, dehydration, electrolyte imbalance, and disruption of a surgical site. Even though antiemetic drugs are vastly improved these days, they can have side effects that some people dislike, one of which is drowsiness. Also, these medications don't work for everyone.

Therapists experienced in massaging patients in nursing homes, hospitals, and hospices will have anecdotes of dramatic improvement in people who are nauseous. That kind of anecdotal evidence is important. Surprisingly, however, there is a dearth of research on this symptom. It is a belief within the massage profession that touch therapies decrease nausea, but the collective story is not yet clear enough to declare this. At best, a therapist could say that some patients were observed to improve. The following results show the potential of massage for nausea management, but the number of studies is insufficient and the strength of them considered to be weak.

An examination by Naseri-Salahshour showed statistically significant improvement from 30 minutes of reflexology for people undergoing hemodialysis,[80] as did Çankaya's research of a 10-minute foot massage following laproscopic surgery.[67] Lively et al. found that a group of bone marrow transplant patients had decreased nausea from 20–30-minute sessions.[81] Cassileth's retrospective study showed a minor improvement in nausea,[25] whereas the chemotherapy patients in Robison's study had significant improvement.[30] Billhult et al. found a 73% improvement in nausea, however, the control group receiving a friendly visit had nearly a 50% improvement,[43] so it is difficult to say whether the improvement was due to the massage intervention or the contact with the therapist. Wang et al. studied patients with malignant ascites. The results indicated improvement in perceived bloating and other variables, but not nausea.[24]

Constipation

Constipation affects a patient's quality of life in a significant way. This small group of investigations shows a trend toward the effectiveness of various bodywork techniques on subjects experiencing constipation. However, for the reasons previously stated, a firm conclusion cannot be made.

The nursing home patients of Cevik et al. had significant improvement in the number of bowel movements, stool consistency and weight, straining, and ability to completely empty the bowels from 45–60-minute abdominal massages for 30 days.[82] Lamas et al. also studied the effects of abdominal massage combined with laxative use in nursing home patients, compared to just laxative use and found a more positive outcome with the group that used massage.[83] Moghadam et al. compared 15-minute reflexology treatment compared with the oral ingestion of a honey and roses mixture called Golghand. Both interventions were effective on the elderly patients, but the Golghand was more effective.[84] Two studies of advanced cancer patients found improvement.[85,86] Lai et al. studied both massage alone and aromatherapy massage: both showed improvement, but the aroma massage group was even better than plain massage.[85] Wang also found improvement using acupressure to

CV12, CV4, and ST25 with a group of hospice patients who had advanced cancer.[86] By the end of a 4-week period, Abbasi et al. reported significant improvement in frequency of defecation and quality of stool with hemodialysis patients using acupressure to LV3, ST36, SP15, and CV6 three times a week.[87]

Depression

The term depression can refer to a clinical diagnosis or it can describe a short-term, situational event caused by a traumatic episode or series of them. The massage research doesn't discern between the two. Most likely the depression referred to in these studies is situational.

The examinations below paint the same cloudy picture as other variables. Two investigations of cardiac patients showed improvement in depression[12,13] while a third indicated none.[46] A single study was done of people with dementia, which had a positive outcome on depression.[18] Three of four studies of cancer patients found improvement.[25,45,63] An investigation of the psychological state of people admitted to the hospital for cardiac catheterization showed no difference between the 20-minute back massage intervention and usual care as measured by the Profile of Mood States tool.[66]

Fatigue

Despite being a major complaint of many patients, fatigue is under-studied. Five studies of cancer patients found improvement,[25,27,30,31,62] as did a study of people following open-heart surgery,[53] and an examination of people having hemodialysis.[88] The study by Vergo examined massage and Reiki: a single session of both modalities improved fatigue, but those receiving Reiki showed greater improvement.[31]

Immune-related research

Over a long period of time, sustained levels of stress can negatively affect the immune system, which is why measuring stress markers is a part of assessing immune

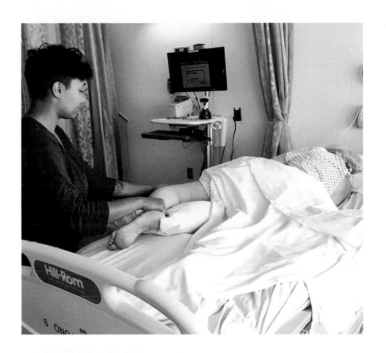

FIGURE 2.3
Resting and gathering energy during massage.

(Photo by Carolyn Tague.)

function.[89] Researchers test a variety of hormones and neurotransmitters to measure stress – cortisol is a commonly used marker of stress in massage studies. Stringer et al. tested cortisol and prolactin as stress markers,[90] and Osaka et al. used a salivary chromogranin A (CgA) test.[26] Kim et al. tested epinephrine and norepinephrine, which are neurotransmitters related to stress.[40]

The reader won't be surprised that the small body of studies had mixed findings. Billhult et al. found no difference in cortisol levels between groups in two different studies.[44,70] However the intervention groups of the Stringer et al. study,[90] which used plain massage oil and aromatherapy massage, both had a reduction in cortisol and the massage group had a reduction in prolactin. The results from the Kim et al. study of a 5-minute pre-operative hand massage showed a drop in cortisol, epinephrine, and norepinephrine levels.[40] The small group of patients with dementia in the Schaub et al. study had a decrease in salivary cortisol.[91] Osaka et al. also achieved lowered CgA levels with a group of cancer patients.[26]

Researchers also measure lymphocytes to directly evaluate immune function. Three studies evaluated lymphoctye levels. Kim et al.[40] and Billhult et al.[44] found no difference in lymphocyte levels between groups. However, another study by Billhult et al. showed that the massage group had less deterioration of natural killer (NK) cells, a type of lymphocyte.[70] Might this imply that less deterioration would translate into improved functioning of the NK cells?

The reader is left with no definitive picture in terms of immune-related research. It doesn't mean that massage has no effect on stress and immune function, but the research does not support the claim at this time.

Use of pain medication and potential cost savings

Pain medication use is of interest for two reasons. One is the negative side effects caused by analgesic drugs. They range from the mundane, like constipation, to the severe, such as addiction. If other less harmful interventions can be part of the pain management regimen, it could temper the byproducts of pain medications. The other reason being the search for less costly means of pain management.

Only three studies in this chapter examined the effect of touch therapies on the use of analgesics. Dhany et al. found that all types of anesthesia use were decreased during the intrapartum period, which is the time from the start of labor to delivery of the placenta. These included epidural, spinal, and general anesthesia.[92] Simonelli et al. researched the effect of a 20-minute massage on opioid use after an unplanned C-section: drug usage was less on days 1 and 2 in the massage group.[57] The third study, by McRee et al., investigated the effects of a 30-minute pre-operative Swedish massage and 30 minutes of gentle, passive touch on anesthetic and narcotic needs. The need for inhaled anesthesia was the same for both groups, however, the massage group needed significantly less narcotic medication during surgery.[39]

If massage does decrease the need for analgesics, does this translate into cost savings? The patients of Mehling et al. had an improvement in pain levels due to an acupuncture and massage intervention after surgery. However, it was noted that no savings were found in medication costs.[45] Two other studies, both retrospective, examined this question as it pertains to integrative medicine in a broad sense, not just massage use. Estores et al. studied inpatient cancer patients' use of integrative medicine, which included massage, tai chi/qigong, meditation/relaxation, or yoga. It showed reduced use of tranquilizing and pain medication by 44% and a "significant reduction in average drug costs per day."[93] Dusek et al. looked back at the charts of hospitalized patients who participated in the Integrative Medicine Program, which consisted of massage therapy, acupuncture, music therapy, and holistic nursing. Patients who received these therapies had reduced pain and a cost reduction of $898 per admission.[94]

This handful of studies is insubstantial and inconclusive.

Length of stay

The one-day cost of a room in a hospital or rehabilitation center is very expensive. Any intervention that could shorten the length of stay would save money for all concerned. The research into this question is miniscule. Five studies were found, two of stem cell transplant patients and three of surgical patients. The patients of Lively et al. who received massage during bone marrow transplantation went home three days sooner than the non-massage group, saving the hospital $2,850 per patient.[81] However, this cannot be cited as strong evidence as the sample size was small and the study methodology lacking. The feasibility pilot study of Lu et al. comparing daily Healing Touch or relaxation therapy to a control group found that both experimental groups had shorter lengths of stay, although this finding was not statistically significant.[95] The three other studies were on surgical patients[35,45,46] and found no difference in length of stay.

Lesser-studied variables

Many other important variables have only received cursory examination to date. Four studies looked at patient satisfaction, which all reported positive outcomes.[14,25,29,36] Quality of life was included in only three studies. Two found an improvement in quality of life, one as it correlated to constipation[85] and the other to hemodialysis.[80] The third, with cancer patients, found no difference.[43]

Other topics included: weaning time from mechanical ventilation; massage for nitroglycerin-induced headache; and the relationship of massage to the rate of engraftment, and total parenteral nutrition (TPN) use for people who have had a stem cell transplant. There is an infinite number of topics to explore.

The study of variables such as nausea, sleep, and anxiety is constructive. But what if research questions were slanted toward the positive instead of being based on the absence of pain, nausea, or fatigue? What might be discovered if joy or connection or having the energy to phone a friend were examined?

Patient populations

This section summarizes patient populations in chart form: studies are grouped by patient populations, from oldest to the most recent. The charts provide thumbnail sketches, allowing the reader to quickly access the study's basic information by noting the sample size, location of the study, use of randomization and control, intervention and who performed it, the variables studied, and the results. To understand the methodological protocols, tools of measurement, statistical analyses, the results in greater detail, and limitations, the full journal article must be read. Some articles can be accessed from the internet, others must be ordered through interlibrary services at hospitals, medical and nursing schools.

The following abbreviations are used throughout the charts:

abdom	abdominal	CCU	Coronary Care Unit	L	left	reflexol	reflexology
ACS	acute coronary syndrome	CNS	central nervous system	M	massage	RR	respiration rate
acupress	acupressure	DBP	diastolic blood pressure	min	minutes	SBP	systolic blood pressure
admin	administration	diff	difference	MT	massage therapist	SCM	sternocleidomastoid
AMI	acute myocardial infarction	Dx	diagnosis	N	number	signif	significant
aroma	aromatherapy	effl	effleurage	neuro	neurological	stat	statistical
avg	average	exper	experimental	NG	nasogastric	SVO_2	venous oxygen saturation
BM	bowel movement	FV	friendly visit	op	operation	TPN	total parenteral nutrition
BP	blood pressure	h	hour	psych	psychological	Tx	treatment
BR	breast	hosp	hospital	pts	patients	w/	with
btw	between	HR	heart rate	QoL	quality of life	wkly	weekly
CA	cancer	ICU	Intensive Care Unit	R	right	wks	wks
CABG	coronary artery bypass graft	improve	improvement	RCT	randomized controlled trial	wt	weight

Chapter TWO

Cardiology

The majority of cardiac studies were of people in critical care units due to surgery, often open-heart. Anxiety, pain, vital signs, and sleep were examined most often. Short-term anxiety consistently improved from the variety of interventions used,[5–14] as did pain[5,6,9,50–52] and sleep.[7,53,71–73] Vital signs were studied more often with cardiac patients than any other group; as reported earlier in the Vital Signs section, the outcomes were mixed. All of the above is in alignment with the conclusions of a *best evidence topic report* by Grafton-Clarke et al. on postoperative pain and anxiety in cardiac patients.[96] (A best evidence topic report is a systematic review of the research on a specific question.)

As would be expected, many of the interventions focused on the feet and hands. However, a couple of the studies gave full or partial body massage to these very complex patients. An older study by Lewis et al.[97] is included because it contains clinical information useful to positioning for a back massage. These researchers examined venous oxygen saturation (SVO_2), which is a marker for how well oxygen is being delivered to peripheral tissue. Lewis et al. found that a 1-minute back rub decreased SVO_2, an undesirable outcome that may indicate that a back rub causes a minor stimulus that increases heart rate and oxygen demand in many critically ill people. The authors also looked at the effect of positioning in relation to the back rub. Both left and right side-lying caused a drop in SVO_2, but turning to the left resulted in an even greater reduction.

In addition, Lewis et al. compared the stress of turning and immediately receiving massage, with turning and receiving the back rub after a 5-minute equilibration period. The positioning followed by a back rub after a 5-minute delay caused less of a drop in SVO_2. Oxygen saturation returned to clinically acceptable levels within five minutes of the back rub. The authors advised that massage can be administered immediately after repositioning if the individual is hemodynamically stable. Unstable patients should be monitored closely and receive delayed or gentle back rub. (Gentle massage is indicated for many reasons in this situation.)

The Grafton-Clarke et al. analysis[96] came to the conclusion that massage is not an effective therapy due to the variety of methodological protocols and the failure of some of the studies to report on analgesic requirements. It is important to report all of the research and analysis but also to bear in mind that people will look at it through different lenses. The perspective of a physician will be different from that of the nurse, massage therapist, or patient. One thing that cannot be denied is that all of studies have one thing in common: feasibility. They show the practitioner that it is possible to deliver massage to very complex patients and their hands-on techniques may help people manage some of their symptoms.

Research can also be valuable for the seeds it plants. Two studies in this group present interesting possibilities: one examined massage's influence on weaning time from mechanical ventilation,[69] the other researched the use of massage for people suffering from nitroglycerin-induced headaches.[51]

Reasonable research claims: Improvement of pain and anxiety show the strongest results from massage therapy. Sleep needs more study, but findings lean toward positive outcomes. Massage techniques cannot lay claim to improving vital signs.

TABLE 2.1 Cardiology patients

Author/Year/ Ref #	Hospital/ Country	Sample	Intervention	Key variables	Results
Lewis et al. 1997 97	Methodist Hospital, Huston, Texas, USA	• 57 male postop cardiac ICU pts • Randomly assigned to right or left side-lying position	• Admin by nurse • Group 1: placed in side-lying & immediately given 1-min back M • Group 2: placed in side-lying for 5 min before 1-min back M	• SVO_2	• L side-lying ↓ SVO_2 more than R side-lying • Position change & immediate back M caused greater ↓ in SVO_2 than delayed back M
Kshettry et al. 2006 50	Abbott Northwestern Hospital, Minneapolis, Minnesota, USA	• 104 open-heart surgery pts. – Exper: N = 53 – Control: N = 51 • RCT	• Admin by MT w/ special training • Exper: Pre-op – guided imagery, 30 min gentle touch or light M Postop days 1&2: 20 min music (pt choice). At discharge from ICU pt given a 2nd gentle touch or light M, guided imagery (usually day 2 postop) • Control: Usual care	• Feasibility • Safety • HR • DBP • SBP • Pain and tension	• Feasible and safe • Exper group signif ↓ pain and tension day 1 postop • No stat diff in HR, DBP, SBP
Albert et al. 2009 46	Department of Cardiovascular Surgery, Cleveland Clinic, Cleveland, Ohio, USA	• 252 open-heart surgery pts – Exper: N = 126 – Control: N = 126 • RCT	• Admin by licensed MTs • Intervention: two 30-min postop massage sessions (legs, arms, back) on days 2 or 3 or days 4 or 5 • Control: usual care	• Feasibility • Mood • Depression • Pain • Anxiety • Length of stay • Physiologic measurements • Atrial fibrillation	• M is feasible • No statistical diff in any measurements except for lower BP
Bauer et al. 2010 5	Department of Surgery, Mayo Clinic, Rochester, Minnesota, USA	• 113 cardiac surgery pts. – Exper: N = 62 – Control: N = 51 • RCT	• Admin by MT • Exper: 20 min postop massage on day 2 & day 4 • Control: usual care/quiet relax time, postop on day 2 & 4	• Pain • Anxiety • Tension	• Signif ↓ pain, anxiety, and tension

continued

TABLE 2.1 Cardiology patients *continued*

Author/Year/ Ref #	Hospital/ Country	Sample	Intervention	Key variables	Results
Nerbass et al. 2010 53	Heart Institute, University of São Paolo School of Medicine, São Paolo, Brazil	• 40 CABG surgery pts – Exper: N = 20 – Control: N = 20 • RCT	• Admin by physiotherapist • Exper: M to neck/ shoulders/back. Light to hard compressions, trigger point therapy, cervical traction, mobilization • Control: Usual care	• Sleep • Pain • Fatigue	• M group improve sleep all 3 days, ↓ complaints of fatigue days 1 & 2 • Pain ↓ signif in both groups all 3 days
Babaee et al. 2012 12	Isfahan Chamran Hospital, Isfahan, Iran	• 72 pts postop CABG – Exper: N = 36 – Control: N = 36 • RCT	• Admin by nurse researcher • Exper: 20 min Swedish M/4 days w/ baby oil on legs, hands, back; days 3-6 post op • Control: Usual care	• Mood measured by anxiety, depression, fatigue, confusion, anger & ability	• Signif improve in mood postop
Braun et al. 2012 14	Monash University Alfred Hospital, Melbourne, Victoria, Australia	• 146 open-heart surgery pts – Exper: N = 75 – Control: N = 71 • RCT	• Admin by MTs • Exper: 20 min individualized M session on day 3 or 4 postop and day 5 or 6 postop • Control: 20 min rest time	• Anxiety • Pain • Muscular tension • Relaxation • Vital signs • Satisfaction	• Signif improve in all variables except vital signs
Oshvandi et al. 2014 71	Ekbatan Hospital Hamedan, Iran	• 60 CCU pts w/ ischemic heart disease – Exper: N = 30 – Control: N = 30 • RCT	• Admin by nurse researcher • 20 min foot M, 2 consecutive nights • Control: usual care	• Sleep quality	• Significant improve in sleep quality
Adib-Hajbaghery et al. 2014 10	Shahid Beheshti Hospital, Kashan, Iran	• 120 male CCU pts w/ Dx of ACS or AMI – Exper: N = 60 – Control: N = 60 • RCT	• Admin by nurse researcher certified in M or supervised assistant • Exper: 60 min whole body M on day 3 postop • Control: usual care	• Anxiety • Vital signs	• Signif ↓ in anxiety • Signif ↓ HR, RR, DBP

continued

TABLE 2.1 Cardiology patients *continued*

Author/Year/ Ref #	Hospital/ Country	Sample	Intervention	Key variables	Results

Bagheri-Nesami et al. 2014 *11*	Mazandaran Heart Center, Sari, Iran	• 80 pts postop CABG
		  – Exper: N = 40
		  – Control: N = 40
		• RCT
			• Admin by nurse researcher
			• Exper: 20 min reflexol to L foot for 4 days
			• Control: 1 min gentle M to L foot w/oil for 4 days
				• Anxiety	• Signif ↓ in anxiety from reflexology

Siavoshi et al. 2017 *72*	Bahman Hospital Neyshabour, Iran	• 90 pts w/chronic heart failure
		• Three-arm study
		  – 1. Acupress: N = 30
		  – 2. Pseudo: N = 30
		  – 3. Control: N = 30
		• Double-blind RCT w/ placebo
			• Admin by nurse researcher
			• 1. Acupress: Heart 7 point on wrist, 5 min/3 days
			• 2. Pseudo: Acupressure 1.5 cm away from Heart 7 point
			• 3. Control: usual care
				• Sleep quality	• Signif improve in quality of sleep in acupressure group

Alimohammad et al. 2018 *8*	Hajar Hospital, Shahrekord, Iran	• 70 pts w/ACS
		  – Exper: N = 35
		  – Control N = 35
		• RCT
			• Admin by nurse and patient companion
			• Exper: 20 min hand/foot M
			• Control: friendly visit
				• Anxiety
				• Vital signs
					• Signif ↓ in anxiety
					• Signif ↓ BP, RR, HR

Boitor et al. 2018 *6*	Medical-Surgical McGill University, Montreal, Canada	• 60 ICU cardiac surgery pts
		• Three-arm study:
		  – 1. M group: N = 20
		  – 2. Hand-holding: N = 19
		  – 3. Control: N = 21
		• RCT
			• Admin by registered nurse
			• Group 1: 20 min hand M
			• Group 2: 20 min hand-holding
			• Group 3: 20 min rest period
				• Pain intensity
				• Pain unpleasantness
				• Anxiety
				• Muscle tension
					• Group 1 signif ↓ in all variables
					• No signif diff btw hand holding and resting

continued

TABLE 2.1 Cardiology patients *continued*

Author/Year/ *Ref #*	Hospital/ Country	Sample	Intervention	Key variables	Results

Imani et al. 2018 *51*	Urmia University of Medical Sciences,Urmia, Iran	• 75 males in CCU
		• Three-arm study:
		  – 1. Exper: N = 25
		  – 2. Placebo: N = 25
		  – 3. Control: N = 25
		• RCT
			• Admin by nurse researcher
			• Exper: reflexol 2x/20 min to head reflexol zone at 3 hr interval
			• Placebo: unspecified point at heel
			• Control: usual care
				• Nitroglycerin (NTG) migraine-type headache intensity	• Signif ↓ in NTG-induced headache intensity after reflexology Tx

Rodrigues et al. 2018 *9*	A.J. Hospital & Research Center, India Institute of Heart Sciences & Omega Hospital Mangalore, India	• 40 pts postop CABG or valve replacement
		  – Exper: N = 20
		  – Control: N = 20
		• Experimental/non-randomized design
			• Admin by researcher
			• Exper: 20 min foot & hand M, 2x daily (morning & evening) days 1–3 postop
			• Control: usual care
				• Pain
				• Anxiety
				• Vital signs
					• Signif ↓ in pain & anxiety
					• Signif ↓ HR on days 1 and 2 postop

Aygin and Sen 2019 *7*	Bezmialem University, Istanbul, Turkey	• 100 cardiac surgery pts
		  – Exper: N = 50
		  – Control: N = 50
		• RCT
			• Admin by nurse researcher (cert acupress practitioner)
			• Exper: beginning day 3 postop for 3 days, acupressure to H7, PC6, GB20, ST6; 2 mins each point, R and L side of body
			• Control: usual care
				• Anxiety
				• Sleep quality
					• Signif ↓ in anxiety
					• Signif ↑ in sleep quality

Bahrami et al. 2019 *13*	Teaching hospital, Tehran, Iran	• 90 older women (age >60) hospitalized for ACS
		  – Exper: N = 45
		  – Control: N = 45
		• RCT
			• Admin by trained researcher
			• Exper: 20 min M and reflexol, 1x. Stimulation to solar plexus, pituitary, brain, heart, intestines, vertebral column, adrenal, kidney
			• Control: usual care
				• Anxiety
				• Depression
					• Signif ↓ in anxiety and depression

continued

TABLE 2.1 Cardiology patients *continued*

Author/Year/ *Ref #*	Hospital/ Country	Sample	Intervention	Key variables	Results

Cheragjbeigi el al. 2019 73	Imam Ali Hospital, Kermanshah, Iran	• 150 pts w/ cardiac & sleep disorder
		• Three-arm study:
		  – 1. Massage: N = 50
		  – 2. Aroma M: N = 50
		  – 3. Control: N = 50
		• RCT
			• Admin by male/female nurses
			• 1. Massage: 20 min, foot/hand M w/sweet almond oil, daily/ 7 days
			• 2. Aroma M: 20 min foot/ hand M using mixture of lavender/ sweet almond oil daily/7 days
			• 3. Control: usual care
				• Sleep quality	• Number of pts w/ sleep disorder ↓
					• M and aromatherapy signif improved sleep quality

Kandemir et al. 2019 69	Cardiovascular surgical unit of a teaching hospital, Istanbul, Turkey	• 85 ICU open-heart surgery pts on mechanical ventilation
		  – Exper: N = 42
		  – Control: N = 43
		• Non-RCT
			• Admin by researcher certified in reflexol
			• Exper: 20–30 min foot rcflcxology
			• Control: usual care
				• Vital signs
				• Weaning time from mechanical ventilation
					• No signif changes in vital signs
					• Mechanical ventilation weaning time shorter for reflexol pts

Taherian et al. 2020 52	Mazandaran University of Medical Sciences, Sari, Iran	• 80 CABG pts
		  – Exper: N = 40
		  – Control: N = 40
		• RCT
			• Admin by trained nurse
			• Exper: 10 min ice M on Hegu point (I I4), L hand
			• Control: 10 min no pressure, on L hand, using glass marble on Hegu point
				• Pain	• Signif ↓ pain from ice M to LI4

Geriatric

This group of studies examines elders in nursing care facilities. Anxiety, constipation, and sleep were the most commonly examined variables. Like other patient groups, geriatric patients had improvement in anxiety from the various interventions.[15–18] Two different abdominal massage protocols[82,83] and one reflexology study were tested on constipation with good results.[84] Sleep improved with twice weekly reflexology sessions over a 4-week period[54] but not from a 3-minute slow-stroke back massage protocol,[78] or a 5-minute hand massage intervention.[17] The curious reader might then wonder whether a 15-minute slow-stroke back massage would be effective instead of a 3-minute one, or a 15-minute foot massage rather than a 5-minute hand massage. The outcomes of these sleep studies may not be due to an inadequacy of massage but might reflect the wrong dosage and frequency.

Reasonable research claims: As of yet, the study of massage and its effect on elderly patients in the hospital or nursing facility is insufficient to stake any scientific claims.

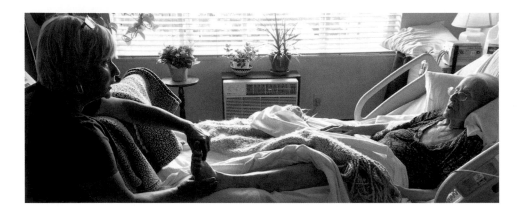

FIGURE 2.4
"Yes, please," a little harder on that spot.

(Photo by Gayle MacDonald.)

TABLE 2.2 Geriatric patients

Author/Year/ Ref #	Hospital/Country	Sample	Intervention	Key variables	Results

Rho et al. 2006 *15*	University Hospital, Seoul, South Korea	• 36 females
		  – Exper: N = 16
		  – Control: N = 20
		• Quasi-experimental control
			• Admin by nurses
			• Exper: 20 min aromatherapy M 3x/ per week for two 3-wk periods, 1-wk break in between
			• Control: usual care
				• Anxiety
				• Self-esteem
				• Blood pressure
				• Heart rate
					• Signif ↓ in anxiety and ↑ self-esteem
					• No signif diff in BP or HR

Cinar et al. 2009 *16*	Long-term nursing home, Izmir, Turkey	• 42 pts
		  – Exper: N = 21
		  – Control: N = 21
		• Experimental study
			• Admin by nurse researcher
			• Exper: 15-30 min back M/3 days
			• Control: Usual care
				• Vital signs
				• Anxiety
					• Signif ↓ in anxiety, HR, and BP
					• No signif diff in RR & body temp

Lamas et al. 2009 *83*	Nursing homes and care centers, Sweden	• 58 pts
		  – Exper: N = 29
		  – Control: N = 29
		• RCT
			• Admin by nurse
			• Exper: laxatives & abdom M
			• Control: laxatives
				• Use of abdom M for constipation management	• Signif ↓ in severity of GI symptoms
					• ↑ in BMs
					• No change in laxative use in either group

continued

TABLE 2.2 Geriatric patients *continued*

Author/Year/ *Ref #*	Hospital/Country	Sample	Intervention	Key variables	Results
Harris et al. 2012 *78*	Four nursing homes in rural southeastern USA	• 40 residents w/ dementia – Exper: N = 20 – Control: N = 20 • Pilot RCT	• Admin by nurse researcher trained in geriatric M • Exper: 3 min, slow-stroke back M at bedtime • Control: usual care	• Sleep	• No stat signif diff btw groups • Dose-finding studies needed
Choi 2015 *17*	• Five nursing home facilities in Seoul and Gyeonggi-do, South Korea	• 72 elderly women • Three groups: – 1. Hand M & music therapy: N = 24 – 2. Hand M: N = 25 – 3. Control: N = 23 • RCT	• Admin by trained research assistants • 1. 5 min hand M w/ chamomile, lavender essential oils w/ jojoba; music via earphones, 2x/wk for 4 wks • 2. Hand M w/ plain oil only • 3. Usual care	• Anxiety • Sleep	• Group 1 ↓ anxiety • No change in sleep btw groups
Rodriguez-Mansilla et al. 2015 *18*	Nursing home, Extremadura, Spain	• 111 elderly residents w/ dementia • 3 groups: – 1. Ear acupress: N = 40 – 2. Massage: N = 35 – 3. Usual care: N = 36 • RCT	• 1. Ear acupress using herbal seeds placed by acupuncturist • 2. M admin by physiotherapist, 20 mins, lower limbs and back • 3. Control: usual care	• Pain • Anxiety • Depression	• Ear acupress and M improved all variables • Ear acupress had greatest improve
Cevik et al. 2018 *82*	Nursing home, Province of Manisa, Turkey	• 22 elderly pts w/ constipation • No control	• Admin by certified MTs • 45–60 min daily abdominal M for 30 days following breakfast	• # of BMs • Consistency & wt of stool • Straining • Ability to completely empty bowels	• Signif improve in all measures

continued

TABLE 2.2 Geriatric patients *continued*

Author/Year/ Ref #	Hospital/Country	Sample	Intervention	Key variables	Results

Fakhravari et al. 2018 54	Nursing homes, Fars Providence of Shiraz City, Iran	• 70 women w/ restless leg syndrome
		  – Exper: N = 35
		  – Control: N = 35
		• Quasi-experimental
			• Admin by researcher
			• Intervention: foot reflexol, eight-20 min sessions/4 wks
			• Control: usual care
				• Sleep quality
				• Restless leg syndrome pain
					• Signif improve in sleep quality and restless leg syndrome pain

Moghadam et al. 2018 84	Bahman Hospital, Gonabad, Iran	• 60 elderly pts w/ constipation in 2 groups
		  – Reflexology: N = 30
		  – Golghand: N = 30 (composition of roses and honey taken orally)
		• RCT
			• Admin by male/female researchers trained in reflexol
			• Reflexol 15 min using sweet almond oil 2x daily/2 wks
			• Golghand 30 min before lunch/2 wks
				• Intensity of constipation
				• Frequency of BM
					• Signif ↑ in # of BMs in both groups, but greater improve from Golghand
					• Signif ↓ in intensity of constipation in Golghand group

Shaub et al. 2018 91	Specialized Geriatric Psychiatry Unit, University Hospital, Switzerland	• 40 dementia pts
		  – Exper: N = 20
		  – Control: N = 20
		• RCT pilot study
			• Admin by nurses & care assistants
			• Exper: 7 hand massages/3 continuous wks.
			• Control: usual care
				• Agitation
				• Biological markers for stress (salivary cortisol and alpha-amylase)
					• ↓ in agitation, but not stat signif
					• ↓ biological stress markers
					• Beneficial for stress

Intensive/critical care

When examining the ICU studies in Table 2.3, the reader should also bear in mind the studies from the Cardiac section, as the majority of these were of patients on a cardiac ICU. The handful of interventions in Table 2.3 varied from back massage, reflexology, abdominal bodywork, and aromatherapy massage. The focus of three of the studies was sleep, with each reporting a positive outcome.[19,74,75] The other two projects examined the issue of nutritional support, which is a key challenge for patients being fed through a nasogastric tube. Lack of caloric intake increases the risk of mortality, malnutrition-related complications, and cost of care. Abdominal massage performed two or three times a day for three days decreased gastric residual volume (GSV), which is a positive outcome. GSV monitoring is used to measure the amount of stomach content: a lesser volume may be a reflection of improved food movement along the intestinal tract and thus quicker transit time of nutrients.[98,99]

Reasonable research claims: The research with general ICU patients is not yet sufficient enough to draw any conclusions.

TABLE 2.3 Intensive care patients (general)

Author/Year/ *Ref #*	Hospital/Country	Sample	Intervention	Key variables	Results
Momenfar et al. 2018 *98*	Fatemeh Zahra Hospital, Ahwaz, Iran	• 60 ICU pts – Exper: N = 30 – Control: N = 30 • RCT	• Admin by researcher trained by sports medicine specialist • Exper: abdom M 20 min, 2x daily for 3 days • Control: usual care	• Gastric residual volume (a reflection of digestive function for pts fed through NG tube)	Signif ↓ gastric residual volume (positive result)
Hsu et al. 2019 *19*	Chi Mei Medical Center, Southern Taiwan	• 60 ICU pts – Exper: N = 30 – Control: N = 30 • Quasi-experimental	• Admin by nurse • Exper: 10 min back M, 3 consecutive nights • Control: usual care	• Sleep quality • Vital signs • Anxiety	• Improved sleep quality and breathing • ↓ anxiety
Kandeel et al. 2019 *74*	6 ICUs affiliated w/ Mansoura University Hospitals, Mansoura, Egypt	• 100 adult surgical ICU pts – Exper: N = 50 – Control: N = 50 • Quasi-experimental design	• Admin by expert MT • Exper: 10 min back M using baby oil/3 consecutive nights • Control: quiet rest	• Perceived sleep quality	• Signif improved sleep quality
Pagnucci et al. 2019 *75*	ICU (med/surg, emergency units), University of Pisa, Italy	• 74 ICU pts – Medical: 17 pts – Surgical: 47 pts ER: 10 pts • Non-controlled clinical study	• Admin by trained nurse • 20 min aroma M using lavender/lemon almond oil and musical sounds	• Sleep quality	• Signif improved quality of sleep
El-Feky et al. 2020 *99*	ICUs affiliated w/ Cairo University Hospitals, Cairo, Egypt	• 60 ICU pts w/ NG tubes in place – Exper: N = 30 – Control: N = 30 • Quasi-experimental	• Admin by nurse researchers • Exper: abdom M 3x/day for 15 min w/ paraffin oil • Control: usual care	• Gastric residual volume	• Signif ↓ gastric residual volume

Maternity

The majority of the maternity-related studies examined pain at various points of the birthing process: during labor,[3,22,23,55,58,60,61] after a planned C-section,[20] and postpartum pain.[56,57] Pain diminished for the women in all of the above circumstances.

Three studies measured the use of pain medication, one during labor[92] and two for postpartum pain.[57,59] Dhany et al. studied over 2,000 charts retrospectively and found an "apparent" decrease in anesthesia use during labor of the women who received massage and aromatherapy.[92] Simonelli reported less opioid use on days 1 and 2 following an unplanned C-section.[57] However, Nia et al. found no difference in analgesia usage between groups of postpartum patients.[59] As with other patient populations, anxiety decreased in each instance.[20–23,55]

First-time mothers can become extremely anxious and fearful from the pain of childbirth, which sets off the release of hormones and neurotransmitters that can exacerbate the pain and prolong labor. Controlling pain and anxiety can have tangible outcomes in the delivery process. Duration of labor is one of the main possibilities and it was explored in four studies. The first-time mothers of Hanjani et al. and Dolatian et al. had shortened duration in all three phases of labor as a result of foot reflexology during labor.[23,61] The first two stages of labor were shortened from massage for the patients of Bolbol-Haghighi et al.,[101] while Valiani et al. found a reduced length of time for the first stage from reflexology.[60]

The other important outcome from controlling anxiety and pain during labor is the potential of improved Apgar scores in the newborn (this score summarizes the baby's health at birth). Three studies rated this aspect and all found improved Apgar scores.[23,60,101]

Two unique questions were posed among this group of studies. How does reflexology affect the rate of hemorrhage during labor? And, can massage affect the quantity of mothers' breast milk? With respect to the first question, Valiani et al. found that the rate of hemorrhage was reduced in the group that received 30 minutes of reflexology two times during labor.[60] Regarding mothers' milk, massage to the neck was compared to massage to the pectoralis muscle. Neck massage significantly increased the quantity of the mother's milk.[102]

Reasonable research claims: Massage "may have a role in reducing pain, reducing length of labor and improving women's sense and emotional experience of labor..."[100]

TABLE 2.4 Maternity patients

Author/Year/*Ref #*	Hospital/Country	Sample	Intervention	Key variables	Results
Chang et al. 2002 *55*	Regional hospital in southern Taiwan	• 60 women in labor, first pregnancy – Exper: N = 30 – Control: N = 30 • RCT	• Admin by nurse researcher and colleague • Exper: 30 min M (abdom, sacral pressure, shoulders/back) at start of each of 3 phases of labor • Control: Usual care	• Pain • Anxiety	• Signif ↓ pain at each stage of labor and ↓ of anxiety in early stage. • 87% reported M was helpful
Valiani et al. 2010 *60*	Hospitals of Isfahan, Iran	• 88 women in labor (1st pregnancy, vaginal birth) – Exper: N = 44 – Control: N = 44 • Quasi-experimental	• Admin unknown • Exper: 30 min reflexol each foot: general zones & ovaries, uterus, fallopian tubes, liver, spleen, kidney, pituitary, solar plexus during active labor; 2x during labor • Control: Usual care	• Pain • Labor duration • Rate of hemorrhage • Apgar score	• Signif ↓ pain, and rate of hemorrhage • Signif ↓ duration 1st phase of labor, but not 2nd & 3rd • ↑ Apgar score

continued

TABLE 2.4 Maternity patients *continued*

Author/Year/*Ref #*	Hospital/Country	Sample	Intervention	Key variables	Results

Dolatian et al. 2011 *61*	Shahid Akbarabadi Hospital, Tehran, Iran	• 120 women in labor (1st pregnancy)
		• 3 groups
		  1. Reflexol: N = 40
		  2. Emotional support: N = 40
		  3. Usual care: N = 40
		• RCT
			• Admin by midwife researcher
			  1. 40 min reflexol at 4-5 cm dilation, pituitary, solar plexus, lumbar/sacral area, genital area zones
			  2. 40 min emotional support
			  3. Usual care
				• Pain at all stages of labor
				• Labor duration
					• Reflexol group ↓ pain and duration of labor at each stage
					• Emotional support group ↓ pain in early labor

Dhany et al. 2012 *92*	General maternity unit in southwest England, UK	• 2,158 pregnant intrapartum patients
		  – Exper: N = 1,079
		  – Comparison: N = 1,079
		• Retrospective
			• Admin by aroma and M staff
			• Exper: M and aroma
			• Comparison: Usual care
				• The need for analgesia during labor	• Aroma and M appear to ↓ intrapartum anesthesia use

Hanjani et al. 2015 *23*	Alborz and Bahonar hospitals, Karaj, Iran	• 80 women in labor (1st pregnancy)
		  – Exper: N = 44
		  – Control: N = 44
		• Quasi-experimental
			• Admin unknown
			• Exper: 20 min each foot, general M w/sunflower oil and specific foot reflexolpituitary, solar plexus, uterus
			• Control: M to other parts of foot
				• Anxiety
				• Pain
				• Labor duration
				• Type of labor
				• Apgar score
					Exper group:
					• Signif ↓ pain & anxiety, immed after, 30, 60, & 120 min
					• Signif ↓ labor duration
					• ↑ rate of natural vaginal delivery
					• ↑ Apgar score

Irani et al. 2015 *20*	Omolbanin Hospital, Mashhad, Iran	• 80 women w/ planned C-sections
		  – Exper: N = 40
		  – Control: N = 40
		• RCT
			• Admin by trained midwife nurse researcher
			• Exper: 5 min M to each hand and foot 4 hrs postop
			• Control: FV 20 min
				• Pain
				• Anxiety
					• Signif ↓ pain and anxiety immediately, 60, and 90 mins after M vs. FV
					
					continued

TABLE 2.4 Maternity patients *continued*

Author/Year/*Ref #*	Hospital/Country	Sample	Intervention	Key variables	Results

Bolbol-Haghighi et al. 2016 *101*	Fatemieh Hospital, Shahroud, Iran	• 100 women in labor
		  – Exper: N = 50
		  – Control: N = 50
		• RCT
			• Admin by midwifery students instructed in M
			• Exper: Minimum 30 min M under belly, thighs, sacrum shoulders & legs
			• Control: usual care
				• Duration of labor
				• Apgar score
					• Signif ↓ in duration of 1st & 2nd stages of labor
					• ↑ Apgar scores

Basyouni et al. 2018 *56*	El-Shatby University Hospital, Alexandria, Egypt	• 70 post C-section pts
		  – Exper: N = 35
		  – Control: N = 35
		• Quasi-experimental
			• Admin by trained researcher
			• Exper: 5 min kneading to each foot & acupress points CV7, LV3
			• Control: usual care
				• Post C-section pain	• Signif ↓ in pain sensations and intensity

Damanik 2018 *102*	Maternal & Child Hospital, Ummi Khasanah Bantul, Panembahan Senapati Bantul, Indonesia	• 54 new mothers (days 1-3 post-delivery)
		  – 2 groups:
		    Neck M: N = 27
		  – Pectoralis M: N = 27
		• Pre-exper design
			• Admin by midwife researcher
			• 15 min M either to the neck or pectoralis muscles 1x day/3 days
				• Quantity of mothers' breast milk	• Signif ↑ in quantity of mothers' milk after neck M vs. pectoralis M

Simonelli et al. 2018 *57*	Large teaching hospital, northeastern USA	• 165 women who experienced unplanned C-section • Three groups • RCT	• Admin by nurses & researchers • Group 1: 20 min M • Group 2: usual care • Group 3: 20 min individual attention	• Pain • Stress • Relaxation • Opioid use	• M group signif ↑ relaxation, ↓ stress, pain, & opioid use days 1 and 2

Yilar and Aktas 2018 *21*	State hospital maternity unit, northwestern Turkey	• 154 women in labor (1st pregnancy), 3-4cm dilated
		  – Exper: N = 77
		  – Control: N = 77
		• Semi-exper, non-randomized
			• Admin by midwife researchers trained in foot reflexol
			• Exper: reflexol 15 min each foot
			• Control: usual care
				• Anxiety	• Signif ↓ in anxiety

continued

TABLE 2.4 Maternity patients *continued*

Author/Year/*Ref #*	Hospital/Country	Sample	Intervention	Key variables	Results
Arnon et al. 2018 *3*	Bnai Zion Medical Center, Haifa, Israel	• 36 women in labor • Qualitative study	• Admin by reflexol therapists during latent and active labor but not delivery	• Assess reflexol Tx on physical & psychological aspects of labor process via open interviews	• 94% felt empowered, ↑ confidence, able to self-manage pain during labor/delivery

Nia et al. 2019 *59*	OB/GYN ward, Razi Teaching Hospital, Ahvaz, Iran	• 68 postpartum pts w/ moderate to severe pain
		  – Exper: N = 34
		  – Control: N = 34
		• RCT
			• Admin unknown
			• Exper: reflexology, 10 min each foot to pituitary, solar plexus, uterine points, & inner arch of foot
			• Control: usual care
				• Pain intensity and duration
				• Analgesia
					• Reflexol group greater ↓ in pain intensity & duration
					• No diff in need for analgesia

Sriasih et al. 2019 *58*	Pembantu Dauh Puri Health Center, Denpasar, Bali, Indonesia	• 70 women in labor
		  – Exper: N = 35
		  – Control: N = 35
		• Quasi-experimental
			• Admin by midwives
			• Exper: M w/ frangipani aromatherapy oil
			• Control: M w/ virgin coconut oil
				• Pain intensity	• Signif ↓ in pain intensity w/ frangipani but not with coconut oil

Akkoz and Karaduman 2020 *22*	Bagcilar Hospital, Istanbul, Turkey	• 60 women in labor
		  – Exper: N = 30
		  – Control: N = 30
		• RCT
			• Admin by nurse researchers trained by physical therapists
			• Exper: 30 min M to sacral area
			• Control: usual care
				• Labor pain
				• Anxiety
					• Signif ↓ labor pain & anxiety
					• ↑ patient satisfaction of labor

Oncology

More studies have been done of people with cancer than most other patient groups, and yet, there is not a clear picture from the research of how massage might best be used. The exceptions are with anxiety[24–31] and pain,[25,29–31,62–64] which universally showed positive outcomes. However, the studies of nausea[24,25,43] and sleep[29,63,76] had mixed findings, which mirrors the feedback heard by therapists who work in the hospital setting. Many patients will have commented about how much better they slept the night after a massage, or they may have experienced near-instant relief of their nausea in the midst of a bodywork session. On the other hand, there will be a substantial number of patients who had no improvement in these side effects.

Immune-related variables also had mixed findings.[26,44,70,90] Other symptoms received almost no examination, such as constipation, fatigue, and vital signs.

A study of massage given just before paclitaxel infusion showed great benefit on chemotherapy-induced peripheral neuropathy for breast cancer patients.[103]

This does not weaken the case for massage on oncology units, it is merely a status report of the state of massage research. The anecdotal information, although not rated as a high level of evidence, is abundant. This explains the widespread adoption of touch therapy programs for hospitalized cancer patients.

Many aspects of the massage experience cannot be translated into data. For example, hope or the feeling of belonging cannot be rated numerically. In order to capture the subjective aspects of the massage experience, methods must also be used that provide the patient with an opportunity to be descriptive. Billhult et al. have performed two such qualitative studies with cancer patients.[104,105] The researchers' systematic use of interviews allowed a richer picture to emerge. Patients who received daily massage therapy while in the hospital expressed a sense of feeling strong and that they became aware that their body had possibilities. Massage gave them an experience of being important and special and contributed to the development of a positive relationship with the staff. Patients felt a new balance between dependence and autonomy.[104] The women receiving massage during chemotherapy shared that it offered them a retreat from the negative feelings associated with chemo infusion.[105] Granted, the above information does not translate into cost savings or symptom management, but it speaks to the whole experience.

Reasonable research claims: At this time, only the effects on short-term anxiety and pain have consistent and sufficient findings. The effects on nausea, sleep, and immune function have varying results and inadequate study.

TABLE 2.5 Oncology patients

Author/Year/ *Ref #*	Hospital/ Country	Sample	Intervention	Key variables	Results
Billhult and Dahlberg 2001 *104*	Oncology clinic, county hospital southern Sweden	• 10 women w/ BR CA receiving chemo • Qualitative study	• Admin by trained hospital staff • 5 M sessions, 20–30 min effleurage (lower or upper extremities) during chemo	• Pts interviewed after completion of all sessions	• M offered a retreat from unwanted, negative feelings associated w/ chemo

Lively et al. 2002 *81*	St. Vincent Mercy, Toledo, Ohio, USA	• 31 women w/ BR and ovarian CA, high-dose chemo & stem cell transplant
		  – Exper: N = 17
		  – Control: N = 14
			• Admin by oncology MT
			• Exper: 20-30 min sessions; M to head w/ focus on SCM & craniosacral techniques; Swedish M to legs
			• Control: usual care
				• Nausea/vomiting
				• Length of stay
				• TPN use
				• Cost-effectiveness
					• ↓ nausea and TPN use
					• Length of stay = 3 fewer days
					• $2,850 total cost savings per pt

continued

TABLE 2.5 Oncology patients *continued*

Author/Year/ *Ref #*	Hospital/ Country	Sample	Intervention	Key variables	Results

Smith et al. 2002 29	Veteran's Administration Medical Center, USA	• 41 hospitalized oncology pts
		  – Exper: N = 20
		  – Control: N = 21
		• Quasi-experimental
			• Admin by nurse certified in hospital M
			• Exper:15-30 min light Swedish M, 3 massages during 1x wk hospitalization
			• Control: nurse interaction
				• Pain
				• Sleep quality
				• Symptom distress
				• Anxiety
					• Signif improve in all variables

Smith et al. 2003 28	Bone marrow transplant (BMT) inpatient unit, Denver, Colorado, USA	• 88 BMT pts
		• Three groups:
		  – 1. Control: N = 30
		  – 2. Therapeutic Touch (TT): N = 31
		  – 3. Massage: N = 27
		• RCT
			• Touch therapies admin by nurse every 3rd day beginning w/ start of chemo until discharge
			• Control: 30 min FV w/ volunteer
			• 30 min TT session
			• 30 min M
				• Time of engraftment
				• Complications (pain, food intake, CNS/ neuro, heart lung, liver skin, circulation)
				• Pt perception of benefits
					• No diff in engraftment rate
					• M group improve in CNS/neuro complications only (disorientation, sleep, personality changes, convulsions, malaise, anxiety, depression, speech impairment)
					• Perceived benefit ↑ for M than FV
					• M & TT ↑ comfort

Cassileth and Vickers 2004 25	Memorial Sloan-Kettering Cancer Center, New York, New York, USA	• 1,290 pts over 3-yr period
		• Retrospective
			• Admin by licensed MTs
			• Sessions were 20 min avg duration for inpatients; 60 min avg for outpatients
			• Pts could choose from:
			  – Swedish M
			  – Light touch M
			  – Foot M
				• Pain
				• Nausea
				• Stress
				• Anxiety
				• Depression Fatigue
					• Swed M and foot M most commonly given
					• Swed M & light touch M had 58% improve in symptom
					• Foot M 50% improve in symptoms
					• Improve for inpatients did not last
					• Effects lasted longer for outpatients

continued

TABLE 2.5 Oncology patients *continued*

Author/Year/ *Ref #*	Hospital/ Country	Sample	Intervention	Key variables	Results
Billhult et al. 2007 *43*	Oncology clinic, county hospital, southern Sweden	• 39 women undergoing chemo for BR CA – Exper: N = 19 – Control: N = 20 • RCT	• Admin by trained hospital staff • Exper: 20 min soft stroke M, 5 sessions • Control: FV by staff	• Nausea • Anxiety • Depression	• M group 73% ↓ in nausea • Control: 49.5% ↓ in nausea • Both groups: no signif change in anxiety/depression
Mehling et al. 2007 *45*	Osher Center for Integrative Medicine, University of California, San Francisco, USA	• 138 cancer pts scheduled to undergo CA-related surgery – Exper: N = 93 – Control: N = 45 • RCT	• Admin by certified MTs & licensed acupuncturists • Exper: acupuncture for pain – LI4, SP6 and ear points related to areas of pain; nausea – PC6, ST36; anxiety – L3, LI4, Yin Tang point • Swed M/foot acupressure for 10–30 mins postop days 1&2 • Control: usual care	• Nausea • Pain • Anxiety • Depression • Health care costs	• Exper group had greater ↓ pain and depression compared to control • No diff btw groups in nausea and anxiety • No diff in health care costs btw groups
Billhult et al. 2008 *44*	Oncology clinic, Goteborg University, Goteborg, Sweden	• 22 women w/ BR CA undergoing radiotherapy – Exper: N = 11 – Control: N = 11 • RCT	• Admin by trained nurse • Exper: 20 min effleurage • Control: 20 min FV	• Circulating lymphocytes (NK, CD4+, CD8+ T cells) • Salivary cortisol • Oxytocin • Anxiety • Depression • QoL	• No signif effect on lymphocytes • No diff btw groups on all other measures

continued

TABLE 2.5 Oncology patients *continued*

Author/Year/ *Ref #*	Hospital/ Country	Sample	Intervention	Key variables	Results

Currin and Meister 2008 *62*	Memorial Health University Medical Center, Medical/Surgical Unit Savannah, Georgia, USA	• 251 in-pts
		• Non-randomized single group, pre-post design
			• Admin by oncology-trained MT
			• 10–15 min light Swedish M
				• Distress as measured by:
				  – Pain
				  – Physical discomfort
				  – Emotional discomfort
				  – Fatigue
					• Signif ↓ in all 4 measures

Stringer et al. 2008 *90*	Christie Hospital Haematology and Transplant Unit, Manchester, UK	• 39 hematology pts • Three groups of 13: – 2 exper arms and 1 control arm • RCT	• Admin by qualified hematology/oncology nurse certified in aromatherapy • Exper arm 1: single 20 min, light stroke M w/ no more than 3 essential oils • Exper arm 2: 20 min light stroke M w/ base oil • Control: rest	• Stress as measured by serum cortisol and prolactin levels • QoL	• Signif ↓ in cortisol in M & aroma groups • ↓ in prolactin in the M only group • Aromatherapy no more effective than oil-based M

Billhut et al. 2009 *70*	Oncology clinic, Goteborg, Sweden	• 30 women w/ BR CA undergoing 5 wks of radiotherapy. None had received chemo
		  – Exper: N = 15
		  – Control: N = 15
		• RCT
			• Admin by nurse trained in M technique
			• Exper: 45 min light pressure, full-body effleurage
			• Control: 45 min FV
				• Circulating lymphocytes (peripheral blood NK cells)
				• Salivary cortisol level
				• HR & BP
					• ↓ deterioration of NK cells
					• No change in cortisol level and DBP
					• ↓ HR and SBP

Osaka et al. 2009 *26*	Palliative Care Unit of Shizuoka Cancer Center, Shizuoka, Japan	• 34 palliative care pts • No control	• Admin by licensed MT • 5 min hand M	• Stress measured by CgA saliva test • Anxiety • Pt satisfaction	• Signif ↓ in salivary CgA levels • Signif ↓ in anxiety • Signif ↑ satisfaction

continued

TABLE 2.5 Oncology patients *continued*

Author/Year/ *Ref #*	Hospital/ Country	Sample	Intervention	Key variables	Results

Jane et al. 2011 *63*	Chang Gung Memorial Hospital, Inpatient Oncology Unit, Taoyuan City, Taiwan	• 72 pts w/ bone metastases
		  – Exper: N = 36
		  – Control: N = 36
		• RCT
			• Admin by nurse trained in M
			• Exper: 37–50 min full-body M/3 consecutive days
			• Control: FV by trained research assistant
				• Pain intensity
				• Mood status Muscle relaxation
				• Sleep quality
					• M group ↓ in pain, ↑ in mood & muscle relaxation
					• M sustained muscle relaxation for 16–18 hrs post
					• Both groups had ↑ relaxation
					• No improve in sleep either group

Lai et al. 2011 *85*	Princess Margaret Hospital, Hong Kong	• 32 advanced CA pts w/constipation
		• 3 groups:
		  – 1. Control: N = 8
		  – 2. Abdom M: N = 11
		  – 3. Aroma abdom M: N = 13
		• RCT
			• Admin by nurses trained in specific abdom technique
			• 15–20 min sessions for 5 consecutive days
			• 1. Control: usual care
			• 2. Plain abdom M
			• 3. Abdom aroma M w/ bitter orange, black pepper, rosemary, marjoram, patchouli in olive oil.
				• Constipation
				• QoL
					• Groups 2 & 3 had improve in constipation
					• Aroma M group had signif improve vs. plain M
					• Positive correlation in constipation and QoL

Robison and Smith 2015 *30*	Christ Hospital, Chemotherapy Infusion Unit, Cincinnati, Ohio, USA	• 58 pts receiving chemotherapy • Pre/post study design	• Admin by oncology-trained MT • 20 min M session to either hands or feet (pt preference)	• Anxiety • Pain • Nausea • Fatigue • Satisfaction	• Signif improve in all variables • High level of satisfaction w/ service

Wang et al. 2015 *24*	Kaohsiung Chang Gung Memorial Hospital, Kaohsiung City, Taiwan	• 80 pts w/ malignant ascites
		  – Exper: N = 40
		  – Control: N = 40
		• RCT
			• Admin by nurse practitioner
			• Exper:15 min abdom M, 2x/day for 3 days
			• Control: FV w/ same nurse, 2x/day
				• Ascites-related symptoms:
				  – Appetite loss
				  – Fatigue
				  – Dyspnea
				  – Bloating
				  – Nausea
				  – Pain
				  – Anxiety/ depression
					• M had greatest improve on:
					  – Depression/ anxiety
					  – Well-being
					  – Perceived bloating
					• No effect on other symptoms

continued

TABLE 2.5 Oncology patients *continued*

Author/Year/ *Ref #*	Hospital/ Country	Sample	Intervention	Key variables	Results
Gentile et al. 2018 64	Outpatient oncology setting, community-based cancer institute, North Carolina, USA	• 572 cancer pts • Retrospective study	• Admin by certified practitioner • 45 min Healing Touch or oncology massage customized to the needs of the patient	• Pain	• Both Healing Touch & oncology massage signif ↓ pain
Kuo et al. 2018 76	Kaohsiung Veterans General Hospital, Kaohsiung City, Taiwan	• 47 women w/ ovarian cancer: – Exper: N = 23 – Control: N = 24 • RCT	• Admin by research nurse • Exper: sleep hygiene practices combined w/ gentle fingertip pressure at acupoints on ear • Control: sleep hygiene practices alone	• Quality of sleep	• Intervention signif ↑ sleep
Vergo et al. 2018 31	Dartmouth-Hitchcock Medical Center, Lebanon, New Hampshire, USA	• 1,585 pt encounters (59% CA pts, 41% non-CA) • Retrospective study	• Admin by oncology-trained MTs • Single session of M or Reiki, varying lengths of time from <15 min to >30 min	• Anxiety • Pain • Depression • Fatigue • Nausea • Well-being	• Signif improve in all variables from Reiki & M • Reiki had greater improve for fatigue & anxiety
Kuon et al. 2019 27	Osher Center for Integrative Medicine, University of California, San Francisco, USA	• 109 hematologic cancer/stem cell pts • Single arm feasibility study	• Admin by oncology-trained MT • Swed M; 20–30 min/1 day per week	• Feasibility • Anxiety • Distress • Fatigue • Nausea • Pain • Tension • Sleep	• Feasible and safe • Signif ↓ in: – anxiety – distress – fatigue – pain – tension • ↑ sleep
Wang et al. 2019 86	Hospice unit medical center, Taiwan	• 30 advanced cancer hospice pts – Exper: N = 15 – Control: N = 15 • Non-randomized, pre/post study design	• Admin by researcher • Exper: 8 min acupress Tx (CV12, CV4, ST25) for 3 consecutive days • Control: usual care	• Constipation	• Signif improve in constipation

Chapter TWO

Procedural interventions

This section includes a broad swathe of procedural interventions, such as wound care for burn patients, hemodialysis, Portacath placement, heart catheterization, and a varicose vein procedure. This grouping is less about comparing studies and more a method of bringing some sense of organization to the research. However, some pattern of benefit can be seen in the diverse procedural groups.

Four of the projects examined massage in conjunction with hemodialysis treatment. Each studied a different variable: sleep,[77] comfort needs (muscle cramps, back pain, headache, nausea),[65] constipation,[87] and nausea,[80] and each had significant improvement. Two studies that examined massage given prior to a heart catheterization procedure found no significant difference between the massage group and the control.[47,66] A large group of burn patients received a 20-minute massage, music therapy, or a combination of both prior to wound care in hopes of quelling anticipatory anxiety.[34] Both interventions significantly decreased anxiety, but the two in combination was most effective. Twenty minutes of massage prior to Portacath placement also significantly decreased anxiety.[33] Hand reflexology given during a varicose vein procedure decreased anxiety and shortened pain duration.[32]

Some studies have value because of the ideas they generate. Such is the research by Dal et al.[106] who examined the use of massage for women post C-section. The question was: could massage of the sacral region after a C-section reduce the need for a urinary catheter by stimulating the need to urinate more quickly? The answer was yes. The group who received 10–15 minutes of effleurage and friction every hour following their surgery had the quickest voiding times. "Massaging the sacral region," wrote the authors, "could be recommended instead of urinary catheter insertion."

Reasonable research claims: There is insufficient research to merit any collective claims.

TABLE 2.6 Procedural interventions

Author/Year/ Ref #	Hospital/Country	Sample	Intervention	Key variables	Results
Okvat et al. 2002 47	Columbia Presbyterian Hospital, New York, New York, USA	• 78 pts scheduled for diagnostic heart catheterization • RCT	• Admin by MT • Exper: 10 min standardized M before procedure • Control: 10 min quiet time w/ MT	• Feasibility of M before procedure • Anxiety • Pain • Vital signs	• M was feasible • No signif diff in pain, anxiety, or vital signs
McNamara et al. 2003 66	Massachusetts General Hospital, Boston, Massachusetts, USA	• 46 pts scheduled for diagnostic heart catheterization • RCT	• Admin by MT • Exper: 20 min back M prior to procedure, side-lying position • Control: usual care	• Vital signs • Pain • Psychological state	• No signif diff btw groups except SBP

continued

TABLE 2.6 Procedural interventions *continued*

Author/Year/ *Ref #*	Hospital/Country	Sample	Intervention	Key variables	Results
Shariati et al. 2012 77	Hemodialysis units in two university hospitals (Imam & Golestan), Ahvaz, Iran	• 48 end-stage renal pts receiving hemodialysis – Exper: N = 24 – Control: N = 24 • RCT	• Admin by nurse researcher & assistant • Exper: 6 min M in areas of acupressure followed by 9 min acupressure to HT7, LI4 in hands & SP 6 in the leg, 1 hr after start of hemodialysis; 3x/ week for 4 wks, • Control: usual care	• Sleep quality – latency – duration – efficiency – disturbance – daytime – functional status • Use of sleep medication	• Signif ↑ in all sleep indices
Dal et al. 2013 *106*	Life Hospital, Dept of Gynecology and Obstetrics, Gazi Magusa, Cyprus	• 60 women post C-section • 3 groups: – Exper 1: N = 20 – Exper 2: N = 20 – Control: N = 20 • Cross sectional study	• Admin by researcher • Group 1: 10–15 min M of the sacral area (effl & friction) every h after C-section • Group 2: 10–15 min M every 30 mins after voiding sensation • Group 3: usual care	• M to sacral region after C-section, instead of employing urinary catheter to avoid urinary retention	• Group 1 void time: avg 3.4 hrs post C-section • Group 2 avg void time: 5.5 hrs post C-section • Group 3 avg void time: 6.2 hrs
Rosen et al. 2013 *33*	Boston Medical Center, Boston, Massachusetts, USA	• 60 pts undergoing port placement – Exper: N – 30 – Control: N = 30 • RCT	• Admin by MT • Exper: 20 min M pre & post surgery • Control: structured attention; positive encouragement	• Feasibility • Pain • Anxiety	• M was feasible • M group signif ↓ preop anxiety • Both M & structured attention were beneficial
Hudson et al. 2015 *32*	University of Surrey outpatient clinic, Guildford, UK	• 100 pts w/ minimal varicose vein surgery – Exper: N = 50 – Control: N = 50 • RCT	• Admin by reflexologist • Exper: under local anesthesia, received intra-op hand reflexology during procedure • Control: usual care	• Pain • Anxiety	• Signif ↓ anxiety • Shorter pain duration

continued

TABLE 2.6 Procedural interventions *continued*

Author/Year/ *Ref #*	Hospital/Country	Sample	Intervention	Key variables	Results

Tabiee et al. 2017 *65*	Shahid Chamran Hospital Hemodialysis Unit, Ferdows, Iran	• 40 hemodialysis pts
		  – Exper: N = 20 pts
		  – Control: N = 20 pts
		• RCT
			• Admin by nurse researchers & male colleague
			• Exper: 15 min back M, pt and family education for 6 consecutive sessions
			• Control: usual care
				• Most common complaints: muscle cramps, back pain, headache, nausea	• Comfort scores signif ↑

Najafi Ghezeljeh and Mohaddes Ardebili 2018 *34*	Motahari Burn and Reconstructive Center, Iran University of Medical Sciences, Tehran, Iran	• 240 burn pts
		• 4 groups
		  – 1. Swedish M
		  – 2. Self-selected music
		  – 3. Combination M & music
		  – 4. Control (usual care)
			• Admin by researchers w/ M qualification
			• 20 min intervention prior to wound care, 1x.
				• Anticipatory anxiety prior to wound care	• Signif ↓ in anxiety both M and music
					• Combination of M and music was most effective

Abbasi et al. 2019 *87*	Three hospitals affiliated to Mazandaran University of Medical Sciences, Mazandaran, Iran	• 74 pts undergoing hemodialysis
		  – Exper: N = 37
		  – Control: N = 37
		• Double-blind RCT
			• Admin by trained researcher and colleague
			• Exper: acupress at LI4, LV3, ST 36, SP15, CV6; 3x/wk for 4wks; 9 min per session
			• Control: acupress 1 cm from above points
				• Constipation	• Signif ↑ in frequency of defecation & stool quality in acupressure group by end of week 4

Naseri-Salahshour et al. 2019 *80*	Arak Dialysis Center, Arak, Iran	• 72 hemodialysis pts
		  – Exper: N = 36 pts
		  – Control: N = 36 pts
		• Double-blind RCT
			• Admin by nurse researcher, qualified reflexologist
			• Exper: reflexol 30 mins on solar plexus and soles of feet 1x/day for 12 days; 1 hr after start of dialysis
			• Control: foot M
				• Nausea	• Severity of nausea ↓ signif in reflexology group at days 3, 6, 9, & 12

continued

TABLE 2.6 Procedural interventions *continued*

Author/Year/ Ref #	Hospital/Country	Sample	Intervention	Key variables	Results

Habibzadeh et al. 2020 *88*	Hemodialysis centers in Taleghani and Imam Khomeini, Urmia, Iran	• 120 male hemodialysis pts
		• 4 trial groups
		  – 1. Control
		  – 2. Foot M w/ chamomile oil
		  – 3. Foot M w/ almond oil
		  – 4. Foot M w/ no oil
		• RCT
			• Admin by nurse researcher
			• Exper: 20-min foot M, 1 hr after start of dialysis, 3x/wk for 8 wks; 24 sessions total
			• Control: usual care
				• Fatigue
				• QoL
					• All 3 interventions improved variables
					• Chamomile oil more effective for QoL
					• Almond oil more effective for fatigue

Surgery

The patients in this group underwent a variety of surgeries, such as a laparoscopic procedure, cataract surgery, surgery for tibial shaft fracture, liver transplantation, and abdominal surgery. The interventions ranged from a 10-minute foot massage to a 20-minute back massage, a 15-minute seated, slow-stroke back massage to a 5-minute hand massage. Sometimes the intervention was given before surgery and sometimes after. The point of connection between most of the studies was the examination of anxiety and pain. In every case, anxiety was significantly lessened[35–42] and pain was reduced in nearly all of the studies that included it.[35,36,42,67,68] As with other groups of studies, the conclusions for vital signs were mixed.[40,67,68] Remaining major variables were under-studied or completely lacking in study, such as nausea and sleep. A single study looked at nausea and found improvement after a laparoscopic cholecystectomy.[67] To be sure, there is ample room to pose research questions in this realm.

Reasonable research claims: Levels of short-term anxiety and pain consistently show improvement. The measurements of vital signs had mixed conclusions. Other variables require more research.

TABLE 2.7 Surgery patients

Author/Year/ Ref #	Hospital/Country	Sample	Intervention	Key variables	Results

Kim et al. 2001 *40*	Kangnam St. Mary's Hospital, Seoul, South Korea	• 59 pts having cataract surgery
		  – Exper: N = 29
		  – Control: N = 30
		• RCT
			• Admin unknown
			• Exper: 5 min hand M just before surgery
			• Control: usual care
				• Anxiety
				• Vital signs
				• Epinephrine, norepinephrine, cortisol
				• Blood sugar
				• Neutrophils, lymphocytes
					• M group:
					  – ↓ anxiety
					  – ↓ epinephrine, norepinephrine, cortisol
					• No diff in vitals, blood sugar, or blood cell levels

continued

TABLE 2.7 Surgery patients *continued*

Author/Year/ *Ref #*	Hospital/Country	Sample	Intervention	Key variables	Results

Mitchinson et al. 2007 *35*	Department of Veteran Affairs hospitals, Ann Arbor, Michigan, and Indianapolis, Indiana, USA	• 645 patients undergoing major surgery
		  – Group 1: N = 220
		  – Group 2: N = 211
		  – Group 3: N = 214
		• RCT
			• Admin by MT
			• Group 1: usual care
			• Group 2: 20 min individualized attention from MT
			• Group 3: individualized back M for 20 min
			• Intervention each evening for up to 5 postop days
				• Short and long-term pain intensity
				• Pain unpleasantness
				• Anxiety
					• Signif ↓ short-term pain & anxiety
					• Pain ↓ more quickly days 1–4 postop
					• No diff in long-term anxiety, length of stay, or opiate use

McRee et al. 2007 *39*	One university hospital and two community hospitals in Tucson, Arizona, USA	• 105 female pts who had undergone laparoscopic gynecological surgery w/ general anesthesia
		  – Exper: N = 54
		  – Control: N = 51
		• RCT
			• Admin by nurse researcher
			• Exper: 30 min preop Swedish M of posterior body
			• Control: 30 min preop gentle passive touch to posterior body
				• Pain
				• Anxiety
				• Anesthetic use
				• Narcotic use
					• No signif diff in inhaled anesthetics during surgery
					• M group used signif ↓ intraop narcotics
					• M group had ↓ postop anxiety

Miller et al. 2015 *37*	Orthopedic unit of a community-based hospital, Norwich, Connecticut, USA	• 25 postop orthopedic pts • Pre/post-test, RCT, cross-over design	• Admin by MT • Exper: 5 min hand/ arm M at the time of oral analgesic admin • Control: oral analgesic alone	• Pain • Anxiety • Pt satisfaction w/ pain management	• Signif ↑ pt satisfaction in M group • No signif diff in pain or anxiety btw M or control

Çankaya and Saritas 2018 *67*	Firat University Hospital, Elazig, Turkey	• 88 pts w/ laparoscopic cholecystectomy
		  – Exper: N = 44
		  – Control: N = 44
		• Semi-experimental
			• Admin by nurse researcher
			• Exper: 10 min classic foot M
			• Control: usual care
				• Vital signs
				• Pain
				• Nausea and vomiting
					• Signif ↓ in pain, nausea, SBP

Ozturk et al. 2018 *42*	Ege University Hospital, Turkey	• 63 female pts, postop hysterectomy
		  – Exper: N = 32
		  – Control: N = 31
		• RCT
			• Admin by nurse researcher trained in reflexology
			• Exper: 10 min reflexol to each foot, postop days 1–3
			• Control: usual care
				• Pain
				• Anxiety
					• Signif ↓ pain & anxiety

continued

TABLE 2.7 Surgery patients *continued*

Author/Year/ Ref #	Hospital/Country	Sample	Intervention	Key variables	Results
Pasyar et al. 2018 *36*	Khatam-Al-Anbia Hospital, Zahedan, Iran	• 66 pts w/ tibial shaft fracture surgery – Exper: N = 33 – Control: N = 33 • RCT	• Admin by MT • Exper: 10 min foot M using sweet almond oil • Control: usual care	• Pain • Anxiety	• Signif ↓ pain and anxiety
Demir and Saritas 2019 *68*	Inonu University Turgut Ozal Medical Centre, Malatya, Turkey	• 84 liver transplant pts – Exper: N = 42 – Control: N = 42 • Quasi-experimental	• Admin by researcher • Intervention: back M 2x/day, postop • Control: usual care	• Pain • Vital signs • O_2 saturation	• ↓ pain • ↓ vital signs • ↑ O_2 saturation
Keramati et al. 2019 *38*	Amiral-Momenin Hospital, Zabol City, Iran	• 60 pts prior to cataract surgery – Exper: N = 30 – Control: N = 30 • RCT	• Admin by researcher w/ M qualification • Exper: 15 min, seated, slow stroke back M, 30 min before surgery • Control: usual care	• Anxiety	• Signif ↓ anxiety
Cavdar et al. 2020 *41*	Ophthalmology Clinic, Manisa Celal Bayar University Hospital, Manisa, Turkey	• 140 cataract surg pts – Exper: N = 70 – Control: N = 70 • RCT	• Admin by nurse researcher • Exper: 10 min hand M just before surgery • Control: usual care	• Preop anxiety • Vital signs • Comfort	• ↓ anxiety • Improved vitals except SVO_2 • ↑ comfort

Summary

This chapter has presented thumbnail sketches of research carried out with people who are hospitalized or in nursing facilities. The advantage to this abbreviated approach is that the reader is exposed to a broad variety of research. One of the downsides is that it doesn't allow for a discussion of the limitations of the studies. Many of these weaknesses were mentioned earlier in the chapter: small sample size, no control group, and weak methodology; however, another common limitation is bias. Patients willing to be part of massage research are favorably biased toward touch therapies, which means that the sample group is not composed of an impartial representation of patients. Improvement in pain is sometimes difficult to show because it is already controlled with analgesia. Another limitation is the lack of description about the massage strokes: what speed and pressure is employed? These are but a short list of the common limitations.

Despite what might be lacking, there is potential in the current research, and momentum is building. The view presented by scientific research, though, is still unclear.

Chapter TWO

Many old questions remain unanswered and new questions have yet to be asked. Research requires a slow, methodical process. It takes time to gather a body of evidence, especially in the field of complementary therapies.

Only two variables, short-term anxiety and short-term pain, have had any significant amount of study. In the majority of cases, both anxiety and pain improved, no matter the modality tested, dosage, frequency or patient population. Sleep and constipation tended toward improvement from the use of massage techniques, although there is not yet enough research to draw a firm conclusion. Nausea, vital signs, depression, and immune-related variables had mixed results as well as insufficient study.

However, it is important to point out that research of massage in hospital patients is stronger than it was two decades ago. Sample sizes are much larger and methodology meets a higher level of evidence. There is also renewed motivation from mainstream medicine to find less harmful methods of symptom management, which in turn promotes research.

This chapter endeavored to make a case for understanding the research as it stands now. This knowledge is important, but as massage educator Tracy Walton points out, it is also essential to recognize that: "Not every element of the therapeutic relationship submits itself to the rigors of scientific study. Many truths about our work remain hidden from the measurement tools of a randomized, controlled clinical trial. What happens during a massage is true – it doesn't need verification from anyone. It is often unexplainable and magical – but true, nevertheless. In fact, there are many mysterious truths about the healing power of touch, and there are many ways of knowing those truths."

The path for massage therapists working in a health care setting is a paradoxical one. They must simultaneously embrace science and yet never lose sight of the art; they must understand the clinical but never at the expense of the mystery and magic; and they must maintain wholeness at the same time as they are dissecting the massage experience.

Test yourself

True or False: Place a "T" next to all true statements and an "F" next to the false ones. Rewrite the false statements so that they are true. There is usually more than one correct way to rewrite the false statements.

1. Nausea and anxiety are the most commonly investigated variables.

2. There is strong evidence that massage reduces the need for pain medication.

3. Massage therapy techniques are generally beneficial for labor pain.

4. A control group generally receives usual care.

5. Research conclusively shows that vital signs improve as a result of massage techniques.

6. A case study is the highest level of research evidence.

7. A variable refers to what is being measured.

8. There is strong evidence that massage reduces the length of stay in a hospital and thus provides significant cost savings.

9. Sleep leans toward improvement as a result of massage, but the evidence is not yet strong enough to ethically claim that it does so.

10. Bodywork techniques support immune function in health care patients.

11. Qualitative studies tend to use interviews to understand a patient's experience.

12. A feasibility study examines whether it is safe and practical to provide massage in a certain circumstance.

References

1. Dodd SJ, Savage A. Evidence-informed social work practice. Oxford Research Encyclopedias: Encyclopedia of Social Work; 2016. Available from: https://oxfordre.com/socialwork/view/10.1093/acrefore/9780199975839.001.0001/acrefore-9780199975839-e-915

2. Ijaz N, Rioux J, Elder C, Weeks J. Whole systems research methods in health care: a scoping review. J Altern Complement Med. 2019; 25(S1):S21–S51.

3. Arnon Z, Dor A, Bazak H, et al. Complementary medicine for laboring women: a qualitative study of the effects of reflexology. J Complement Integr Med. 2018; 16(1):1–7.

4. Kahn J. Research matters. Massage Magazine. 2001; 92:65–9.

5. Bauer BA, Cutshall SM, Wentworth LJ, et al. Effect of massage therapy on pain, anxiety and tension after cardiac surgery: a randomized study. Complement Ther Clin Pract. 2010; 16(2):70–5.

6. Boitor M, Martorella G, Maheu C, et al. Effects of massage in reducing the pain and anxiety of the cardiac surgery critically ill – a randomized control trial. Pain Med. 2018; 19(12):2556–69.

7. Aygin D, Sen S. Acupressure on anxiety and sleep quality after cardiac surgery: a randomized controlled trial. J PeriAnesthesia Nurs. 2019; 34(6):1222–31.

8. Alimohammad HS, Ghasemi Z, Shahriar S, et al. Effect of hand and foot surface stroke massage on anxiety and vital signs in patients with acute coronary syndrome: a randomized clinical trial. Complement Ther Clin Pract. 2018; 31:126–31.

9. Rodrigues JW, Sams LM. Effectiveness of foot and hand massage on postoperative pain, anxiety, selected physiological parameters among postoperative open-heart surgery patients in cardiothoracic intensive care units of selected hospitals of Mangaluru. Int J Appl Res. 2018; 4(5):461–74.

10. Adib-Hajbaghery M, Abasi A, Rajabi-Beheshtabad R. Whole body massage for reducing anxiety and stabilizing vital signs of patients in cardiac care unit. Med J Islam Repub Iran. 2014; 28:47.

11. Bagheri-Nesami M, Shorofi S, Zargar N, et al. The effects of foot reflexology massage on anxiety in patients following coronary artery bypass graft surgery: a randomized controlled trial. Complement Ther Clin Pract. 2014; 20(1):42–7.

12. Babaee S, Shafiei Z, Sadeghi MMM, et al. Effectiveness of massage therapy on the mood of patients after open-heart surgery. Iran J Nurs Midwifery Res. 2012; 17(2 Suppl1): S120–S124.

13. Bahrami T, Rejeh N, Heravi-Karimooi M, et al. The effect of foot reflexology on hospital anxiety and depression in female older adults: a randomized controlled trial. Inter J Ther Massage Bodywork. 2019; 12(3):16–21.

14. Braun LA, Stanguts C, Casanelia L, et al. Massage therapy for cardiac surgery patients – a randomized trial. J Thorac Cardio Surg. 2012; 144(6):1453–59.e1.

15. Rho KH, Han SH, Kim KS, Lee MS. Effects of aromatherapy massage on anxiety and self-esteem in Korean elderly women: a pilot study. Int J Neurosci. 2006; 116(12):1447–55.

16. Cinar S, Eser I, Khorshid L. The effects of back massage on the vital signs and anxiety level of elderly staying in a rest home. Hacettepe University Faculty of Health Sciences Nursing Journal. 2009; 14–21.

17. Choi N. The effects of hand massage using aroma essential oil and music therapy on anxiety and sleeping for elderly women in the sanatorium. Intern J Bio-Sci and Bio-Tech. 2015; 7(5):151–8.

18. Rodriguez-Mansilla J, Gonzales Lopez-Arza MV, Varela-Donoso E, et al. The effects of ear acupressure, massage therapy and no therapy on symptoms of dementia: a randomized controlled trial. Clin Rehabil. 2015; 29(7):683–93.

19. Hsu WC, Guo SE, Chang CH. Back massage intervention for improving health and sleep quality among intensive care unit patients. Nurs Crit Care. 2019; 24(5):313–9.

20. Irani M, Kordi M, Tara F, et al. The effect of hand and foot massage on post-cesarean pain and anxiety. JMRH 2015; 3(4):465–71.

21. Yilar EZ, Aktas S. The effect of foot reflexology on the anxiety levels of women in labor. J Altern Complement Med. 2018; 24(4):352–60.

22. Akkoz CS, Karaduman S. The effect of sacral massage on labor pain and anxiety: a randomized controlled trial. Jpn J Nurs Sci. 2020; 17(1):1–9.

23. Hanjani SM, Tourzani ZM, Shoghi M. The effect of foot reflexology on anxiety, pain, and outcomes of labor in primigravida women. Acta Med Iran. 2015; 53(8):507–11.

24. Wang TJ, Wang HM, Yang TS, et al. The effect of abdominal massage in reducing malignant ascites symptoms. Res Nurs Health. 2015; 38(1):51–9.

25. Cassileth B, Vickers AJ. Massage therapy for symptom control outcome study at a major cancer center. J Pain Symptom Manage. 2004; 28(3):244–9.

26. Osaka I, Kurihara Y, Tanaka K, et al. Endocrinological evaluations of brief hand massage in palliative care. J Altern Complement Med. 2009; 15(9):981–5.

27. Kuon C, Wannier R, Harrison J, Tague C. Massage for symptom management in adult inpatients with hematologic malignancies. Glob Adv Health Med. 2019; 8:1–6.

28. Smith MC, Reeder F, Daniel L, et al. Outcomes of touch therapies during bone marrow transplant. Altern Ther Health Med. 2003; 9(1):40–9.

29. Smith MC, Kemp J, Hemphill L, Vojir CP. Outcomes of therapeutic massage for hospitalized cancer patients. J Nurs Scholarship. 2002; 34(3):257–62.

30. Robison J, Smith C. Therapeutic massage during chemotherapy and/or biotherapy infusions: patient perceptions of pain, fatigue, nausea, anxiety, and satisfaction. Clin J Oncol Nurs. 2015; 20(2)E1–7.

31. Vergo MT, Pinkson BM, Broglio K, et al. Immediate symptom relief after a first session of massage therapy or Reiki in

hospitalized patients: a 5-year clinical experience from a rural academic center. J Altern Complement Med. 2018; 24(8):801–8.

32. Hudson BF, Davidson J, Whitely MS. The impact of hand reflexology on pain, anxiety and satisfaction during minimally invasive surgery under local anaesthetic: a randomised controlled trial. Int J Nurs Stud. 2015; 52(12):1789–97.

33. Rosen J, Lawrence R, Bouchard M, et al. Massage for perioperative pain and anxiety in placement of vascular access devices. Adv Mind Body Med. 2013; 27(1):12–23.

34. Najafi Ghezeljeh T, Mohaddes Ardebili F. Comparing the effects of patients preferred music and Swedish massage on anticipatory anxiety in patients with burn injury. Randomized controlled clinical trial. Complement Ther Clin Pract. 2018; 32:55–60.

35. Mitchinson AR, Kim HM, Rosenberg JM, et al. Acute postoperative pain management using massage as an adjuvant therapy: a randomized trial. Arch Surg. 2007; 142(12):1158–67.

36. Pasyar N, Rambod M, Kahkhaee FR. Effects of foot massage on pain intensity and anxiety in patients having undergone tibial shaft fracture surgery: a randomized clinical trial. J Orthop Trauma. 2018; 32(12):482–6.

37. Miller J, Dunion A, Dunn N, et al. Effect of a brief massage on pain, anxiety, and satisfaction with pain management in postoperative orthopaedic patients. Orthop Nurs. 2015; 34(4):227–34.

38. Keramati M, Sargolzaei MS, Moghadasi A, et al. Evaluating the effect of slow-stroke back massage on the anxiety of candidates for cataract. Int J Ther Massage Bodywork. 2019; 12(2):12–17.

39. McRee L, Pasvogel AE, Hallum AV, et al. Effects of preoperative massage on intra- and postoperative outcomes. J Gynecol Surg. 2007; 23(3):97–103.

40. Kim MS, Cho KS, Woo H, Kim JH. Effects of hand massage on anxiety in cataract surgery using local anesthesia. J Cataract Refract Surg. 2001; 27(6):884–90.

41. Cavdar AU, Yilmz E, Baydur H. The effect of hand massage before cataract surgery on patient anxiety and comfort: a randomized controlled trial. J Peri Anesthesia Nurs. 2020; 35(1):54–9.

42. Ozturk R, Sevil U, Sargin A, Yucebilgin MS. The effects of reflexology on anxiety and pain in patients after abdominal hysterectomy: a randomised controlled trial. Complement Ther Med. 2018; 36:107–12.

43. Billhult A, Bergbom I, Stener-Victorin E. Massage relieves nausea in women with breast cancer who are undergoing chemotherapy. J Alter Complement Med. 2007; 13(1):53–7.

44. Billhult A, Lindholm C, Gunnarson R, Stener-Victorin E. The effect of massage on cellular immunity, endocrine and psychological factors in women with breast cancer: a randomized controlled clinical trial. Auton Neurosci. 2008; 140(1–2):88–95.

45. Mehling WE, Jacobs B, Acree M, et al. Symptom management with massage and acupuncture in postoperative cancer patients: a randomized controlled trial. J Pain Symptom Manage. 2007; 33(3):258–66.

46. Albert NM, Gillinov AM, Lytle BW, et al. A randomized trial of massage therapy after heart surgery. Heart Lung. 2009; 38(6):480–90.

47. Okvat HA, Oz MC, Ting W, Namerow PB. Massage therapy for patients undergoing cardiac catheterization. Altern Ther Health Med. 2002; 8(3):68–75.

48. Goldberg DS, McGee SJ. Pain as a global public health priority. BMC Public Health. 2011; 11:770.

49. Clark SD, Bauer BA, Vitek S, Cutshall SM. Effect of integrative medicine services on pain for hospitalized patients at an academic health center. Explore (NY). 2019; 15(1):61–4.

50. Kshettry VR, Carole LF, Henly SJ, et al. Complementary alternative medical therapies for heart surgery patients: feasibility, safety and impact. Ann Thorac Surg. 2006; 81(1):201–5.

51. Imani N, Shams SA, Radfar M, et al. Effect of applying reflexology massage on nitroglycerin-induced migraine-type headache: a placebo-controlled clinical trial. Agri. 2018; 30(3):116–22.

52. Taherian T, Shorofi S, Zeydi A, et al. The effects of Hegu point ice massage on post-sternotomy pain in patients undergoing coronary artery bypass grafting: a single-blind, randomized clinical trial. Adv Int Med. 2020; 7(2):73–8.

53. Nerbass FB, Feltrim MI, Souza SA, et al. Effects of massage therapy on sleep quality after coronary artery bypass graft surgery. Clinics (Sao Paolo). 2010; 65(11):1105–10.

54. Fakhravari AA, Bastani F, Haghani H. The effect of foot reflexology massage on the sleep quality of elderly women with restless leg syndrome. JCCNC. 2018; 4(2):96–103.

55. Chang MY, Wang SY, Chen CH. Effects of massage on pain and anxiety during labour: a randomized controlled trial in Taiwan. J Adv Nurs. 2002; 38(1):68–73.

56. Basyouni NR, Gohar IE, Zaied NF. Effect of foot reflexology on post-cesarean pain. IOSR–JNHS. 2018; 7(4):1–19.

57. Simonelli MC, Doyle LT, Columbia M, et al. Effects of connective tissue massage on pain in primiparous women after cesarean birth. J Obstet Gynecol Neonatal Nurs. 2018; 47(5):591–601.

58. Sriasih NGK, Hadi MC, Suindri NN, et al. The effect of massage therapy using frangipani aromatherapy oil to reduce the childbirth pain intensity. IJTMB. 2019; 12(2):18–24.

59. Nia GB, Montazeri S, Afshari P, Haghighizadeh MH. Foot reflexology effect on postpartum pain: a randomized clinical trial. J Evolution Med Dent Sci. 2019; 8(39):2976–81.

60. Valiani M, Shiran E, Kianpour M, Hasanpour M. Reviewing the effect of reflexology on the pain and certain features and outcomes of the labor on the primiparous women. Iran J Nurs Midwifery Res. 2010; 15(Suppl1):302–10.

61. Dolatian M, Hasanpour A, Montazeri S, et al. The effect of reflexology on pain intensity and duration of labor on primiparas. Iran Red Crescent Med J. 2011; 13(7):475–79.

62. Currin J, Meister EA. A hospital-based intervention using massage to reduce distress among oncology patients. Cancer Nurs. 2008; 3(3):214–21.

63. Jane SW, Chen SL, Wilkie DJ, et al. Effects of massage on pain, mood status, relaxation and sleep in Taiwanese patients with metastatic bone pain: a randomized clinical trial. Pain. 2011; 152(10):2432–42.

64. Gentile D, Boselli D, O'Neill G, et al. Cancer pain relief after healing touch and massage. J Altern Complement Med. 2018; 24(9–10):968–73.

65. Tabiee S, Momeni A, Saadatjoo SA. The effects of comfort-based interventions (back massage and patient and family education) on the level of comfort among hemodialysis patients. Mod Care J. 2017; 14(3):1–6.

66. McNamara ME, Burnham DC, Smith C, Carroll DL. The effects of back massage before diagnostic heart catheterization. Altern Ther Health Med. 2003; 9(1):50–7.

67. Çankaya A, Saritas S. Effect of classic foot massage on vital signs, pain, and nausea/vomiting symptoms after laparoscopic cholecystectomy. Surg Laparosc Endosc Percutan Tech. 2018; 28(6):359–65.

68. Demir B, Saritas S. Effects of massage on vital signs, pain and comfort levels in liver transplant patients. Explore (NY). Nov 12, 2019. Available from: https://doi.org/10.1016/j.explore.2019.10.004.

69. Kandemir K, Oztekin SD. How effective is reflexology on physiological parameters and weaning time from mechanical ventilation in patients undergoing cardiovascular surgery? EuJIM. 2019; 26:43–9.

70. Billhult A, Lindholm C, Gunnarsson R, Stener-Victorin E. The effect of massage on immune function and stress in women with breast cancer: a randomized controlled trial. Auton Neurosci. 2009; 150(1–2):111–15.

71. Oshvandi K, Abdi S, Karampourian A, et al. The effect of foot massage on quality of sleep in ischemic heart disease patients hospitalized in CCU. Iran J Crit Care Nurs. 2014; 7(2):66–73.

72. Siavoshi M, Vahidi Sabzevar A, Talebi S, et al. The effect of acupressure on sleep quality in patients with chronic heart failure. J Biomedicine Health. 2017; 2(1):21–7.

73. Cheragjbeigi N, Modarresi M, Rezaei M, Khatony A. Comparing the effects of massage and aromatherapy massage with lavender oil on sleep quality of cardiac patients: a randomized controlled trial. Complement Ther Clin Pract. 2019; 35:253–8.

74. Kandeel NA, El-Hady MM, Tantawy N. The effect of back massage on perceived sleep quality among adult patients in intensive care units. AJNR. 2019; 7(3):278–85.

75. Pagnucci N, Tolotti A, Cadorin L, et al. Promoting nighttime sleep in the intensive care unit: alternative strategies in nursing. Intensive Crit Care Nurs. 2019; 51:73–81.

76. Kuo HC, Tsao Y, Tu HY, et al. Pilot randomized controlled trial of auricular point acupressure for sleep disturbances in women with ovarian cancer. Res Nurs Health. 2018; 41(5):469–79.

77. Shariati A, Jahani S, Hooshmand M, Khalili N. The effect of acupressure on sleep quality of hemodialysis patients. Complement Ther Med. 2012; 20(6):417–23.

78. Harris M, Richards KC, Grando VT. The effects of slow-stroke back massage on minutes of nighttime sleep in persons with dementia and sleep disturbances in the nursing home: a policy study. J Holist Nurs. 2012; 30(4):255–63.

79. Hu RF, Jiang XY, Chen J, et al. Non-pharmacological interventions for sleep promotion in the intensive care unit. Cochrane Database Syst Rev. 2015 Oct 6; (10):CD008808.

80. Naseri-Salahshour V, Sajadi M, Abedi A, et al. Reflexology as an adjunctive nursing intervention for management of nausea in hemodialysis patients: a randomized clinical trial. Complement Ther Clin Pract. 2019; 36:29–33.

81. Lively BT, Holiday-Goodman M, Black CD, Arondekar B. Massage therapy for chemotherapy-induced emesis. In Rich GJ, (ed). Massage Therapy: The Evidence for Practice. Edinburgh: Mosby; 2002. pp. 85–104.

82. Cevik K, Cetinkaya A, Gokbel K, et al. The effect of abdominal massage on constipation in the elderly residing in rest homes. Gastroenterol Nurs. 2018; 41(5):396–402.

83. Lamas K, Lindholm L, Stenlund H, et al. Effects of abdominal massage in management of constipation: a randomized controlled trial. Int J Nurs Stud. 2009; 46(6) 759–67.

84. Moghadam TM, Shareinia H, Moghadam HM, et al. Comparison the effect of Golghand and foot reflexology on constipation in elderlies. IJPR. 2018; 25(3):1–9.

85. Lai TKT, Cheung MC, Lo CK, et al. Effectiveness of aroma massage on advanced cancer patients with constipation: a pilot study. Complement Ther Clin Pract. 2011; 17(1):37–43.

86. Wang PM, Hsu CW, Liu CT, et al. Effect of acupressure on constipation in patients with advanced cancer. Support Care Cancer. 2019; 27(9):3473–8.

87. Abbasi P, Mojalli M, Kianmehr M, Zamani S. Effect of acupressure on constipation in patients undergoing hemodialysis: A randomized double-blind controlled clinical trial. Avicenna J Phytomed. 2019; 9(1):84–91.

88. Habibzadeh H, Dalavan OW, Alilu L, et al. Effects of foot massage on severity of fatigue and quality of life in hemodialysis patients: a randomized control trial. IJCBNM. 2020; 8(2):2–12.

89. Dhabhar FS. Enhancing versus suppressive effects of stress on immune function: implications for immunoprotection and immunopathology. Neuroimmunomodulation. 2009;16(5):300–17.

90. Stringer J, Swindell R, Dennis M. Massage in patients undergoing intensive chemotherapy reduces serum cortisol and prolactin. Psychooncology. 2008; 17(10):1024–31.

91. Schaub C, Von Gunten A, Morin D, et al. The effects of hand massage on stress and agitation among people with dementia in a hospital setting: a pilot study. Appl Psychophysiol Biofeedback. 2018; 43(4):319–32.

92. Dhany AL, Mitchell T, Foy C. Aromatherapy and massage intrapartum service impact on use of analgesia and anesthesia in women in labor: a retrospective case note analysis. J Altern Complement Med. 2012; 18(10):932–8.

93. Estores IM, Arce L, Hix A, et al. Medication cost savings in inpatient oncology using an integrative medicine model. Explore (NY). 2018; 14(3):212–15.

94. Dusek JA, Griffen KH, Finch MD, et al. Cost savings from reducing pain through the delivery of integrative medicine program to hospitalized patients. J Altern Complement Med. 2018; 24(6):557–63.

95. Lu DF, Hart LK, Lutgendorf SK, et al. Effects of healing touch and relaxation on adult patients undergoing hematopoietic stem cell transplant: a feasibility pilot study. Cancer Nurs. 2016; 39(3):E1–E11.

96. Grafton-Clarke C, Grace L, Roerts N, Harky A. Can postoperative massage therapy reduce pain and anxiety in cardiac surgery patients? Interact CardioVasc Thorac Surg. 2018; 28(5): 716–21.

97. Lewis P, Nichols E, Mackey G, et al. The effect of turning and back rub on mixed venous oxygen saturation in critically ill patients. Am J Crit Care. 1997; 6(2):132–40.

98. Momenfar E, Abdi A, Salari N, et al. Studying the effect of abdominal massage on the gastric residual volume in patients hospitalized in intensive care units. J Intensive Care. 2018; 10(6):47.

99. El Feky HAA, Ali NS. Effect of abdominal massage on gastric residual volume among critically ill patients at Cairo University Hospitals. Inter Acad J Health, Med, Nurs. 2020; 2(1):36–53.

100. Smith CA, Levett KM, Collins CT, et al. Massage, reflexology and other manual methods for pain management in labour. Cochrane Database Syst Rev. 2018 Mar 28; 3:CD009290.

101. Bolbol-Haghighi N, Masoumi S, Kazemi F. Effects of massage therapy on duration of labour: a randomized controlled trial. J Clin Diagn Res. 2016; 10(4):QC12–15.

102. Damanik L. The effectiveness of neck massage, in increasing puerperal mother's breast quantity from day one to day three in Bantul. HSJ. 2018; 12(6):599.

103. Izgu N, Metin ZG, Karadas C, et al. Prevention of chemotherapy-induced peripheral neuropathy with classical massage in breast cancer patients receiving paclitaxel: an assessor-blinded randomized controlled trial. Eur J Oncol Nurs. 2019; 40:36–43.

104. Billhult A, Dahlberg K. A meaningful relief from suffering experiences of massage in cancer care. Cancer Nurs. 2001; 24(3):180–84.

105. Billhult A, Stener-Victorin, E, Bergbom I. The experience of massage during chemotherapy treatment in breast cancer patients. Clin Nurs Research. 2007; 16(2):85–99.

106. Dal U, Korucu AE, Eroğlu K, et al. Sacral region massage as an alternative to the urinary catheter used to prevent urinary retention after cesarean delivery. Balkan Med J. 2013; 30(1): 58–63.

Additional resources

Association of Massage Therapists (Australia) Massage Research Database: https://www.amt.org.au/amt/classified-research-database.html.

Burns P, Rohrich RJ, Chung K. Levels of Evidence and their role in Evidence-Based Medicine. Available from: https://www.ncbi.nlm.nih.gov/pmc/articles/PMC3124652/.

Cochrane Library: www.cochrane.org.

Cumulative Index of Nursing and Allied Health Literature: https://www.ebscohost.com/nursing/products/cinahl-databases/cinahl-complete.

Dryden T, Moyer C, eds. Massage Therapy: Integrating Research and Practice. Windsor, Ontario: Human Kinetics; 2012.

Evidence-based Practice for Health Professionals: Levels of evidence. Available from: https://libguides.nvcc.edu/c.php?g=361218&p=2439383.

Field T. Social touch, CT touch and massage therapy: A narrative review. Developmental Review. 2019; 51:123-45.

Fulton B. The Placebo Effect in Manual Therapy: Improving Clinical Outcomes in Your Practice. Edinburgh: Handspring Publishing; 2015.

Lewith G, Jonas WB, Walach H, eds. Clinical Research in Complementary Therapies E-Book: Principles, Problems and Solutions. Edinburgh: Churchill Livingstone; 2011.

Massage Therapy Foundation: https://massagetherapyfoundation.org.

Menard M. Making Sense of Research (2nd edition). Toronto: Curties Overzet Publications; 2009.

Murad MH, Asi N, Alsawas M, Alahdab F. New evidence pyramid. BMJ Journals. Available from: https://ebm.bmj.com/content/21/4/125.

National Center for Complementary and Integrative Health: https://nccih.nih.gov.

National Institute for Health and Care Excellence: https://www.evidence.nhs.uk.

PubMed: https://www.ncbi.nlm.nih.gov/pubmed/

Research Council for Complementary Medicine: http://www.rccm.org.uk.

Touch Research Institute: http://pediatrics.med.miami.edu/touch-research

University theses: https://www.proquest.com/products-services/pqdtglobal.html

Health practitioners are the peacemakers of a new generation.

Senator Mark O. Hatfield, State of Oregon

Bodyworkers who enter the hospital to apply their skills, whether as employees, independent contractors, volunteers, students on a clinical rotation, or as private contractors hired by the patient or family, will encounter an atmosphere that is very different to that in other massage settings. It is more regulated, standardized, hierarchical, complicated, unpredictable, and team-oriented. Therapists will work in conjunction with a wide variety of other health care providers, which decreases the sense of autonomy but increases the feeling of community. Concepts that massage therapists are taught in school, such as confidentiality, Standard Precautions, liability, and scope of practice, are applied more stringently than in other massage environments. Many factors that therapists can control in a private practice, spa, or wellness center, such as time, noise, and interruptions, are out of their control in a hospital.

Learning to function in a hospital is analogous to traveling in a foreign land. The people in this territory speak an unfamiliar language, dress to fit their special environment, and have habits, roles, and characteristics that express their values. As with travelers who adapt to local customs, bodyworkers who embrace the ways of hospital culture will find their journey more harmonious and enriching.

Each health care institution has standards that reflect its uniqueness. For instance, a medical center run by a religious order will have some principles that differ from those of a hospital funded by the county government, and the environment of a teaching hospital will be unlike that of a community hospital. However, there are also practices and values shared by all hospitals. The purpose of this chapter is to outline those standards.

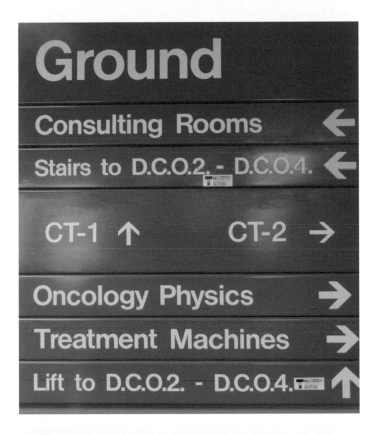

FIGURE 3.1

Being in a hospital is like traveling in a foreign land.

(Photo by Andrew Secretan.)

Professional appearance

Professional appearance describes dress, grooming, hygiene, body adornments or any combination of those. Meeting professional appearance requirements is usually a condition of service in medical facilities. One way to fit in is through common dress. Practitioners may possess exquisite massage skills, and yet, if their attire and grooming deviates significantly from the institutional norm, they may never make it past the proverbial front door. The following are typical norms when working in health care facilities.

Chapter THREE

Clothing

- ID badge.
- Shoes with closed toes and heels. The shoes should also be clean and present no safety hazard.
- Socks.
- Long pants or skirt that falls near the knee. No shorts or miniskirts, even in the summer. Sweat pants and leggings are not typical within hospital culture.
- Shirt or blouse with a collar. No tank tops, halter-tops, or spaghetti straps. Scrubs, lab coats, or polo shirts are often worn in hospitals. Wearing a shirt in a particular color will help the staff recognize massage therapists more easily. Some therapists prefer to wear street clothes in the medical setting to convey a more relaxed mood. There are pros and cons to this.
- Shirt sleeves should not extend beyond the elbows for hygiene reasons.
- Fabrics should not be see-through nor should undergarments be exposed. Necklines should not be low-cut.
- Clothes should be clean and wrinkle free. Launder all clothing items after each shift.
- Clothing with logos or silk screen designs are often not acceptable for the hospital setting (e.g., T-shirts with brand names).

Grooming and personal hygiene

- Do not use scents of any kind, such as perfume, scented soaps, lotions, shampoos, or deodorants. These scents can trigger nausea for some patients.
- Maintain short-trimmed, clean nails. This is part of a professional image as well as a Standard Precaution (see Chapter 5).
- Beards, mustaches, and sideburns should be neat and trimmed.

Accessories and adornments

- Do not wear items that dangle, such as necklaces and long earrings, and tie back long hair.
- Consult with management about visible tattoos, body or oral piercings, plugged ear gauges, and hair sculptures.
- No type of nail enhancement should be used. This includes artificial nails, acrylics, tips, wraps, appliqués, gels, or any additional items applied to the nail surface.
- Proprietary insignias, pins, or buttons are usually not allowed.
- Do not chew gum!

A human resources manager recounted her experience of interviewing a group of touch practitioners for the hospital's first massage position. A number of people did not make it onto the short list because of how they were attired. They were probably fantastic bodyworkers but appeared more appropriately dressed for attending the weekend farmers' market.

First impressions matter. Dress and grooming tell an interviewer, the staff, or clinical massage instructor many things. One is that the therapist is willing to adhere to institutional policy, which is important down the road with regard to massage precautions, documentation, and Standard Precautions. It can also signal to patients that the practitioner is clean, professional, and willing to put them at ease.

Hospital dynamics

Bodyworkers often enter the hospital scene believing that the most difficult and challenging aspect will be in relating to people who are seriously ill. They are often anxious beforehand about the odors, tubes, machines, or incisions – fears that usually turn out to be unfounded. Commonly, angst doesn't arise from learning to be with patients, but from two other necessities: 1) mastering the art of interacting with the doctors, nursing staff, social workers, or myriad of other staff workers; and 2) settling into the rhythms and pace of the hospital itself.

Hospital life waxes and wanes unpredictably, making it difficult for touch therapists to create the restful or sacred space they desire. Nurses may need to come in and out of the room giving medications, attending to intravenous (IV) lines, or taking vital signs. Doctors' rounds, family visitors, or a consultation with the nutritionist may intrude. Ten minutes into the massage, the patient may be whisked away for an MRI (magnetic resonance imaging) scan. Although receiving massage might seem like a high priority to the patient, massage can't always be accommodated in the way the therapist and patient would like. Not only is the bodyworker unable to control the physical environment, but the patient also has minimal influence on their surroundings.

To the uninitiated, the health care setting appears confusing and disorderly. Figuring out which of the multi-colored-clad staff are nurses, doctors, students, physical therapists, or respiratory therapists is difficult. In the past, there was the doctor and the nurse, each of whom could be easily identified. In today's health care environment, nearly every one of the many specialists who provides direct care wears scrubs, making it difficult to recognize the many staff members and their accompanying responsibilities.

Bodyworkers new to the hospital environment often feel slighted when starting out because everyone goes about their duties with hardly an upward glance. This business-as-usual approach is taken as a snub, when it is the farthest thing from the truth. Nurses are thrilled for their patients to receive massage, but their workload is so staggering and stressful that they have little spare energy to attend to other health care team members.

Bodywork practitioners should expect to take the initiative in learning each hospital's routines, especially if they are volunteering or working independently. They may have to ask where the linen is, what to do with a full urinal, or where to lock up their valuables. Whether this is the best way to orient novices or anyone else is questionable, but it is a reality in today's rapid-paced work life. Students will have a clinical supervisor to assist them with this orientation, and therapists employed by the hospital may have a brief training session, but hospital massage therapists need to be bold about asking questions and being self-directed.

Eventually, rapport and trust will be established, and the staff will begin to recognize the massage therapist as an individual, then as a member of the health care team that they and the patients look forward to seeing. The bodyworker will literally be greeted with big smiles and open arms. But the transition from outsider to insider can be bumpy and long.

Team care: Working with staff

Massage therapy, on the whole, is a solitary business. Even the practitioner who is employed by a large spa or resort, shares office space with a group of bodyworkers, or is involved with an interdisciplinary group of practitioners, generally operates independently. In this model of care, the client and therapist are free to make treatment decisions on their own. In the medical setting, patients are cared for by a team. The physician or nurse practitioner is the lead decision-maker, while the patient's nurse oversees the treatment plan and coordinates the various care providers, often including massage therapists. Massage is just one of many services that must all fit together into a coherent whole.

When massage is a new concept within a hospital unit, integration into the team won't happen immediately. The respect of and acknowledgment by other professionals must be earned. Touch practitioners can foster this by becoming familiar with the roles of other staff, staying within the bodyworker's own scope of practice, and clarifying the proper channels of decision-making. They also have a responsibility to educate other staff who often don't realize the potential of massage in the acute care setting or don't understand what patient information a practitioner will need. It becomes the responsibility of the massage therapist to ask the right questions of team members so that sessions are safe for patients. Even if the nurse is busy, and stopping her to obtain information seems like an imposition, bodyworkers must fulfill their obligation to the patient by asking for the necessary medical data.

Chapter THREE

Info Box 3.1 Unanticipated benefits

The Mayo Clinic in Rochester, Minnesota has found unanticipated benefits from having a massage service. Because the massage therapists spend more one-on-one time with patients than the rest of the care team combined, and often with the patient unclothed, the therapists contribute: "novel and critical diagnostic information to the care teams."[1] Here is one example.

A woman who had undergone a partial small intestine resection two days prior to a massage session was complaining of back pain from prolonged time in bed. The surgical team ordered the massage hoping to improve the patient's comfort. The practitioner observed warmth in the left lower quadrant, which the patient said was tender. The therapist stopped the massage and reported the patient's symptoms to the nursing staff. It was discovered that the patient had intestinal leakage and infection in the abdomen.[1]

While touch practitioners do not have the luxury of independent action in a hospital, they have the opportunity to be part of a group from whom they can learn and seek support. They are in an atmosphere that is professionally stimulating and personally expansive. As a team member, the touch therapist learns to play a specific role and yet comes to see the broader view. This bigger picture includes the roles played by other staff members, the patient's family and medical history, and institutional and even societal needs. The bodyworker's part is an important element of a larger whole and the care given intersects and overlaps with a multitude of other forces. For the hospital practitioner, massage therapy is no longer a solitary business.

The majority of staff interactions will be with the nursing personnel, which includes nurse practitioners (NPs), registered nurses (RNs), licensed practical nurses (LPNs), and certified nursing assistants (CNAs). Regional differences exist in the use of nursing staff. In some areas, LPNs do not work in acute care settings but will be found in long-term care facilities. Massage therapists will also engage with physical and respiratory therapists, social workers, unit secretaries (sometimes known as ward clerks), and housekeepers.

Engagement with medical staff

The medical staff, which can include physicians, nurse practitioners, or physician assistants, are responsible for prescribing a patient's treatment. Massage practitioners will commonly cross paths with them during rounds, but on the whole, there is not a great deal of one-on-one interaction between massage providers and physicians. It might occur occasionally if the hospital requires medical approval for massage. However, even if referral for massage service comes from the medical staff, the physician is seldom the one who gives the touch therapist details about the patient.

Interacting with nursing staff

By and large, both RNs and LPNs provide direct patient care under the instruction of the medical staff. They also coordinate other health care practitioners such as physical therapists and nutritionists and document the patient's condition. Registered nurses, because of lengthy and in-depth training, also take on administrative responsibilities, oversee other nursing personnel such as LPNs and CNAs, and tend to patients requiring high-tech care. Massage practitioners commonly interact with nurses in the following ways:

- To triage the patients, gaining input on who is most in need or would most benefit.
- To obtain permission to give massage.
- To collect pertinent patient data.
- To inform of changes in the patient's condition.
- To report medical devices or equipment that need attention.
- To confer about unfamiliar health conditions.
- To obtain assistance with hospital furniture or positioning a patient.
- To get assistance with linens and lotion, if the nursing assistant is unavailable.

Therapist's journal 3.1
Benefits to the nursing staff

Partnering with a Hospital-Based Massage Therapy (HBMT) program has provided benefits not only to our patients, in the form of physical comfort, but to our nursing staff through the sharing of knowledge. Each new generation of nurses entering the workforce brings with them an ever-increasing base of knowledge regarding non-pharmacological options; however, the more experienced nurse may not understand or embrace these ideas. We find that HBMT students are eager and willing to share their expertise with these nurses, as they interact to coordinate patient care. Their demonstration of competence in a health care setting encourages nurses to consider massage therapy as an option for patient needs. Recognizing this level of professional knowledge in HBMT-trained massage practitioners led us to make it the gold standard for employment as a massage therapist in our facility.

Cathrine Weaver MSN, HN-BC, INFF, RN
Integrative C.A.R.E. Services Coordinator
Baptist Health Lexington, Lexington, Kentucky

The role of the nursing assistant/medical assistant

The nursing or medical assistant aids patients with less technical tasks, such as activities of daily living (ADLs), positioning, lifting, transfers, and recording vital signs. Massage practitioners should not get massage approval or clinical details from these assistants; however, they may help the massage therapist in a variety of ways, such as:

- Providing extra bedding, sheets, towels, pillows or personal items, such as lotion.
- Positioning the patient.
- Assisting the patient onto the commode or to the bathroom.
- Changing sheets due to a bowel or bladder accident or vomiting.
- Removing a urinal, bedpan, or emesis basin.

Social workers and chaplains

Social workers offer psychosocial supportive care that can include counseling, education, and referrals to other services, such as housing, financial assistance, and legal aid. Chaplains attend to people's spiritual care. Both sets of professionals can make bodywork practitioners aware of people who might benefit from touch therapy due to isolation, emotional difficulty, or just because a patient is having a really hard day. The massage practitioner who receives a referral through these departments must still confer with the patient's medical or nursing staff member to obtain clinical information.

Tip 3.1 Networking within the medical setting

Very often a bodywork practitioner in a medical setting must build a practice within that agency. One way to create a network is to contact members of the patient's interdisciplinary team after a session to report how it went. Team members appreciate the live contact via phone or by visiting their office. Over time, these connections will increase the likelihood of referrals.

Unit secretaries and housekeepers

Unit secretaries are known by many other titles, such as ward clerk or health unit coordinator. These staff members can help a massage therapist in the following ways:

- Obtaining supplies that are in locked cabinets.
- Paging staff members.
- Supplying information about patient or staff location.

Do not forget to cultivate a relationship with the housekeepers, who are also known as cleaning staff, environmental workers, and in The Netherlands, care supporters. This last designation, care supporters, is perhaps the most accurate, as they are part of the patient care team. Often, they are able to help in a variety of situations, such as:

- Finding bedding.
- Taking care of spills on the floor, including broken glass. (Never clean up spills yourself, as body fluids may be involved.)

Chapter THREE

Educating staff

Medical and nursing staff are often unfamiliar with massage as it is practiced in a hospital. They are unacquainted with the training of a massage therapist and neither understand what they do, nor their relevance to hospital dynamics. Staff also aren't aware of the wide range of touch modalities that can be employed with complex patients. Initially, they may not realize that there is always a way to provide skilled, comforting touch if the patient so desires. In addition, they may not understand why touch therapists request certain clinical information about the patient prior to starting the session.

Establishing rapport with the staff takes time – sometimes years when a program is just starting. One way to get to know staff and introduce the service is to offer short taster sessions at staff meetings or as part of a special "staff hour." Giving seated massage to personnel at such events will give the practitioner a chance to educate staff about what their discipline offers to the hospitalized patient. By integrating some of the comfort-oriented techniques into the seated sessions with

---

Tip 3.2 Massage sessions for staff

It is tempting to offer massage sessions to staff during spare moments: while waiting for a patient to use the commode, finish consulting with the doctor, or conclude a family visit. Often, there is not enough time to see another patient during the wait, and rather than letting the time go to waste, therapists may want to use these few minutes to offer a brief neck or shoulder massage to a staff member. However, rather than just jumping in and spontaneously offering a short massage while the nurse finishes her charting, communicate with the manager about the best way to incorporate staff massage into the schedule.

The reader may wonder why it isn't a good idea to utilize their time in this efficient way; however, misperceptions can arise when one staff member is seen to be receiving a massage at their station and others aren't able to receive the same benefit. There may also be funding parameters that only allows massage for the patients, even disallowing care for family members.

---

the staff, therapists will help them quickly understand that everyone is a potential candidate for massage. In addition, comfort and relaxation is provided to a group of people who are often stressed out and overworked.

Once rapport is established, a therapist will have more influence to suggest other ways to educate staff, such as presentations at staff meetings held by nurses, physicians, and pastoral care or social workers. Topics that give staff insight into hospital massage therapy include the following. (The agenda will be different for a nurses' meeting than one with social workers.)

- Benefits of massage and touch therapy, including symptom management.
- Difference between massage received at a spa, wellness clinic, or from a private practitioner.
- Types of touch modalities appropriate in the hospital setting.
- Adjustments needed for people who are hospitalized.
- The reasoning behind the questions therapists ask the nursing staff.
- Recent research.
- Training standards specific to working in a hospital.

Relating to patients: Patient-therapist boundaries

At first glance, the standards of behavior expected of staff toward patients may seem as if they are meant to create distance between the two. In reality, these standards are in place for two reasons: 1) to help caregivers establish a relationship in which the patient is free to focus on himself; and 2) to create equality of care. This model of relating doesn't exclude compassion and care – in fact, it will make compassion and care all the more possible.

Because massage creates a close bond between patient and therapist, it is imperative that bodyworkers maintain healthy emotional boundaries. Nina McIntosh points out in *The Educated Heart* that: "For [patients] to relax and drop their guard, they need the security and safety of sturdy boundaries. A safe environment is predictable, consistent, and focused on [the patients]."[2] Emotional boundaries are often crossed because massage therapists are trying to meet unconscious needs of their own, such as the common desire to be a hero. Or, the patient may bring to mind a special family member that they miss or someone with whom they have unresolved grief. Perhaps the patient's loneliness strikes a chord deep within the practitioner.

One beginner therapist stepped over the bounds with an elderly woman who brought to mind her grandmother. Meaning only to be helpful, she visited the woman after her shift and even offered to do several tasks outside the hospital. Her own grandmother, after all, was the same age, and the therapist hoped that others were doing these things for her. While the offer to help ostensibly seemed like a kindness, in the end the situation became a messy tangle. The patient developed expectations the practitioner could not meet and thus the safe environment that allowed the patient to focus on herself was gone. The massage therapist had made the mistake of trying to fix aspects of the patient's life, forgetting that the job of professional care providers is to help patients find their own healing resources. The focus in this case had shifted from healing the patient to meeting each other's needs.

The question of whether to share personal information can be a boundary conundrum. On one hand it can diminish the patient–therapist relationship, causing patients to feel a need to care for the practitioner. This takes attention away from the reason they are in the hospital: to focus on their own healing. For example, Heidi, a nursing home resident, would always ask her massage therapist how she was feeling at the start of each session. If the therapist answered, "I'm a little tired" or "My back is sore," Heidi tried to take care of the therapist, urging her not to work too hard or too long. The therapist learned to tell Heidi that she was always "fine." Otherwise, Heidi focused on the practitioner instead of on herself.

Sometimes an innocent comment can unintentionally become disastrous. For instance, without thinking, a therapist who was working with an ovarian cancer patient made a comment about her sister having been through the same treatment. The next question out of the patient's mouth was: "How is she?" This backed the therapist into a corner because her sister had died. Conversely, there are times when the practitioner's personal story can be supportive for the person who is ill. The question therapists must ask themselves is: "Am I sharing this to support the patient's process or my own?" For example, if the massage therapist had successfully been treated for the same or a similar condition, it is often helpful to share just that much with the patient. The patient feels relief knowing that there is an unspoken understanding based on their shared experience.

Those new to hospital work frequently muddy the waters by making the following gestures. Although these actions are meant to be compassionate and caring, they cross the bounds of a professional relationship.

- Calling the nurses' station to check on the patient.
- Exchanging addresses or phone numbers.
- Calling the patient outside of work to see how they are.
- Giving gifts, which can cause the patient or family to feel they need to reciprocate.
- Accepting tips or other money. Tips sometimes are literally forced on a therapist, in which case, the money could be given to a person in charge who can then return it to the patient or family member with an explanation of the hospital's policy. Some hospitals handle this situation by donating the money to the hospital foundation.
- Offering to come to the hospital on personal time to visit or give massage.
- Singling out certain patients for extra attention.
- Visiting patients at home after they are discharged, for other than professional reasons.

Sturdy boundaries benefit not only the patients but care providers as well. Hospitals can be stressful places, and only with well-established boundaries can practitioners thrive in such an environment. Without them, they would be in perpetual exhaustion, overloaded by the desire to fix problems that have no solution. Chapter 4 will help the reader explore more deeply the topic of the therapeutic relationship with patients.

Chapter THREE

The following suggestions will help practitioners to be mindful of the therapeutic container:

- Only work your scheduled shift time. Don't stay longer in order to be with a patient or family that is special to you.
- Follow the nurse's example and maintain a team approach to the care of each patient. No one patient belongs to a specific therapist.
- Stay within the scope of your task and don't spend time with patients or family in other ways.
- Don't accept family contact information or invitations to socialize outside of the hospital.
- Be mindful of making comments that might influence decisions of the family.
- Be careful not to provide support in place of family caregivers or health care staff.
- When sharing your own personal stories, be sure it is for the patient's benefit and not your own.

Equality of care

Massage practitioners in private practice have the choice of choosing to work with only certain populations. This is not an option when working in a public organization. Ideally, in medical settings, care is given to everyone on an equal basis: poor and rich, old and young, thin and fat, grumpy and cheerful, women, men or gender fluid, gay, straight or bisexual, a person of faith or non-believer.

There are always certain people the staff love to care for. They are the cooperative, optimistic ones who make the care providers feel they are great at their jobs, who are inspirational, or who light up the room. But it is the person who is irritable and seems ungrateful that may be in even greater need of attention. Sometimes the staff will comment on how difficult a patient is. However, when the touch therapist encounters this same person, he finds a sweet and vulnerable soul. Maintaining an open mind about each individual, no matter what other staff members have said, is important to providing equal and heartfelt care.

Therapist's journal 3.2
The grumpectomy

Oftentimes the nurses will ask me to see a patient they're having a hard time with. Either the patient is demanding and excessively pushing the call button, or is confused, restless or irritable. Working with the irritable patients is my favorite. I jokingly refer to this as performing a "grumpectomy" and tell the nurses: "If you want me to perform a grumpectomy, it is going to cost you some chocolate out of your candy stash."

One gentleman in particular comes to mind. He was snapping at everyone that walked into the room and nothing the staff did made him happy. I went to his room, knocked on the door, introduced myself and asked him how he was doing. Of course, he snapped: "Not good!" I asked him, "What's going on?" and I listened while he listed all the typical frustrations that people experience while being in hospital. When he was done, I said, "That is very frustrating, do you think a massage will help you feel better?" He replied grumpily back, "I don't know if anything will make me feel better." I said that we could try it, and if he didn't like it then he could tell me to stop. Then he said in a grumpy tone, "OK, what do you want me to do?" I gave him choices. Would you like your feet, back or neck massaged? How are you most comfortable, lying on your side or sitting up like you are? Would you like some aromatherapy or music turned on? By the end of the intervention the patient was relaxed and in a better mood with the staff.

When people are in the hospital, they are told what is going to happen to them and when, creating a feeling of powerlessness. By taking the time to listen and give the patient choices, it restores some sense of control. Meanwhile, the massage releases the stress and muscle tension, which, in turn, relaxes the patient. Everyone is happy. The patient is in a better mood, the nurses are not getting snapped at, and I get some chocolate.

Tammy R. Walker BCTMB
Swedish American Hospital, Rockford, Illinois

It might be daunting at first to work with types of people a therapist is unfamiliar with, such as a patient in a coma, or the person who has undergone gender reassignment surgery, someone who is deaf, a person who is paralyzed below the neck, or a patient who is in the prison system. These experiences can really stretch a therapist: learning to work equally with all patients expands a practitioner's comfort zone. She becomes a greater asset to herself, the hospital, and her colleagues because she is able to provide service to a wider variety of patients.

Ideally, all patients would have access to massage. However, with a service such as massage therapy for which the funding is limited, equality of care is not possible in every instance. Until full funding is available, the therapists involved with the massage therapy program must strive to the best of their ability to provide a level of care that is just and fair. When prioritizing patients on any given shift, therapists must take into consideration a complex set of variables: clinical needs and acuity level, social support, the patient's ability to access touch therapy through private means, massages already received during the patient's stay, length of stay, and the collective atmosphere on the unit. The symptoms and factors that are frequently used as gauges by therapists to help prioritize their limited time are: pain, anxiety, fatigue, social isolation, end of life, failure to thrive, and a new diagnosis. (See Chapter 11 for additional insights about triaging patients.)

Patient privacy and confidentiality

Protecting patient privacy is an obligation of all workers within a medical institution. The United States put the Health Insurance Portability and Accountability Act (HIPAA) of 1996 in place to ensure national standards of privacy and security regarding patients' health information.[3] The United Kingdom has a similar set of regulations that are part of the Data Protection Act 1998 and the NHS Care Record Guarantee.[4] Research of health care systems around the globe will find comparable confidentiality policies. The guiding principles within these regulations have the following commonalities:

- Confidential information must be protected against improper disclosure during reception, storage, transmission and disposal.

- Access to confidential information must be on a need-to-know basis. Recipients must respect that it is given to them in confidence.

- Disclosure of identifiable or confidential information must be limited to a required purpose. Disclosing information must be justified and documented.

- Patients have the right to know how their health information may be used and what disclosures have been made.

- Patients have a right to obtain a copy of their own health records and request corrections.

- Patients have a right to restrict the use of their health information and to request confidential communication of their health information.

Info Box 3.2 Examples of protected information

Name
Address (or any part of the address)
Names of relatives
Names of employers
Email or internet protocol (IP) address
Telephone or fax number
Date of birth
National identity number
Finger or voice prints
Photographs
Vehicle information
Medical record number

Examples of other information that must remain privileged include discussions with or conversations overheard from other health care workers and information told by the patient or their family. Personal information about the patient should not be discussed among the health care team; only that which may be relevant to the patient's treatment or psychosocial well-being should be talked about. For example, discussing such things as the patient's political beliefs, past drug use, or sexual history among the staff would be irrelevant to the patient's care and, therefore, a breach of confidentiality.

The one occasion a massage therapist would be ethically bound to break a patient's confidence is if the person's safety or well-being were in jeopardy. Robert, for example, was preparing to massage someone with an extremely low platelet count. Just before he entered the room, the patient had a spontaneous nosebleed, which the patient had packed with toilet paper. However, the blood continued flowing down her throat. The therapist asked the woman if she had notified the nurse of the bleed. "No, I will after the massage," she responded. As the reader will learn in future chapters, patients with a low platelet count have very slow coagulation times and are at risk for brain or retinal bleeds, both of which are extremely serious. Quite appropriately, Robert excused himself and left the room to report the patient's nosebleed to her nurse.

If there is a need to discuss an experience outside the hospital, such as during school clinical rounds, professional meetings, or in professional literature, omit using names or descriptions that might reveal a patient's identity, such as the diagnosis, age, date of admission, ethnicity, or name of the hospital.

Tip 3.3 Social media awareness

Nowadays therapists must also be mindful of how and what they communicate via social media. It goes without saying that information about specific patients should never be discussed. It is essential to be aware of your privacy settings, and who has access to what you post online. In addition, posts from the institution's intranet should remain in the private domain.

Because of confidentiality, independent contractors, friends, and even family members wishing to give massage usually will not have access to the same medical information that a hospital massage therapist will. For example, if an independent contractor asks the nurse about the patient's platelet count, it probably would not be given out unless there is a physician's order for the massage and the patient has signed a release form. That data is available only to staff, hospital volunteers, or therapists who have a contract with the hospital. However, a touch practitioner working privately can get the general information from the patient and/or the family.

When massage is being given on a more informal basis to a friend or family member, the lines can become blurred and facts that the patient would prefer to remain private can unknowingly be passed along to others within the social circle. Giving out general information about the patient to other friends or family, such as "She's not feeling well" or "He's very upbeat," is acceptable. However, no specific facts should be given unless the patient has consented. Examples of such precise information may include that a cancer has metastasized, the patient is having trouble with his bowels, or that he lost his job.

It is often tempting to call family and friends to announce changes in the patient's health status, but patients must be allowed to convey the specifics of the situation in their own way and time. An extreme example of violating a friend's privacy is the woman who put an announcement in the church bulletin of her friend's upcoming surgery for breast cancer. The patient, who was sitting in church on Sunday when the notice was read out, was horrified. Of course, the woman was only trying to be helpful, but she failed to understand that everyone has a unique feeling about her body and health status.

The following guidelines will safeguard confidential information:

- View or listen to confidential information only when necessary to fulfill responsibilities. Wanting to know isn't a good enough reason for listening in on privileged conversations.
- Share confidential information only with those who need to know to fulfill patient care responsibilities.
- Have private discussions in private places.
- Keep confidential information such as medical records safe and secure so that others cannot see them or take them.

- Be sure that unauthorized people cannot view confidential information on the computer. Log out of the computer before leaving it unattended.
- Do not display confidential information, such as a patient's name, on appointment schedules or public sign-in sheets.

The regulations concerning privacy are explicit and seemingly simple, but mastering them requires acute vigilance. People sometimes unintentionally breach a confidence when first confronted with these new protocols. Although innocent mistakes may be made in the learning process, it is important that health care providers remain committed to protecting patient privacy. Everyone deserves control of the information that is made public about his or her health.

Liability

Liability is an unavoidable fact of life within health care and greatly influences the attitudes and behaviors of those who work in it. When practicing in this arena, touch therapists must adopt a high level of awareness. The actions of private bodywork practitioners reflect only on themselves, whilst those of the hospital massage therapist impact the entire institution, which is ultimately responsible, or liable, for the care and safety of patients.

Massage therapists working in medical settings do not have the same latitude in decision-making and implementing interventions as private practitioners. It is the physician or nurse practitioner who decides on the overall medical and surgical treatment plan and writes the orders to be carried out by the nursing staff, physical therapists, nutritionists, and all of the many other professional caregivers, including massage therapists. Because massage is commonly thought of as an extension of nursing, the touch practitioner often works under the direction of the patient's nurse.

Adhering to the nurse's or doctor's instruction is imperative with regard to liability. It is important to check with the appropriate staff, usually the nurse, before proceeding with anything that is outside the agreed-upon scope of practice. For example: a therapist new to hospital work

thought that a patient had the beginnings of a pressure sore. Without conferring with the nurse, the therapist went ahead and treated the sore as taught in massage school. This action, however, was outside that hospital's job description for massage, which was to provide comfort-oriented touch only. Acting outside the agreed-upon job description jeopardizes the staff's trust in the massage therapist.

Even though health care employees are covered by the hospital's group liability insurance program, it is prudent for therapists to have a personal professional liability insurance policy. This is true whether they are volunteers, employees, or independent contractors, and regardless of whether the massage is intended for relaxation or as a treatment measure. While the institution accepts major liability for patients' care, each licensed worker employed by the facility is individually liable for performing his duties in accordance with the regulations and limitations of his licensing board or governing body.

Scope of practice

In the hospital, the scope of practice for massage therapists is more limited than in a typical private practice. In the privacy of their offices, therapists may offer advice on various other subjects, such as nutritional supplements, essential oils, and guided imagery. When working in a medical setting, bodyworkers must refrain from crossing clinical boundaries and offering information or guidance that is outside their identified discipline and/or job description. There are several reasons for this: it may conflict with the treatment plan set out by the physician, stray into the responsibilities of other members of the health care team, or go against the patient's or institution's beliefs.

It is easy to make suggestions that could be construed as medical advice. Because hospital patients' situations can be much more complex than those of clients seen in private practice, massage therapists are not in possession of all the salient information. A well-meaning suggestion, which might be appropriate in other settings, could prove to be harmful to the patient or cross the line into another care provider's purview. Examples of crossing clinical boundaries would be:

- Suggesting a diagnosis to the patient.
- Recommending that the patient eat certain foods.
- Recommending that a patient place ice on a painful joint without knowing the effect this may have on their skin.

Instead of offering advice or information to patients on subjects outside of their scope of practice, therapists might work to become skillful at questioning the patient. For example, a bodyworker might query, "Have you spoken to the nutritionist about that?" Or, "Is your nurse practitioner aware of that?" The following story illustrates how a bodyworker can unintentionally drift beyond her scope of practice. A newly licensed massage therapist had just finished working with a postpartum patient who was a first-time mother. The massage therapist was an older woman who had raised several children and was an experienced parent. After the session was over, the practitioner pulled up a chair and discussed breast-feeding, one mother to another, offering advice along the way. To be sure, the therapist meant only to be helpful, but she also may have presented information that conflicted with what the lactation specialist had given, thereby confusing the patient and stepping on the toes of the person assigned to help mothers with breast-feeding.

The scope of practice will differ between countries. In Europe, the UK, and many Commonwealth countries, it would be considered typical to educate patients about essential oils, whereas in the US it would generally be outside a massage therapist's scope of practice. Guided imagery is another example: within some hospitals, it would be readily acceptable for the bodywork practitioner to lead the patient through breathing or visualization practices, whereas other institutions would frown on this. When wanting to integrate new complementary activities or disciplines such as aromatherapy or visualization techniques into a hospital massage practice, it is best to have the support of the nurse manager or other administrator beforehand. Depending on the hospital's culture, the approval to include new practices may be immediate and on-the-spot, or it may require a number of committee meetings with final approval by a hospital governing body.

Etiquette toward patients, visitors, and staff

The following courtesies toward patients, family, and staff should be observed:

- If the patient's door is shut, knock before entering. If it is partially or fully open, still knock on either the door or door frame, or in some way get permission from the patient to enter the room.

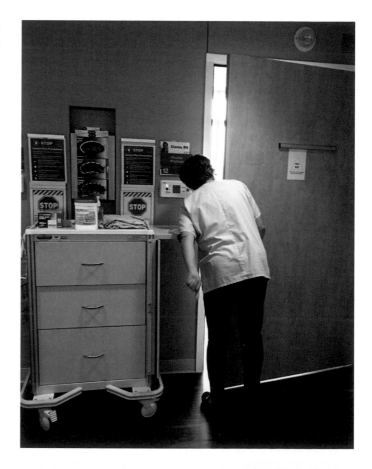

FIGURE 3.2
Asking permission to enter the patient's room.

(Photo by Gayle MacDonald.)

- Clarify with the patient how they prefer to be addressed: by first name, a nickname, Mr, Ms, Mrs, Dr, or by gender-neutral pronoun. Until it is clear, use a formal label, such as Mr Lopez or Ms Jones.

- If the curtain is pulled around the bed, it often means that the nurse is performing care that requires privacy, such as changing a dressing or assisting the patient with the bedpan. Most often, it is best to wait outside until the curtain has been opened.

- Only sit on the patient's bed with his or her permission. (Generally, professional caregivers do not sit on a patient's bed.)

- If a doctor needs to consult with the patient during a massage session, ask the patient if they would like you to step out or to remain in the room. Check with the doctor to ascertain their preference too. Sometimes the doctor needs a lengthy period of privacy to discuss the situation at hand; other matters take only a minute and can be accomplished while the therapist remains in the room and even continues the massage.

- Nurses may need to interrupt the massage to perform tasks. As they become accustomed to having massage therapists on the unit, they will be willing to postpone nonessential responsibilities until the bodywork session is complete. The massage can often continue even through essential tasks, such as attending to IVs, giving blood products, or taking vital signs. Ask the nurse and patient if it is OK to continue the massage.

- Visits by family and friends are important. If they arrive during a massage, some visitors will wait in the hall, while others will want to be with the patient. Welcome them into the room in some way, perhaps by eye contact, a smile, or a "Come on in."

- Conduct yourself with gentleness and courtesy in all parts of the hospital, such as the hallways, elevators, and cafeteria. It is impossible to know which of the people you encounter will be facing the most difficult of circumstances: a parent who is dying from cancer, a spouse who has a ruptured aneurysm in the brain, or a child whose feet were just amputated because of a bacterial infection.

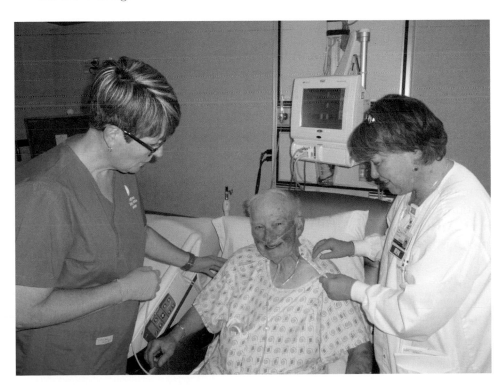

FIGURE 3.3
The massage can often continue even through essential nursing tasks.

(Photo by Carolyn Jauco-Trott.)

General etiquette in health care settings

Some of the following guidelines exist for hygiene reasons, some are aimed at avoiding clutter in work areas, and some are intended for both.

- Consume food and beverages in the staff lunchroom, never on the unit, at the nurses' station, or in patients' rooms. This includes use of personal drinks bottles.
- Store personal items in designated areas. Do not take them into patients' rooms or leave them at the nurses' station.
- Store food in designated areas.
- Change clothes in an area set aside for this purpose, such as a staff locker room.
- Do not use the patient's toilet.

Conflict of interest

Conflict of interest can occur when an individual is involved in multiple types of service. The most common example in the massage realm is the practitioner who is employed by the hospital but also has a private practice. Without vigilance, it would be easy to overlap or be perceived to be overlapping the two. By observing the following guidelines, conflicts of interest can be avoided:

- If a patient or staff member initiates a query or conversation about the therapist's private massage practice, the therapist is free to answer the query.
- No promotion of the therapist's private practice should occur.
- If the patient or staff member initiates a request for the therapist's business contact information, the massage therapist may give the information, including a business card. However, outside massage treatments should be conducted from the therapist's place of business.
- There will be times when therapists step out of their official role as a hospital employee and provide massage to a friend, family, or private client who is hospitalized. During those instances, the touch therapist should consider dressing in "street clothes" without

their hospital identification badge. Records should be kept in the therapist's own private documentation system.

Summary

Without a doubt, the customs and conventions of medical institutions are stricter than those of the massage profession in general. The hospital setting is less flexible and requires greater standardization and accountability. In order to be comfortable in the hospital, massage practitioners must come to grips with two paradoxes. The first is that of being simultaneously sensitive to the patient and insensitive toward the standard operating procedures inherent in a large health care facility. There is, however, still infinite space for the massage therapist to provide skilled touch that is creative, inspired, and heartfelt. The second paradox is how to accept hospitals for what they are and yet strive to make them more humane places to be. No easy solutions exist for these dilemmas. The immediate answer lies in the therapist's ability to embrace opposing energies – to hold both sides at once.

Test yourself

True or False: Answer true or false to each of the following statements. Rewrite each of the false statements to make it true. There is usually more than one correct way to rewrite the false statements.

1. The massage therapist makes the decisions about a patient's massage treatment plan.

2. Massage therapists are typically part of a team that works under the direction of the nursing staff.

3. Nurses typically coordinate the patient's care with physical, occupational, respiratory, and other types of therapists.

4. Once a therapist has completed their slate of patient sessions for the day, it is OK to spend extra time with patients who are special to them.

5. Wait until a patient is being discharged before exchanging emails or phone numbers.

6. Shirt sleeves should not extend beyond the elbows for hygiene reasons.

7. One of the patients you are massaging goes to the same church as your best friend. You should only share with your friend that the patient was admitted to the facility.

8. During a patient's massage session, the patient tells the therapist that he is a prostitute who specializes in S&M. This information should be passed on to fellow hospital massage therapists who might also be called on to work with this patient.

9. Wear freshly laundered clothes for each hospital shift.

10. In the health care setting, a massage therapist's scope of practice includes suggesting information about exercise and stretching.

11. A practitioner should never bring their own food or water into a patient's room. Instead, it should be left at the nurses' station.

12. Acrylic nails should only come to the tip of the finger.

References

1. Mallory MJ, Hauschulz JL, Do A, et al. Case reports of acupuncturists and massage therapists at Mayo Clinic: new allies in expediting patient diagnoses. Explore: The Journal of Science and Healing 2018;14(2)149–51.

2. McIntosh N. The Educated Heart: Professional Guidelines for Massage Therapists, Bodyworkers and Movement Teachers. Philadelphia: Lippincott Williams & Wilkins; 2003.

3. Health and Human Services. HIPAA for Professionals. 2017. Available from: https://www.hhs.gov/hipaa/for-professionals/index.html

4. National Health Service England. Confidentiality Policy. 2016. Available from: https://www.england.nhs.uk/wp-content/uploads/2019/10/confidentiality-policy-v5.1.pdf

…compassion triggers the momentary yet timeless connection of souls. Without it, there is technique or technology – interesting but not healing.

Rosalyn Bruyere[1]

In order to be truly skillful, a massage therapist must be adept at building a therapeutic relationship with each patient. This way of relating refers not only to addressing muscle tension or physical pain, but also allows for the psychosocial and sometimes spiritual interactions with a patient to be acknowledged. It is a whole-person, patient-centered relationship.

Experts define the **therapeutic relationship** as one in which: "Patients perceive themselves to be in a caring, supportive, nonjudgmental, and safe environment, often during a time of stress. Typically, the professionals in this type of relationship relate in a way that is warm, friendly, shows genuine interest, empathy, and the wish to facilitate and support. This atmosphere creates a climate that leads to more effective communication as well as improvement in patient satisfaction, adherence to treatment, quality of life, levels of anxiety and depression, and a decrease in health care costs."[2]

Boundaries and scope of practice, as discussed in Chapter 3, are foundational. Building on from there, how does the provider–patient relationship become a space of healing and not a space of stasis, or worse, a negative experience? How does a practitioner embrace not only the body, but the mind, heart, and soul? Successful providers master two specific skills in the art of therapeutic relationships: authentic communication and skillful compassion.

Author's note

Before going on, it is important to say that a therapeutic relationship is specific to professional situations. While the strategies from this chapter may have relevance in one's personal life, relationships with families and friends are significantly different and are best not professionalized.

Authentic communication

Everyone has experienced an interaction with a health care provider who is not truly present, i.e., not paying full attention. "How are you?" is often unconscious small talk, asked while the provider's focus is elsewhere. Experiences such as these often leave the client feeling like an inconvenience at best, or ignored and unheard at worst. Establishing habits that eliminate mindless interactions is one pro-active way of developing therapeutic relationships with each patient. For example, in a hospital room, if needing to accomplish tasks prior to the intake questions, a skillful option is for the therapist to first confirm with the patient that the service is wanted, and if so, then explaining the process including any setting up or paperwork to be completed prior to the start of the session. The provider can then assure the patient they will have time to fully check in with them in just a moment. This way, when asking the question "How are you?", the therapist is present, face to face and able to apply the therapeutic active listening skills discussed below. If possible, quietly pull up a chair next to the patient's bed to complete the intake questions. This gives the indication that the touch therapist has time to listen and is truly present.

Tip 4.1 Mastering the art

Developing one's gifts for creating healthy therapeutic relationships will both promote the patient's own healing process and often help prevent the practitioner from experiencing caregiver burnout. According to Drs Chou and Cooley of the Academy of Communication in Healthcare, practitioners that master the art of building therapeutic relationships with their patients are personally more fulfilled in their work and find more successful outcomes in those they serve.[3]

Understanding patients under stress

Patients are often under tremendous stress. In some situations, their stress response may be difficult for therapists to handle, and so recognizing stress responses of patients is a very helpful first step in creating a therapeutic

Chapter FOUR

relationship. Acute stress may present as restlessness, darting eyes, or twitching feet, and in a health care setting may be complicated by medications, isolation and decreased physical movement. While medications may be given specifically to reduce anxiety, some medications can increase the depth of emotions. However, not all stress presents outwardly: if stress has become chronic, the behaviors are likely to be quite different. Long-term stress may present as fatigue, confusion, anger and/or lethargy.

Assessing for stress level and whether it is acute or chronic can add tremendous advantage in building effective therapeutic relationships with patients who most certainly can benefit from whole-person support. Recognizing and normalizing the stress response without becoming frustrated or reactive is a useful ability to develop.

Holding space

Holding space is the concept of being with a client, fully present but without trying to fix them. Holding space means neither judging nor advising. It is the practice of being attentive. Holding space is being centered on the "spectrum of caring" presented below and in Table 4.1, and is the foundation of authentic communication within therapeutic relationships. The practices of holding space include:

- Deep inhalations which indicate a visceral comprehension of what was shared.
- Attentive silence and stillness.
- A gesture of recognition, such as placing one's hand on one's heart.
- No words are needed.
- Using gentle eye contact which is not too demanding, but is at the ready to listen.

Other than the logistics of charting and interacting with medical staff, the most common concern bodyworkers express about working in medical settings is over what to do in an intensely emotional patient situation. New practitioners in the field often ask: "How can I stay professional and strong when really I feel the need to cry?" Holding space is one strategy for these times.

For example, what should a touch therapist do when a client shares that her very best friend died unexpectedly? Or, how should a therapist respond when a patient at the end of life describes their fear of pain and expected death? Some massage practitioners will deny or dismiss their client's emotions because it is too uncomfortable and "outside the scope of practice." Some providers will feel the client's suffering so deeply that they offer their own personal experiences and solutions in order to help "fix" a situation that is too hard to bear. Instead, they could just hold space.

Therapeutic active listening

Another fundamental element of authentic communication is therapeutic active listening. According to researchers: "… listening was seen by patients as creating the conditions to promote healing and recovery."[2] In traditional active listening practice often used in psychotherapy, the therapist restates a client's report. An example might be: "I hear you say that your low back has been hurting since being in the hospital on the air mattress." In order to expand this technique to *therapeutic* active listening, the practitioner will include restating and clarifying any emotions or feelings that were shared in addition to the "facts". For example: "I hear you say that you have low back pain now and you suspect that it's from the air mattress. I am also sensing frustration when you say 'it's really hard to sleep here'". Simply being heard and understood can be therapeutic. Also, allowing the patient time to expand on or correct what the clinician repeated will likely improve the quality of the assessment and treatment plan. This is especially important for clients speaking in a second language or when colloquialisms may not be clearly understood between therapist and patient.

Practitioner vulnerability

Another important aspect of authentic communication is responding with a willingness to be vulnerable and honest. If a client's story is particularly moving, an authentic response means acknowledging one's reaction in a controlled way. The practitioner's response should be short and not fall into over-sharing of personal issues. However, the therapist can and should be human. For example, a patient once shared with a touch practitioner that she is "horrible" at making decisions, and is now faced

Therapist's journal 4.1
How to touch someone

Before you lay a hand,
you must lay your thoughts aside,
and breathe into yourself,
and gather your intentions –

Why are you here?

Now it's time to pay attention!
to the person sitting here, in front of you,
ready to receive your care.

Who is this person?

You have no idea, and they might not say –
they might not even know,
for what the mind forgets, the body remembers.

This person's body has a history –
perhaps loving, perhaps harsh.
Hands to this person may be
wonders or weapons.

Suppose you have a warrior in front of you,
a survivor,
a child,
a mother,
a lover.

You must be gentle, yet strong.
You must go slow, and flow.

Most importantly, you must breathe –
breathe into your heart, your hands,
your heart-hands.

Remember –
what you feel, he feels,
what you feel, she feels.

Feel the warmth of the space between you.
Only *now* may you begin...
...the laying on of hands.

by **Allison Young** CMT

with what type of treatment to have for advanced cancer. If the touch practitioner personally identifies with, in this case, challenges of decision-making under difficult circumstances, that common experience can be shared. No words are needed, but if the therapist senses it to be appropriate to share their own vulnerability as a means of connecting, the practitioner might briefly disclose part of their own experience. For example, in this case the practitioner might say something like: "I am really bad at making decisions myself. I can imagine with a decision this important, it's very stressful." Being human and allowing one's self to be imperfect, and broken in one's own unique ways, builds a bond and helps both to feel less isolated and closer to the mutually healing experience of being understood. The guideline for personal disclosures in these situations however is always "less is more".

Motivational interviewing

The therapeutic relationship is intended to be patient-centered. However, practitioners often automatically respond by giving advice when patients share something of their situational challenges. A common reply might be: "Maybe you should…", or, "I know another client who had similar issues and they…" These are therapist-centered responses. While they are well-intentioned and might be helpful, these bits of advice could also feel like yet another person imposing unhelpful clutter in an already stressful situation.

Motivational interviewing is a patient-centered strategy used widely in integrative medicine and other health care practices that can empower the client to discover their own answers, motivation and commitment.[4] It engages people in their own health care,[3] and because a provider never has all the answers to life's presenting problems, the burden and risk in finding the answer to the patient's problem is removed from the practitioner.

This strategy is useful on many levels. It can be used when trying to help a patient who is working to improve a symptom, such as anxiety. There are always many options toward a solution – the key is, what motivates the patient and what are they willing to commit to? It is immaterial what the therapist believes they should do.

The bodyworker is there to listen, ask questions when appropriate and help the patient frame a plan that motivates them.

For example, practitioners often struggle with what to say when a patient questions the worth of continuing treatment, or concludes that they are not prepared for dealing with financial crisis due to loss of work. What does one say when the patient has extensive family issues which take priority even over their own health? It is perfectly acceptable, and is actually more appropriate, *not* to provide answers. When conversation is expected, motivational interviewing is a best practice that may help clients identify their own solutions or initiate a transformation. In the above circumstances, the therapist could include motivational interviewing by asking the patient to consider their sources of information. For example, a skillful question might be: "Do you feel comfortable asking a few people on your health care team more about the options you have?" This type of question draws attention to the patient's immediate resources for decision-making, and is open enough to allow for the emotional aspects possibly associated with asking for input, or interacting with medical staff. Affirming the goals of the team for the client's best outcomes is inherent in the question, which also makes it skillful.

Sample motivational interviewing questions

Below are sample motivational interview style questions which may be appropriate for medical settings when patients engage in telling their story. They may be asked during a first appointment or as conversation unfolds at the bedside session. As these are intensely personal questions, complete attention and holding space for an authentic response is crucial. Without genuine interest in the client's answers, the questions could be felt as intrusive or inappropriate. A key component of skillful questions is that they are open-ended – this means there is not a quick yes or no answer and that further conversation is welcomed.

1. What brings you joy? Where do you find happiness? At home, what do you do for fun?

2. Where do you find purpose? What gives you meaning? What are you learning about yourself?

3. What are your goals? What are your goals for when you are back home?

Unfortunately for many chronically ill patients, they can become medicalized and overly identified with their conditions. Asking patients about their joy, meaning, or goals is intended to activate the inner drive and remind them of who they are outside of the medical setting. For example, a newly admitted stroke survivor in a rehabilitation facility requested massage therapy for pain relief. During the first intake, the touch therapist asked: "If you had one goal to accomplish this week, what would it be?" This question opened up the full spectrum of the patient's goals and also helped set expectations that were attainable. The patient responded with: "I need to send my brother a birthday card." The therapist was then able to offer extra focus on the patient's hands and arms and connected that the massage might help "get the hands ready" to write.

The search for meaning can be from moment to moment or the quest of a lifetime. Therapists of any discipline who help patients to recognize their own goals, are mastering therapeutic relationships.

Skillful compassion

People in the various health care disciplines are generally thought to be compassionate by nature. Experience and research show, however, that compassion can also be taught and therefore is a skill that can be improved, regardless of the starting point. Working with seriously ill patients, in environments that are often hectic and stressful, can be very emotionally demanding. Being skillful in expressions of compassion serves patients, their families, staff members and practitioners themselves by allowing for true human emotions without overstepping professional boundaries or scope of practice. The Spectrum of Caring chart (see Table 4.1) was developed specifically for practitioners working with medically complex patients and clients in health care settings. It bears repeating that these skills may inform personal relationships, but the agreements between family and friends are different in important ways. The Spectrum of Caring guidelines below are for the presenting psychosocial needs of a client within a given session of touch therapy.

If authentic communication is the outward behavior that builds therapeutic relationships, skillful compassion is the internal counterpart. Where is one's heart and mind in any given client interaction? Is there judgment of any kind regarding why the patient is in the hospital? Is the mind busy solving all the person's problems? Skillful compassion is the inner balance of being fully present and not ever assuming one has solutions to another's concerns.

Journaling exercise 4.1
What is helpful to me?

Take a moment to consider a time when you personally have been in a difficult situation, e.g. physically or perhaps in a challenging relationship. What type of support was most helpful to you? Did you appreciate others sharing similar experiences so you could learn from them or perhaps feel less alone? Did you appreciate someone bringing you food, taking care of tasks but otherwise giving you space to be alone? Did you find the best support in a group that shared together over time? Perhaps you felt best supported by an expert, professional provider that took charge of the situation and gave you instructions as to what to do.

In reflecting on your experiences, it is likely obvious that different situations need different and often multiple supports. However, it may also occur to you that you have strong personal preferences for what actually feels supportive to you. If you can do this exercise with a few colleagues and share your responses, you will probably find that different people prefer different types of support. What is helpful to one is not necessarily helpful to another. How does this relate to skillful compassion and healthy therapeutic relationships?

Skillful compassion is offered through listening for and acknowledging the emotional aspects of what a patient shares, and holding space for whatever is expressed without attempting to fix it. For many bodyworkers, this is the appropriate limit to the conversation – holding space is enough. Simply acknowledging the conversation in some way before proceeding to the hands-on work, and again at the close of the session is a good rule of thumb

and helps build a therapeutic relationship. For example, a comment such as: "Thank you for sharing some of your story with me," shows gratitude and conveys that the patient was heard.

Internally however, the therapist is wise to stay curious without judgment. Recognize any emotional response is one's own and not the patient's. When patients significantly trigger the practitioner's own emotions, it is best to keep a balance between professional knowledge and heartfelt reaction.

If the ideal outward expressions of healthy therapeutic relationships are excellence in treatment, authentic communications and skillful compassion, the Spectrum of Caring is like a GPS tracking device for the practitioner's internal terrain. Each column in Table 4.1 offers a variation of attitudes and behaviors that fall on the spectrum of caring.

Sympathy

Start with the column labeled "Sympathy." Sympathy here means the provider has an understanding and recognition of the client's difficult situation, and will feel relatively distant from the client.

Empathy

On the opposite end of the spectrum is the response labeled "Empathy." When in empathy, the therapist recognizes and understands the problematic situation but also feels it more deeply. There is an emotional and sometimes visceral experience in the practitioner. For some, there is a kind of meshing or melding with the emotions of the client.

Compassion

While both sympathy and empathy provide a quality of holding space and are certainly expressions of care, there is yet a third, middle way that has the potential to be of better service to the patient and to sustain the clinician. The middle way, to overtly borrow from the Buddhist tradition, is the response of compassion. Definitions and translations can

Chapter FOUR

TABLE 4.1 Spectrum of Caring[9]			
Symbol[†]			
Spectrum	SYMPATHY	COMPASSION	EMPATHY
Location	Brain	Spirit	Heart
	Pity ←———— Holding space ————→ Overwhelm		
Definition	Sameness of feeling; agreement	Sympathetic consciousness of another's distress	Ability to share another's feelings
Description	Perceiving another's situation/ emotions as painful, tragic, horrific, etc. Needing to be fixed, changed, corrected	Meeting another where they are. Being present to all that is. Allowing the emotions and story to be heard/ person to be seen	Being fully connected emotionally to another's emotions or "story". Feeling what you think they feel
Energy (provider's)	Giving away. Pouring out. Can turn into "fixing"	Holding space. Being with. Trust	Melding. Merging. Can turn into "fixing"
Energy (patient receives)	Heavy weight on them	Supportive. Empowering	Melding. Merging. Diverted
Dos	Acknowledge your heart's mind and your mind's heart	Stay present. Don't run away. Help facilitate another's finding their own answers/solutions	Feel what you feel and track what is yours and what is another's
Don'ts	Assume you can fix or solve another's "problems", situations or behaviors	Preach about how it will all work out or that "it's for the best" (passive fixing)	Take on the emotions of another or add your own emotional reactions to another's
Skillful communication	Listen only!	"What do you need?"	"How can I help?" *
Shadow side	Pity. Arrogance. "Fixer"	Disengaged. Philosophic/spiritual righteousness	Boundaryless. Manipulative
Flipside	They/we still show up!	Patients tend to resonate with truth. There is a bigger context to our lives	Burnout. Unable to work. Quit and "go live on a mountain"

†See Question 5 in the Test yourself section at the end of the chapter.
*This is a skillful question for empathy, but not necessarily the best; may lead to breaking boundaries.

confuse the core meaning: here, consider the definition of compassion as the response of understanding, recognizing, and feeling another's difficulties and emotional states. Compassion stays fully present to all that is, without feeling within one's self the need to fix or change the other person. Compassion is a practice of acceptance with an awareness that healing is always a potential. Compassion is neither being on the sidelines nor a superhero. It opens the space to facilitate a client's own discovery of what they need, in any given moment. Compassion allows for feelings of brokenness or rawness but also the sense of freedom in being seen and acknowledged: in a word, accepted. It is a space that understands to the core that transformation, if not cure, is possible no matter the circumstances.

As doctor Wayne Jonas says, "healing emerges in the space between people – in the collective mind – and its benefits can go either way".[5]

Examples of skillful compassion in patient–practitioner conversation

- "I can sense the frustration you are experiencing and I can feel that this is a tough situation for you." Eye contact and pausing are helpful here.

Journaling exercise 4.2
Where are you on the Spectrum of Caring?

Please spend some time journaling your thoughts about the questions below.

The Spectrum of Caring was developed as a guide or framework to help the professional caregiver look inward. *Sustainability* and *resilience* are hot topics in health care as clinician burnout rates and attrition appears to be at an all-time high. While systems and workload demands are prime factors, one's philosophy and world view play a part. What do you believe your role is in health care? How do you define "healing?" Why do you believe people get sick or have pain? One's answers to these questions will give an insight into a therapist's perspectives and presumptions. The suggestions on the Spectrum of Caring guideline are intended to help the therapist navigate closer to center when interacting with patients and clients.

Tip 4.2   Patients in trouble

In clinical environments, all staff are required to report if a patient suggests any kind of harm to self or others. Suicide rates for seriously ill people are substantially higher than in the general population. If a patient states, in any terminology, the thought or intention of doing harm to themselves or others, notify the patient's nurse of what you heard directly after the session. Follow all medical center protocols for any additional steps including noting the statement verbatim in the patient's chart.

- "I can really understand that this is also an emotional time for you. Do you feel like you have the support you need?"
- Have a list of the departments to which you can refer patients. In the hospital, these would include chaplains, social workers, case managers and of course the nurses.

Diversity, equity and inclusion

Health care environments should serve all people in need equally. It is the responsibility of every provider, regardless of discipline, to educate one's self and continually engage in self-reflection around issues of diversity, equity, and inclusion. Aptitude for successfully engaging any and every person who is on the referral list is a core skill in building therapeutic relationships with clients. The beauty of building these skills is that they are often both "good medicine" for the patient, and increase the fulfillment experience of the therapist.

Typically, recognizing the impact of culture on an individual depends very much upon which culture that person identifies with. The daily impacts of a society's culture are a given to those in underrepresented minority groups and are often completely invisible to those in privileged or majority groups. The conversation about bias between groups is not usually easy, but it is imperative for therapeutic relationships.

Dr Linda Clever explains: "Everyone has attitudes. They live in you and tend to persist unchecked unless you take charge… Grounded in emotion, attitudes show up in your body language, words, and behaviors. Attitudes are your outlooks at the same time that they mirror you."[6] It is imperative in the building of therapeutic relationships that practitioners examine their own biases, assumptions, prejudices, and attitudes. Behavior follows thought. Health disparity, with its unfortunate foundation in prejudice and socioeconomic inequities, is a dedicated field of study within public health. Inward examination and reexamination of one's attitudes throughout one's professional career is required for those who seek to build truly therapeutic relationships.

Embedded in any relationship is the reality that people have differences. How differences are welcomed or shunned is a core question in the study of diversity, equity and inclusion. Culture is defined in different ways and changes over time. Around the globe, culture is a cause

Chapter FOUR

Journaling exercise 4.3
Topics for further research and reflection

Select one or more of these topics to research and journal your thoughts on what you find.

- Implicit bias, automatic reactions. We all have them – take the self-test at: https://implicit. harvard.edu/implicit/iatdetails.html.
- Microaggressions: "Brief, everyday exchanges that send denigrating messages to a target group such as people of color, women, and gays."[7]
- Privileges: Everyone has these too, based on gender, sexual orientation, able-bodiedness, religion, race, nationality, language, age, economic ability, geographic location.
- Being an ally: Recognizing and acting to "call out", or "call in"[8] others' microaggressions or behaviors that foster inequity or exclusion.

Tip 4.3 Habits for successful therapeutic relationships in health care settings

1. Set appropriate expectations at each session.
2. Hold space: listen and allow silence and stillness.
3. Stay aware of internal reactions and feelings of "need to fix." Hold reactions gently, breathe.
4. Ask skillful questions instead of giving answers.
5. Be human.
6. Be curious about cultural differences and include them in conversation. Accommodate cultural-based needs in delivery of services as appropriate and if possible.
7. Look for assumptions or implicit biases, and consider if they would be any different if the client was from a different demographic, such as ethnic or racial.
8. Give credit to the health care team whenever possible for their thoughtfulness in referrals and support.
9. Track whether emotions are leaning either toward pity or a sense of melding, and consider if a response could be balanced in compassion.
10. Provide closure with each patient. Show gratitude; don't over-promise the future.

for celebration but unfortunately often used as reason for discrimination and unequal treatment. One serious example of the impact of cultural inequity is seen in health care disparities. Among different minority cultural, ethnic, socioeconomic and other demographics, data show significant adverse outcomes in life expectancy, disease rates, and death in childbirth, compared to majority populations. Decidedly, important structural changes are needed to correct these inequities. There is no excuse for waiting, however – each professional provider can do their part to be the change.

Self-care

One important reason to establish self-care practices is to help discharge emotional energy that does not serve the professional caregiver and in turn does not serve those being cared for. What constitutes effective self-care is rarely studied. When asked about self-care practices, many providers talk about what they like to do on their days off. "Time in nature", "playing with kids or pets", "a hot soak" are often on top of the list. These are wonderful

options and all highly recommended. For professional caregivers though, daily self-care is a must.

It is relatively easy to incorporate simple activities into a work shift in any medical center setting. Washing hands with intention is one example. Instead of washing hands while thinking of the next tasks, practitioners can use the time to clear the mind with simple breathing exercises. If a session was particularly impactful, the time washing hands could be used to also acknowledge whatever is in one's heart. Naming the emotion and expressing gratitude for the awareness and experience can help close a session internally. Drinking water as a ritual throughout a work day can also be an intentional act of self-care. Perhaps one says a favorite positive word or a mantra before each sip. Perhaps the clinician visualizes a favorite body of water during each hydration. It is not likely that a water bottle can be carried during sessions, but water bottle "closets" or places where personal belongings can be kept may provide the opportunity to store a special water bottle. Colorful and meaningful stickers could be placed purposefully as self-care reminders. The possibilities are endless, the benefit is crucial.

Summary

While compassion and listening skills are hoped for in all health care professionals, specific skills and behaviors can be developed and improved to promote truly therapeutic relationships with clients. Culturally informed skills of holding space, therapeutic active listening, and motivational interviewing along with the Spectrum of Caring framework may improve the quality of therapeutic relationships. Personal relationships aside, skillful compassion does not attempt to solve problems but engages patients in discovering their own inner wisdom and guidance. The tools of authentic communication, skillful compassion and excellence in discipline-specific care are more effective for client relationships, as well as for increasing the resilience of providers. Appreciating differences, acknowledging individual expression of cultural identities and efforts to include each person and family are embedded practices within successful therapeutic relationships. Self-care is a necessity and is best practiced daily, including through small habits integrated into the work schedule.

Test yourself

Journal your thoughts on the following questions.

1. My philosophy:

   A   What is my philosophy of: Health? Health care? Healing?

   B   What are my perspectives on illness and disease?

2. Reflect on a particularly challenging client interaction.

   A   What was your intention in the communications?

   B   Where did you fall on the Spectrum of Caring?

   C   What behaviors or communications could help "hold space" in a centered, compassionate place for this client?

3. In what ways do you feel included in your work community? In what ways do you feel excluded in your work community?

4. What specific behaviors could you incorporate to help your underserved minority clients feel more included?

5. In the top row of the Spectrum of Caring (Table 4.1) are three blank boxes. Draw a symbol that for you represents each heading of the spectrum: sympathy, compassion and empathy.

References

1. Carlson R, Shield B (Editors). Healers on Healing. New York: Putnam; 1989.

2. Kornhaber R, Walsh K, Duff J, Walker K. Enhancing adult therapeutic interpersonal relationships in the acute health care setting: an integrative review. J Multidiscip Healthc. 2016; 9: 537–46. Available from: https://doi.org/10.2147/JMDH. S116957.

3. Chou C, Cooley L. Communication Rx: Transforming Healthcare Through Relationship-Centered Communication. New York: McGraw Hill Education; 2018.

4. Miller WR, Rollnick S. Motivational Interviewing: Helping People Change. New York: The Guilford Press; 2013.

5. Jonas W. How Healing Happens: Get Well And Stay Well Using Your Hidden Power to Heal. New York: Lorena Jones Books; 2018.

6. Clever L. The Fatigue Prescription: Four Steps to Renewing Your Energy, Health and Life. Berkeley: Viva Editions; 2010.

7. Sue DW, Capodilupo CM, Nadal KL, Torino GC. Racial microaggressions and the power to define reality. Am Psychol. 2008; 63(4), 277–9. Available from: http://dx.doi.org/10.1037/0003-066X.63.4.277.

8. Adapted from Oregon center for education equality: what did you just say? Responses to racist comments collected from the field. Interrupting Bias: Calling Out vs. Calling In. www.seed the way.com. Available from: https://www.showingupforracial-justice.org/surj-values.html

9. Tague C. Spectrum of Caring (5th edition). Tague Consulting; 2019.

Chapter FOUR

Additional resources

Academy of Communication in Healthcare. www.achonline.org.

Adams C, Jones P. Therapeutic Communication for Health Professionals (3rd edition). New York: McGraw Hill; 2011.

Baron, D. What's Your Pronoun? Beyond He and She. New York: Norton; 2020.

Benjamin B, Sohnen-Moe C. The Ethics of Touch. Tucson: Sohnen-Moe Associates; 2014.

Douglas M, Pacquiao D, Purnell L (Editors). Global Applications of Culturally Competent Health Care: Guidelines for Practice. Switzerland: Springer; 2018.

Enact Leadership. www.enactleadership.com.

Hick SF, Bien T. Mindfulness and the Therapeutic Relationship. New York: The Guildford Press; 2010.

Khan S. When patients discriminate. Available from: https://opmed.doximity.com/articles/when-patients-discriminate?_csrf_attempted=yes

Kinzbrunner B, Policzer J. End-of-Life Care: A Practical Guide. New York: McGraw Hill; 2011.

Koloroutis M, Trout M. See Me as a Person: Creating Therapeutic Relationships With Patients and Their Families. Minneapolis: Creative Health Care Management; 2012.

Lambert MJ, Barley DE. Research summary on the therapeutic relationship and psychotherapy outcome. Psychotherapy: Theory, Research, Practice, Training, 2001; 38(4):357–61. Available from: https://psycnet.apa.org/record/2002-01390-002

Merchey J. Building a Life of Value: Timeless Wisdom to Inspire and Empower Us. Beverly Hills: Little Moose Press; 2005.

Mitchell A. The Therapeutic Relationship in Complementary Health Care. Churchill Livingstone; 2003.

Pan C. Lost in translation: Google's translation of palliative care to 'do-nothing care.' GeriPal Geriatrics and Palliative Care Blog. 2019. Available from: https://www.geripal.org/2019/05/lost-in-translation-googles-translation-of-palliative-care.html

Patterson K, Grenny J, et al. Crucial Conversations: Tools for Talking When Stakes are High (2nd edition). New York: McGraw Hill; 2012.

Santorelli S. Heal Thy Self: Lessons on Mindfulness in Medicine. New York: Three Rivers Press; 1999.

UNESCO. Universal declaration on cultural diversity, Paris, v.1: resolutions. 2001. Available from: http://unesdoc.unesco.org/images/0012/001246/124687e.pdf#page=67

University of California, Davis. LGBTQIA resource glossary. 2019. Available from: https://lgbtqia.ucdavis.edu/educated/glossary

University of California, San Francisco. Implicit bias and health care disparities resources. Available from: https://diversity.ucsf.edu/resources/strategies-address-unconscious-bias/

Wasserman J, Palmer R, Gomez M, et al. Advancing health services research to eliminate health care disparities. AJPH 2019; 109:S64–9. Available from: https://doi.org/10.2105/AJPH.2018.304922.

Wheeler D J, Zapata J, Davis D, Chou C. Twelve tips for responding to microaggressions and overt discrimination: When the patient offends the learner. Med Teach. 2019; 41:10, 1112–7. Available from: https://doi.org/10.1080/0142159X.2018.1506097.

Wilber K. Integral Psychology: Consciousness, Spirit, Psychology, Therapy. Boston: Shambala; 2000.

The agenda, if you were to have one, is to be with the patient, not to give a massage. Massage therapists may have to drop techniques in favor of just being there. It's amazing how putting our attention on someone can shift things.

Dawn Nelson,

author of *Compassionate Touch*

One of the biggest learning curves for the massage therapist who is new to working in health care institutions is that of infection control practices. For the experienced therapist the task is to stay mindful of these habits and to not let down their guard. As the therapist reads more deeply into this chapter, they will understand the need for the hygienic vigilance needed in hospitals, long-term care facilities, and rehabilitation centers. This diligence has been unequivocally reaffirmed by the global COVID-19 pandemic.

The World Health Organization (WHO) estimates that each year millions of patients are affected by health care-acquired infections (HAIs). These are infections picked up in any setting: hospital, long-term care, ambulatory, or home care. The term nosocomial refers to infections that occur specifically in hospitals.[1] In Europe, approximately 5–6% of patients develop an HAI[2]; in the US, the rate is 3%.[3] WHO estimates that the average in developing countries is 10%. HAIs can affect anyone, but most typically they are seen in patients who are immunocompromised, elderly, and post-surgical. Adding to those risks is the failure of health care staff to wash their hands, overuse of antibiotics, indwelling catheters, and long-term stays in health care facilities.[1]

HAIs add to the patient's length of stay, which then increases the cost of care and also results in further complications and even deaths. The United States Centers for Disease Control and Prevention (CDC) estimates that HAIs are responsible for 1.7 million infections and 99,000 deaths per year in the US.[4] In addition to patients being infected, thousands of health care workers also acquire an infectious disease while on the job.

The threat of microbes that are resistant to treatment is especially a concern in this day and age. People, animals, and goods now travel with ease around the world,

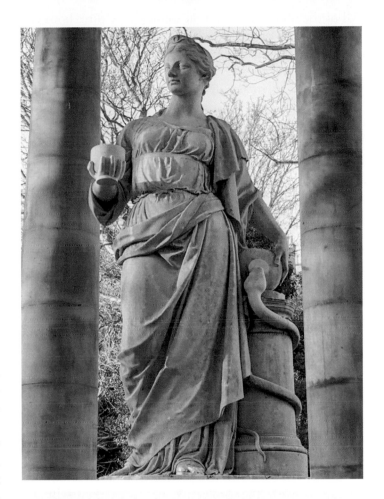

FIGURE 5.1
Hygeia, Greek goddess of health and cleanliness; her name is at the root of the word *hygiene*.

which means that infections are bound by no borders. The United Nations report, "No Time to Wait: Securing the Future from Drug-Resistant Infections," states that drug-resistant diseases cause at least 700,000 deaths per year globally. By 2050, this figure could increase to 10 million deaths globally per year if no action is taken, including 2.4 million of those deaths in high-income countries.[5] To address this, a partnership of nations, international organizations, and non-governmental organizations has come together to create the Global Health Security Agenda.[6]

Protective practices: a high priority

All of the above information sounds very dire, however, over the past number of years, improvement has been made in reducing the number of HAIs. In US acute care hospitals and long-term care facilities, there has been a decrease in methicillin-resistant *Staphylococcus aureus* (MRSA) and *Clostridioides difficile* (C. diff) events as well as a reduction in abdominal surgical site infections, central line-associated bloodstream infections, and catheter-associated urinary tract infections. However, the data for inpatient rehabilitation centers in the US are not as positive: no improvement has occurred except for C. diff events.[3]

Influential health organizations, such as the WHO, CDC, the National Health Service (NHS) in the UK, and the European Centre for Disease Prevention and Control (ECDC) have made protective precautions a high priority. These practices are organized into two levels. The first tier, known as Standard Precautions, is designed for the care of all patients, regardless of their diagnosis or presumed infection status. The second tier, Transmission-Based Precautions, is used only when caring for specified patients known or suspected to be infected by specific pathogens. There are three types of Transmission-Based Precautions: Airborne, Droplet, and Contact Precautions.[7]

The purpose of this chapter is to acquaint massage therapists with the protective practices they will use when working with the patient in a health care setting. These include **handwashing**, **gloving**, **masking**, and **gowning**. In addition, material is presented on protecting patients who are immunosuppressed, proper handling of bedding and work clothes, exposure to body fluids, and when to stay home during illness.

Gowning, masking, and gloving is not as simple as 1-2-3. It takes a significant amount of time to become proficient at the individual components, let alone using all the protective gear together. For example, a massage therapist who came from a nursing background and had a great deal of experience in the ICU setting was massaging a patient who was under Contact Precautions. In the middle of the session, she moved her glasses from her face and placed them on top of her head. Suddenly she realized what she had done, that the person had C. diff, and that she had just contaminated her glasses and thus her hair.

There is an emotional component when first learning to follow these protective practices and anxiety is common at the beginning. Who can blame a therapist for having an emotional response when confronting the reality of exposure to bacterial infections or touching people who have weeping around lesions or dried body fluids on their gown?

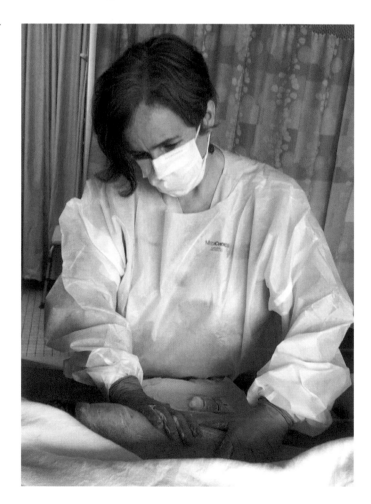

FIGURE 5.2
Total presence is possible, even while being masked, gloved, and gowned.

(Photo by Gayle MacDonald.)

Massage therapists also worry that personal protection equipment (PPE) places a barrier between them and the patient that will preclude connecting on a deep level. It doesn't have to. This work is about being present, no matter what the circumstances. Gloves will not get in the way of compassion. A mask and gown will not prevent the transmission of kindness. Softness can be maintained in the midst of seemingly rigid rules.

Standard Precautions

The infection control practices introduced in the 1980s were termed Universal Precautions, which referred specifically to bloodborne micro-organisms. In the mid-90s, the infection control practices were expanded to include all body fluids.[8] The new techniques became known as **Standard Precautions** and applied to all patients regardless of their diagnosis or presumed infection status.

Info Box 5.1 Potential pathogenic substances

The following are examples of body fluids, tissues, and substances that may carry pathogens.[9,10,11]

- Blood
- Breast milk
- Cerebrospinal fluid
- Feces
- Nasal secretions
- Pericardial fluid
- Peritoneal fluid
- Perspiration
- Pleural fluid
- Saliva
- Semen
- Sputum
- Synovial fluid
- Tears
- Urine
- Vaginal secretions
- Vomitus
- Wound exudate

When studying information sources about infectious spread of disease, it is easy to get confused if the resource only focuses on bloodborne pathogens. Practitioners in the health care setting must remain aware that bacteria and viruses can be spread via feces, nasal secretions, saliva, sweat, tears, urine, and vomit. Standard Precautions are meant to be applied to all body fluids.

Those in private massage practice sometimes adopt a casual attitude toward adhering to Standard Precautions. For example, they might think nothing of stroking over an area of skin that is scabbed. The hospital massage therapist, on the other hand, would don gloves for such a situation. Paranoia is not called for when following these protocols, but serious care, attention, and diligence must be applied. It is better to be too careful than too casual. Close adherence to these practices then allows therapists to relax and be fully present with their patients.

Author's note

Before diving into the specifics of infection control techniques, it should be said that despite hygienic practices appearing to be a black and white topic, there are a multitude of beliefs, preferences, experiences, cultural influences and research that affect how the seemingly same protective practices are implemented. Gloving is an example. For instance, some hospitals mandate that all staff wear gloves when engaged with a patient, even to enter the person's room. Other institutions have an encouraged-but-not-required glove usage policy, while others only require gloving when there is a risk of contact with a transmissible substance. These policies are influenced by a variety of factors, such as emphasis on scientific research and cultural impacts. Bodyworkers touch the body and specifically the skin: that experience of touching skin is paramount to practitioners and one they don't want to give up unless necessary.

Masking is another practice that is influenced by cultural beliefs. In Asian countries it is good manners to wear a mask, even in public, out of consideration for yourself and others. On the other hand, it is not part of the North American or European mindset.

It isn't the mission of this book to override the policies within any given health care system. We have presented the common guidelines followed by large organizations, such as the World Health Organization, the National Health Service, Centers for Disease Control and Prevention, and the European Centre for Disease Prevention and Control.

Infection control techniques

The protective practices in this chapter are presented with an eye toward ease of learning. First, each of the components – handwashing, gloving, masking, and gowning – are addressed singly. This will allow the newer practitioner the opportunity to master those skills one at a time. However, in real life, they are often used in combination, such as gloving and gowning, which complicates the process. Following the material on each isolated component, the precautions are taught in combination: gowning, masking, and gloving.

The concept of "**clean to clean, dirty to dirty**" is central to the use of protective practices; once it becomes second nature, it will enable practitioners to master the use of protective barriers. An example of the application of clean to clean, dirty to dirty can be found in the handwashing section: turning the taps off with a paper towel. The hands, after being washed, are considered to be "clean." The taps, which have been touched by many unwashed hands, are "dirty." Therefore, the therapist is taught to turn off the taps with a paper towel, which is clean. Another example will be found when learning to unglove. Practitioners will notice that the protocol for ungloving calls for them to never contact the skin, which is "clean," with the outside of the glove, which is "dirty." The clean to clean, dirty to dirty concept also will be put to use when the practitioner is removing a combination of protective barriers, such as gloves and gown. Understanding this idea is a priority.

Hand cleaning

The link between handwashing and the spread of infection was only realized in the mid-1800s by a Hungarian physician, Ignaz Semmelweis. Semmelweis had been assigned to oversee an obstetrics clinic in a Vienna hospital, where he noticed that women who gave birth in the doctor-run maternity ward developed infections significantly more often than the women who gave birth on the ward run by midwives. His investigation found that the doctors were often coming to the birthing process directly from having performed an autopsy. Semmelweis theorized that those who had done an autopsy arrived with "cadaverous particles" on their unwashed hands. Midwives, on the other hand, did not perform autopsies and so were not exposed to infectious material from the dead bodies. Semmelweis thus instituted a rule requiring doctors to handwash with chlorinated lime prior to patient contact, which reduced the rate of deaths from infections dramatically, but was punishing on the hands.[12]

Florence Nightingale also advocated for handwashing at about the same time in the war hospitals during the Crimean War (1853–56). At that time, people believed that infections were caused by foul odors referred to as miasmas. Her handwashing protocol also reduced infections.[13] However, both Nightingale's and Semmelweis's practices were unable to gain traction in their time. It wasn't until the 1980s when the CDC became concerned about a string of foodborne infection outbreaks and HAIs that a set of nationally endorsed hand hygiene policies were rolled out. Other countries followed soon after.[12] Today, it seems obvious that the hands are the most common way to pass contagion, making handwashing the most basic Standard Precaution. But the health care field is still trying to reach the pinnacle of success in terms of handwashing adherence.

All bodyworkers are required to handwash, even those who give therapies through clients' clothing, such as Reiki practitioners or polarity therapists. This is necessary because contagious particles can survive in the bedding or on clothing. Sometimes these organisms are shed from the patient's body, but studies also show that patient footwear, such as non-skid socks or disposable shoe coverings, become contaminated from walking on the floors, most especially to the bathroom. Patients then return to bed, foot covers still on, transferring pathogens such as

MRSA and VRE to the bedding. This can spread to the hands of touch practitioners.[13a–c]

Massage therapists in private practice are accustomed to washing their hands before and after working with each client. In the hospital, it is also necessary to wash after contact with surfaces in the patient's room, such as the overbed table or telephone, as well as after handling the patient's personal items, such as a razor or laptop computer. Handwashing after such minimal contact might seem excessive until the reader considers the research concerning the transmission of pathogens from the floor to common objects such as blood pressure cuffs, call buttons, and phone cords. The micro-organisms are then transferred to overbed tables, side rails, and the patient's hands, and thus there is the potential to infect the hands of care providers.[13d]

Envision the scenario: A massage therapist enters a patient's room to explain the massage service to him. The patient had a peripherally inserted central catheter (PICC) line removed from his arm a few hours before, leaving patches of dried blood on his gown and bedding and a smaller amount on his arm. Since then, the patient has used his razor and cologne, drunk from his water bottle, and eaten from the tray still on the overbed table. As the therapist is at hand, the patient asks if she could move his lunch tray and place his cologne on the bathroom shelf, all of which he has touched since the PICC line was removed. Imagine if the massage therapist then enters the room of another patient, with her hands unwashed. Perhaps she touches that next patient briefly in greeting or is asked to hand her a cup of water. Now the micro-organisms from the previous patient are introduced into this next room. Objects that commonly come into contact with the floor, such as blood pressure cuffs, call buttons, and phone cords, can also transfer pathogens to the hands of care providers.[13d]

Health care facilities contain patients who can have weeping skin conditions, blood around incision sites, antibiotic-resistant bacterial infections that reside on the skin, in the lungs or digestive tract, and unknown viral infections, to name just some potentially contagious scenarios. Handwashing is the first line of defense for the practitioner, for other patients, and for staff members.

Hand hygiene should be performed in the following situations.[14]

- On arrival at work and before going home.
- Between patients and between tasks with individual patients.
- When the hands are visibly dirty.
- Before putting on and after removing gloves, mask, and gown.
- After coughing, sneezing, or blowing your nose.
- After using the toilet.
- Before and after food/beverage break.

Antimicrobial soap and water procedure

Liquid soap should be used rather than bar soap – bar soap harbors micro-organisms.[15] Before beginning, be certain that all abrasions and cuts on the hands and forearms are covered with a waterproof dressing.

1. Remove wristwatch, any bracelets etc. and rings. Ensure your forearms are bare below the elbows.
2. Stand so that clothing does not touch the sink or get splashed.
3. Wet hands and forearms with warm water. Water that is too hot or too cold can cause skin to crack or chap, increasing the risk of infection. Keep the hands lower than the elbows with the fingers pointing down.
4. Soap hands and forearms, working soap into a lather.
5. Before and after giving a massage, wash the entire surface of the hands and forearms for about 30 seconds. Be sure to include:
   - Fingertips and fingernails (Figure 5.3A)
   - Palm to palm (Figure 5.3B)
   - Backs of the hands (Figure 5.3C)
   - Spaces between the fingers (Figure 5.3D)
   - Thumbs, wrists, and forearms (Figure 5.3E)
6. Do not touch the sides of the sink.
7. Rinse well with the fingers pointing downward (Figure 5.3F). Do not shake water off the hands, as splashing spreads germs.

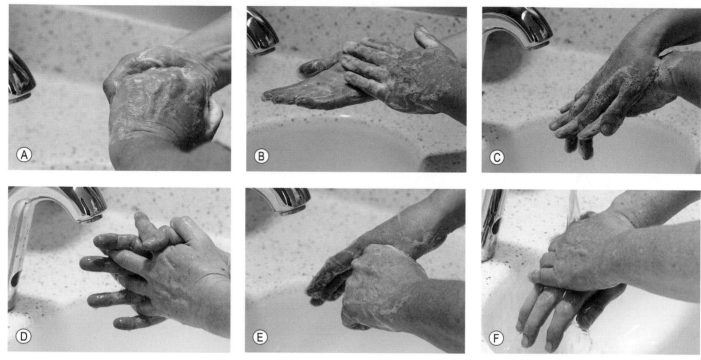

FIGURE 5.3A–G
Correct handwashing procedure.

(Photos by Richard Welander.)

8. Dry thoroughly with a single-use paper towel and then use the towel to turn off the faucet. This protects your hands from dirty faucets. Drying the hands thoroughly is as important as washing them. If the hands are still damp, more germs will attach themselves to the skin (Figure 5.3G).[16]

9. Use soap and water to clean hands after massaging a patient with *C. difficile* or norovirus: handrubs are not effective against either.[15]

Procedure for use of handrubs

Waterless, alcohol-based handrubs are easier, faster, and more effective than soap and water in disinfecting the hands in most circumstances. Guidelines for hand hygiene released by the CDC, NHS, and WHO recommend their use because they improve adherence to hand hygiene. However, not all handrubs are equally effective. Those used in health care settings are more potent than commercially available products. The information presented in this section refers to handrubs found in medical settings, which contain at least 60% alcohol.

The following guidelines should be observed when using handrubs:

- Apply only to visibly clean skin. (Handwash with soap and water if the hands are soiled, such as from massage lotion.)

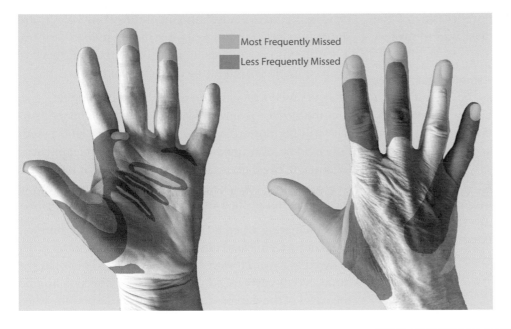

FIGURE 5.4
The most commonly missed areas when handwashing.

(Adapted by Sharon Fisher.)

- Apply to the palm of one hand and rub hands together, covering all surfaces of the hands and fingers until the hands are dry.
- Use handrubs immediately after leaving a patient's room.
- If used immediately after applying hand cream, the handrub may be less effective.
- Handrubs do not eliminate the need to use gloves.
- Handrubs do not eliminate the need to handwash with soap and water. After activities such as eating, using the toilet, or blowing the nose, practitioners should wash their hands with soap and water.
- Do not use handrubs after attending to a person with *C. difficile*. Handwashing with soap and water is required to kill the *C. difficile* spore. Alcohol-based handrubs are also ineffective against norovirus (viral gastroenteritis). Also use soap and water after massaging patients known to have had diarrhea within the previous 48 hours.[15]

Gloving

Gloving has evolved over the centuries. In 1758, gloves made from the intestines of sheep were used during surgery, autopsies, and vaginal examinations for the purpose of protecting the practitioner. Over time, rubber

---

Info Box 5.2 Antibiotic-resistant organisms[17]

The following are some of the antibiotic- or antimicrobial-resistant organisms that the CDC has posted as urgent or serious threats. With the exception of C. diff, hatnd cleaning can be accomplished by using a handrub or soap and water washing before and after patient contact. When caring for a patient with or suspected of having C. diff, only soap and water cleaning is acceptable.

- *Clostridioides difficile* (C. diff)
- Carbapenem-resistant Enterobacteriaceae (CRE)
- Fluconazole-resistant *Candida* species
- Methicillin-resistant *Staphylococcus aureus* (MRSA)
- Vancomycin-resistant *Enterococcus* species (VRE)
- *Candida auris* (C. auris)
- Drug-resistant *Streptococcus pneumoniae*
- Drug-resistant tuberculosis

---

replaced sheep innards and their use expanded to protect health care workers (HCWs) caring for people with communicable diseases such as smallpox, diphtheria, or meningitis. In the mid-1950s, *The Lancet*, a highly respected British medical journal, suggested using gloves as a way to protect nurses' skin from frequent handwashing with harsh chemicals, such as chlorinated lime and chlorhexidine. It wasn't until the 1970s that the US National

Communicable Disease Center, the predecessor of the CDC, advocated for the use of PPE as a way to protect HCWs and patients.[18]

Since the 1980s, it has been advocated that gloves should be worn any time there may be contact with blood, body fluids, mucous membranes, or broken skin, including the HCW's, such as a torn cuticle or cut finger. Some institutions have implemented a policy of "Always glove, no matter what." If used correctly, always gloving might be the best way forward, in light of the way droplets from speech, sneezing, or coughing can settle onto hard surfaces, such as telephones or overbed tables; the high incidence of antibiotic resistant bacteria, which can reside on patients' skin, in bedding, and on floors; and the research highlighting hospital floors as an underappreciated reservoir of pathogens that can then be transmitted to furniture, bedding, and patients' personal items.

However, there is concern within some segments of the nursing profession that the broad use of gloves is unintentionally affecting hand hygiene practices. They are not advocating the abandonment of gloving, but instead, believe staff should be trained to use gloves when the clinical situation indicates the need for use. One supporter writes that: "The use of … gloves has been associated with a significant potential for cross-contamination and transmission of health care-associated infections. This is because they are often used when they aren't needed, put on too early, taken off too late or not changed at critical points."[19] Both positions, always glove and glove as needed, have merit. Practitioners will need to follow their institution's guidance. It is, however, a sticky wicket for touch therapists in light of the research regarding transmission of pathogens to patients' personal items and bedding.

Two types of gloves are commonly used in hospitals: latex, which are made from rubber, and nitrile, a synthetic rubber material. Latex gloves are preferable when handling sharp devices, such as needles or blades, because they have greater resistance to punctures and have resealing properties when a puncture occurs.[15] However, hospitals use fewer latex gloves due to frequent allergic responses by patients and staff. For the task of giving massage, nitrile gloves provide good protection against chemicals and body fluids, without the potential for allergies. Nitrile gloves mold to the hand in a similar way to latex and can be worn for an extended amount of time. Vinyl gloves are sometimes found in hospitals, but mostly in food services. They are also a synthetic, nonlatex material, but they are not as durable or well-fitting as latex or nitrile.

Gloves used for giving massage should be snug fitting so that the surface is unwrinkled. The feel of a smooth surface will be more pleasurable to both patient and practitioner. Some lubricants, especially oils and petroleum-based lotions, will cause gloves to stretch. Not only is it difficult to massage with misshapen gloves, but the protective quality of the glove is diminished and often leads to tears in the glove.

It is tempting when a therapist has a small cut on their hand or torn cuticle to use a liquid skin protectant in order to avoid gloving. However, these products do not offer the same level of safety as gloves because the protection around the edges of the skin product is not reliable, especially when lotions, waxes, or oils are being used. For touch practitioners, the safest practice is to glove if the skin on their hands is not intact. This is true whether the patient's skin is broken or not: micro-organisms can be introduced to the therapist from contact with the patient's skin. Bacteria and fungi can thrive in folds and niches of the skin, such as the occiput, webs of the toes and fingers, around the axilla, the antecubital space, and the trunk.[20] All of these are places that a bodyworker commonly comes into contact with.

Practitioners sometimes worry that the patient will be offended if they glove to give the massage. Because of this, therapists sometimes fail to glove in situations where they should. Other times, massage therapists realize part way into an encounter with a patient that they should have gloved and, rather than stopping to glove, they carry on, not wanting to break the mood. A massage student participating in an obstetrics (OB) rotation did just that. While massaging the upper legs of a woman in labor, the student noticed that there was dried blood in the vicinity. However, she chose not to stop and glove. It is important that care providers follow infection control practices regardless of any imagined judgment others might have and regardless of whether they have to disturb the mood.

Always glove for the following situations:

- To touch any part of the patient where there is a possibility of contact with any body substances, cuts or scabs.

- To remove a urinal, bedpan, or emesis basin that has been used. Gloving the one hand is usually sufficient.
- If the therapist has a cut, open sore, scratch, abrasion, scab or a noncontagious rash on the hands. (Do not give bodywork sessions with any kind of contagious rash, even with gloves. Wait until the condition has cleared.) A method of determining if an area is open or intact is to wipe the area in question with alcohol. If it stings, it is open and should be covered with a glove.
- When any area of the patient's gown or linen is contaminated by body substances, even if the substance has dried. (Before starting the massage, a nursing assistant might be able to change the gown.)
- When a patient is receiving chemotherapy or has received it in the prior 72 hours.
- If steroidal cream has just been applied to the area that will be massaged.
- If the patient has herpes, gloving is the most prudent action, even when working at sites distant from the outbreak. Herpes is most contagious when the sores are open and wet, but it can also be transmitted when there are no sores and the skin appears healthy.[21] The virus can survive on other surfaces from a few hours up to eight weeks.[22] (See the Glossary for further information).
- If the patient has shingles, exposure to the virus that causes it, varicella zoster virus (VZV), can cause chickenpox in those who are not immune. Shingles itself cannot be passed directly from one person to the next. Therefore care, in the form of gloving, needs to be taken when working with a patient population that is immunosuppressed in case any of them are not immune to chickenpox. The contagious period is when the rash has vesicles; after the blisters crust, the virus no longer has the potential of being communicable.[23]
- Never reuse gloves for another patient.
- Do not use a set of gloves for more than one activity. For instance, if a urinal must be moved, change gloves before touching the patient.

Procedure for donning (putting on):

1. Remove rings and bracelets to avoid puncturing or tearing the glove.
2. Wash hands and forearms.
3. Dry thoroughly. Putting gloves onto damp hands can create skin problems.
4. Putting on gloves:[24]
   A. Take glove from box, touching only a restricted area corresponding to the wrist.
   B. Don the first glove.
   C. Take the second glove with the bare hand, touching only the area of the glove corresponding to the wrist.
   D. To avoid touching the skin of the forearm with the gloved hand, turn the external surface of the second glove on the folded fingers of the gloved hand.
5. If wetness is felt or anything suggests that the gloves are leaking, immediately remove them, re-wash the hands, and put on new gloves.

Procedure for doffing (removing):

1. The outside of the glove is contaminated!
2. Remove the first glove by grasping the external surface at the wrist or palm and pulling it off (Figure 5.5A). Wad this glove into the palm of the gloved hand.
3. Remove the second glove by sliding bare fingers inside the glove and pulling up (Figure 5.5B). Touch only the inside of the glove. Do not touch the outside of the glove with the ungloved hand. (Remember: "clean to clean, dirty to dirty.") Fold the second glove over the first dirty glove as it is removed (Figure 5.5C).
4. Discard used gloves in the appropriate receptacle. Sometimes this will be inside the patient's room, for example, if the person is under Contact Precautions. At other times it will be outside the patient's room. Dispose of gloves after each use.
5. Wash and dry hands thoroughly.

Masking

It is often necessary to don a mask before entering the room of a patient who is immunosuppressed or whose illness is contagious via airborne or droplet transmission. A facemask, when worn correctly, can block

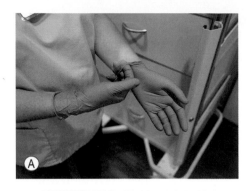
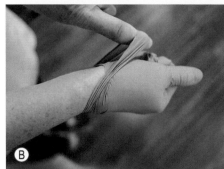
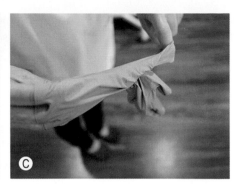

FIGURE 5.5A–C
Correct procedure for removing gloves.

(Photo by Richard Welander.)

large-particle droplets, splashes, sprays, and splatter. They also help reduce exposure to viruses and bacteria from the wearer's own saliva and respiratory secretions to others. However, even when worn properly, masks do not block very small airborne particles that may be transmitted by coughs and sneezes, due to the loose fit between the mask and face.[25]

If masking is necessary, there will be instructions on the patient's door. Masks should be changed between patients, or if they become wet during the massage as moisture causes them to become ineffective: "A wet mask becomes a great wick that draws in moisture and debris."[26] Sometimes care providers will hang the mask from their neck. However, this puts them at risk of breathing in the virus or bacteria from the patient. Cross contamination can also occur when a mask is placed in a pocket or on a counter. Once finished with a mask, it should be placed it in the appropriate trash receptacle.[15]

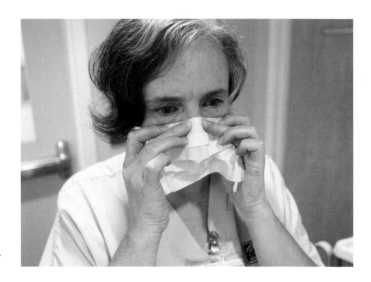

FIGURE 5.6
Affixing the flexible band of the mask to the bridge of the nose.

(Photo by Richard Welander.)

Donning
1. Place mask over the nose and mouth.
2. Affix flexible band over bridge of nose (Figure 5.6).
3. If the mask has strings that tie at the back, tie the top set first and then the bottom strings. In this way, a tight fit is created over the mouth and nose. <u>Be sure the mask is pulled down under the chin</u> as shown in Figure 5.2.

Doffing (reverse the process):
1. The front of the mask is contaminated! Avoid touching it.

2. Untie the bottom strings, touching only the strings.
3. Untie the top strings, touching only the strings.
4. Place into a trash receptacle.
5. Wash and dry hands or apply handrub.

Use of gowns or aprons

In some parts of the world, a gown is used as part of the personal protection equipment, and in other regions a disposable apron is worn. A gown or apron may be used to protect the immunosuppressed patient from microorganisms that may be on the clothes of those entering the room. Gowning also may be required to protect staff when working with patients who are subject to Airborne Precautions, such as in cases of tuberculosis (TB), or Contact Precautions, such as with antibiotic-resistant bacteria.

Donning:

1. Wash and dry hands. (Ensure your forearms are bare below the elbows).
2. Fully cover torso from neck to knees.
3. Fasten the neck and waist.
4. Fasten at the back. Be certain the gown or apron overlaps at the back so that all clothing is covered, as in Figure 5.7.

Doffing:

1. The sleeves and front of the gown are contaminated!
2. Undo neck attachments, then waist. (Paper gowns with Velcro attachments are common.)
3. Pull down on the sleeve of the gown to start the removal process.
4. Reach up toward the shoulders (Figure 5.8A) and pull off the gown at the same time, folding it inward (Figure 5.8B). Roll it up into a ball (Figure 5.8C).

5. Place the gown in a covered container.
6. Wash and dry hands or apply handrub.

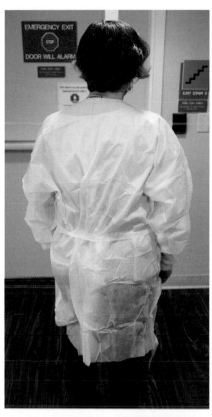

FIGURE 5.7
The gown or apron should overlap at the back so that all clothing is covered.

(Photo by Richard Welander.)

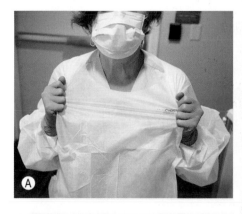

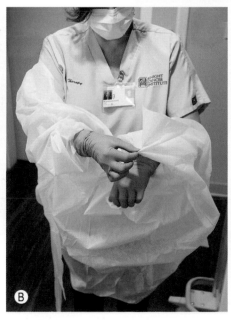

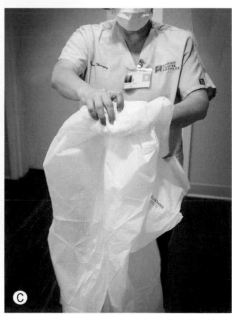

FIGURE 5.8A–C.
Correct procedure for removing gowns.

(Photos by Richard Welander.)

Gowning, masking, and gloving in combination

In situations such as an Airborne or Contact Precautions, a therapist would need to gown, mask, and glove. Further information about these precautions is given below. Observe the following order when it is necessary to gown, mask, and glove.[27,28]

Donning:

1. Wash and dry hands or apply handrub.
2. Gown or apron.
3. Mask.
4. Glove. Extend to cover wrist and tuck in sleeves of gown (Figure 5.9).

Doffing:

1. Reverse the order.

Transmission-Based Precautions

Transmission-Based Precautions are designed for dealing with patients who are known or suspected to be infected with highly transmissible pathogens. There are three types: Airborne, Droplet, and Contact Precautions. Just as with Standard Precautions, these practices also include handwashing, gloving, masking, and gowning, but they are carried out for different reasons.

Transmission-Based Precautions protect staff and visitors from pathogens shed by patients and are specific to the type of disease or condition involved. Some diseases may have multiple routes of transmission and will require a combination of precautions. A sign on the patient's door, as in Figure 5.10, will specify which protocols to follow.[29]

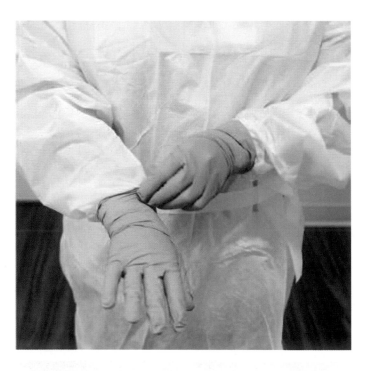

FIGURE 5.9
Gloves should be extended over the wrists.

(Photo by Richard Welander.)

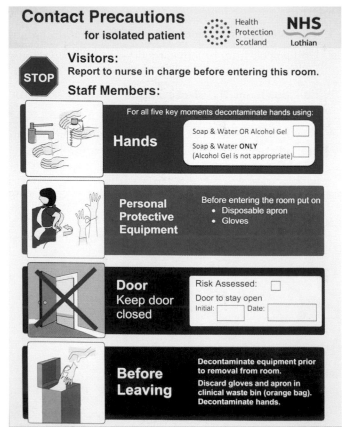

FIGURE 5.10
A typical Contact Precautions sign.

(Photo by Andrew Secretan.)

An isolation cart (also known as an isolation trolley), containing gloves, masks, and gowns often will be positioned outside the door to these patients' rooms (Figure 5.11). The steps listed below are typical when massaging a person who is in isolation:

- Protective gear should be put on outside the room as in Figure 5.11.
- Depending on the type of isolation, the gear will mostly likely be taken off just before leaving the room and discarded in a closed container in the room.

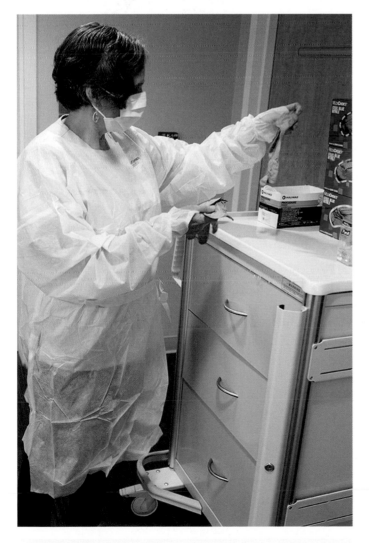

FIGURE 5.11
Donning protective gear from the isolation cart.

(Photo by Richard Welander.)

- Hands should be washed in the patient's room.
- Once outside the room, the hands should be cleaned again.

The following are common types of isolation and the precautions usually taken.

Airborne isolation

According to the CDC, airborne transmission occurs by dissemination either through the residue of small particle droplets containing pathogens that have evaporated and remain suspended in the air for long periods of time, or dust particles containing the infectious agent. Pathogens carried in this manner can be dispersed widely by air currents and may be inhaled by someone in the same room or some distance away, depending on environmental factors. Therefore, special air handling and ventilation are required to prevent airborne transmission. Tuberculosis is an example of airborne disease in which hospitals isolate patients in rooms with negative airflow pressure, thereby keeping the TB bacteria inside the room. Measles, chickenpox, and disseminated herpes zoster are examples of other airborne diseases. Airborne Precautions can involve the use of a special mask or respirator in addition to gowning and gloving.

Droplet isolation

Droplet transmission involves contact with droplets generated during coughing, sneezing, or talking. Certain types of influenza, bacterial meningitis, pneumonia, diptheria, whooping cough, streptococcus (group A),

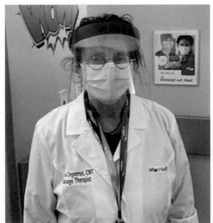

FIGURE 5.12
Massage therapist wearing mask and face shield in compliance with COVID-19 Droplet Precautions.

pharyngitis, scarlet fever, mumps, rubeola, rubella, and COVID-19 are examples of diseases that can be transmitted through droplets. Many of these agents do not remain suspended in the air and generally travel only a short distance, 3 feet or less.[30] However, some viruses, such as that which causes COVID-19, are known to travel well beyond 6 feet.[30a]

Massaging a patient who is under Droplet Precautions requires the use of a mask and in some instances, a face shield (Figure 5.12). Going forward, if Universal Pandemic Precautions become the norm, use of a face shield will become commonplace.

Contact isolation

Transmission by contact can occur directly or indirectly. Direct contact involves transmission from one person's body to another's. Transmission by indirect contact can happen through contaminated instruments, needles, dressings, contaminated hands, surfaces in the patient's room, or gloves that are not changed between patients.

The following are some conditions that warrant the use of Contact Precautions:

- Antibiotic-resistant bacterial infections such as VRE (vancomycin-resistant *Enterococcus*), CRE (carbapenem-resistant Enterobacteriaceae), MRSA (methicillin-resistant *Staphylococcus aureus*), and *C. auris* (*Candida auris*).

- Enteric infections such as certain forms of *Escherichia coli (E-coli)* or hepatitis A.

- Skin infections that are highly contagious or that may occur on dry skin, including cutaneous diphtheria, herpes simplex, conjunctivitis, lice, and impetigo.[30]

- Airborne droplets, mentioned in the previous section, can settle on hard surfaces, including floors, remaining viable for days or longer, if not cleaned properly. Even if a patient is not posted as requiring Contact Precautions, practitioners should heighten their awareness regarding the hard surfaces in all patient rooms, as well as the entire facility. Those surfaces may contain viable bacteria or viruses that are transmissible, for example via a lotion bottle placed on the overbed table, handling a patient's personal items, or even touching surfaces at the nurses' station.

Contact Precautions involve handwashing, gloving, and gowning before entering the patient's room. After the massage, protective barriers should be taken off in the room and placed in a covered container before leaving. After removing the gloves and handwashing, it is important to not touch surfaces in the room that may potentially carry the pathogen, such as the overbed table or bathroom door handle.

Items in the room of someone subject to Contact Precautions should not be taken out of the room nor should other items be brought in from elsewhere. For example, Marta was working with a patient who had VRE, an infectious antibiotic-resistant bacteria. Marta preferred to sit while massaging her patient's feet, however, there was no chair in the room. Without thinking, she left the room and brought in a chair that she had found outside in the hallway. The chair was then potentially harboring the VRE. This mistake is obvious in hindsight, but easy to do in the moment. Also, avoid taking items such as notebooks or lotion holsters into the room. Pocket-sized items, such as pens, should remain in the therapist's pocket. Lotion containers, once in the room, must remain in the room.

Reverse isolation

The purpose of reverse isolation, also known as protective isolation, is to protect vulnerable patients from germs carried by staff and visitors.[31] Typically this would be people who are immunocompromised, such as those who have undergone organ or bone marrow transplantation or those in critical care units. Precautions may be as simple as a 30-second handwashing before entering the room, or they may entail completely masking, gowning, and gloving. In addition, having living plants and fresh food and flowers in the room often will be restricted. Protection isolation precautions vary from hospital to hospital depending on special air handling and ventilation technology. A lengthy handwashing is standard, but masking, gowning, and gloving requirements will differ. Instructions will be clearly posted on the patient's door.

Linen handling [32]

It may be necessary to obtain additional sheets, towels, or blankets for draping, warmth, or to cover soiled areas.

The recommended procedure for handling linen is as follows:

1. Before collecting clean linen, wash and dry hands or apply handrub.

2. Remove the necessary items from the linen closet or cart. Only take as much as is needed for each patient. Remaining linen cannot be taken into another room for use.

3. Do not let clean linen touch your clothing.

4. If any linen falls onto the floor, discard it into the soiled linen hamper, as it is considered contaminated.

5. Do not shake out linens when unfolding. This can stir up a cloud of microbes into the air, even if the linen is clean.

6. Consider any unused linen as dirty and place it in the soiled hamper. Do not replace it in the closet or on the cart.

7. When handling soiled linen, do not let it touch your clothes.

8. When discarding used linen in the hamper, simply place it in. Never plunge your hands and forearms down into the hamper to compact the soiled linen.

9. Do not throw used linens on the floor.

10. Wash and dry hands after handling used linen.

The patient's linen or gown may become contaminated with a variety of body substances, such as urine, feces, wound exudate, or blood, requiring the therapist to glove while massaging. Ideally, linen or gowns that contain areas of contamination should be changed before starting the massage session. If this is not possible, a clean towel or draw sheet can be placed over the area to make for a more pleasing appearance. Gloves should still be worn in this circumstance.

Exposure to body fluids

Bodyworkers typically do not engage in health care tasks that put them at risk for encountering body fluids. They will seldom be involved with changing linens, cleaning up spills, or handling needles. With diligent adherence to Standard Precautions, touch practitioners will be safe, however, if contact occurs with body substances, immediately wash the area with soap and water. If the exposure was caused by a sharp object, save the object for possible testing. Report the incident to the charge nurse or other supervisor. He or she will advise you on any further steps that should be taken.[33]

Handling of work clothes

The purpose of the following guidelines is for the protection of the patient, the practitioner, and those who live with the practitioner.

- Ideally a therapist would put on clean work clothes at the health care facility rather than at home.

- Do not smoke, and try to avoid smokers after putting on hospital clothes. Many patients are often highly sensitive to odors and can become nauseated in their presence.

- When bringing clean clothes from home, place them in a container that is used only for that purpose. For example, do not place hospital work clothes in a backpack or sports bag that is also used to carry personal items such as water bottles, books, and pens.

- Change clothes in an area designated for this purpose, such as a staff locker room. If at all possible, do not change in areas such as a utility room, public restroom, or staff lunch room.

- After finishing at the health care facility, change out of hospital work clothes, including shoes. Research shows evidence of pathogens on the floors throughout hospitals. Presumably, the same is true for nursing homes and rehabilitation facilities. Do not wear clothes to another work site or around the home. This protects those the touch therapist lives with as well as other people who receive bodywork from them.

Miscellaneous precautions

Fingernail length

Those who have direct patient contact must maintain short fingernails.[14] Long fingernails are more likely to tear gloves or accidentally scratch or gouge a patient, and they can trap micro-organisms which can only be removed with vigorous brushing. Long nails also prevent the fingertips from being adequately cleaned, and hospital-acquired infections have been traced back to health care workers with long fingernails.

The following guidelines apply to fingernails:

- Maintain the nails at fingertip length.
- Do not use nail polish as it can flake off nails and enter and contaminate wounds.
- No type of artificial nail should be worn.

Rings

Ring wearing can create a twofold problem: protective gloves are more easily torn and bacteria counts are higher on the hands of care providers who wear rings. NHS guidelines advocate no rings with jewels, stones, ridges, or grooves as they may harbor bacteria and prevent good hand hygiene.[14] A plain band may be worn, but ensure that the area under the ring is included when hands are cleaned.

Lotion

There are a variety of hygienic practices with regard to lotion. Some hospitals require the use of single-serve lotion containers provided by the hospital for patients' personal use. Whilst these lotions usually lack good glide and are not ideal for massage, this ensures that hygiene standards are followed, which is the priority.

Other institutions allow the massage department to buy specially formulated lotions that are supplied in bulk. Therapists then dispense what they need for a single session into a clean paper cup. This arrangement gives the therapist a good product to work with, and it prevents bacteria from being transferred from one patient's room to another's. (Sometimes, in order to secure this arrangement in a hospital, approval must be made through risk management or the epidemiology department.)

Lotion can also be decanted from the bulk container into four or eight ounce bottles that are taken from room to room. There are two potential problems with this method: 1) the outside of the lotion bottle must be cleaned thoroughly between patients; and 2) the inside of the bottle also cannot be cleaned to hospital standards.

Several additional steps need to be observed to be certain the lubricant does not contribute to an infection problem:

- Ideally, massage practitioners should not take the same lotion bottle from patient to patient. If that is the practice, then wash the bottle for 30 seconds between patients just as you would your hands.
- It is best in terms of infection control to use a single portion of lotion. When the massage is over, leave the remaining lubricant with the patient.
- Use the hospital's lotion for immunosuppressed patients. Lotions belonging to the therapist may have been sitting out, carried around in a backpack, or stored in a cupboard for a period of time, thereby increasing the growth of bacteria in the lubricant or causing them to be rancid.
- Bulk lotion should be stored in a refrigerator.
- Only place lotion bottles on tables or counters, never on the floor.
- Do not use a container that requires the fingers to be dipped into it, unless the container will be disposed of after each patient.
- Clarification should be made with the infection control officer regarding the use of holsters for lotion bottles. Some institutions do not allow their use because they cannot be cleaned between patients' rooms. Perhaps if holsters were washed at the end of each shift (as with hospital work clothes), it would satisfy the issue of potential transmission.

Notebooks and other items from outside

When taking objects into a patient's room, the therapist must think through the potential for cross-contamination, especially when the items are being taken from room to room. For example, it is common to have a notebook to record patient information which is taken into the room, or sometimes a music player is available for patient use. When any of these articles are set down on a surface in the room, it creates the possibility of bacteria or viruses attaching to them, therefore, these objects need to be cleaned between patients with an antiseptic wipe. Some institutions advise setting the item on a clean pillowcase rather than directly onto a surface in the patient's room. If this is to be the practice, also clean the object before taking it to another person's room. Other health care facilities discourage or disallow providers taking items from room to room. Notebooks are stored outside the room and music is enjoyed on the patient's personal media device or the hospital's media system. Confer with the facility's infection control officer to establish a policy about this issue.

Kneeling on the floor

Don't. Massage therapists often kneel or sit on the floor in their private practice setting. However, it is probably apparent by now that contaminants will come to rest on floors. Micro-organisms can adhere to the therapist when kneeling and then be transported from one area to another.

When to stay home

The massage therapist who has a fever, flu, is within the first four days of a cold, or is infected by other communicable diseases, such as conjunctivitis or herpes, should stay at home. Be mindful that influenza is communicable one day before symptoms appear and approximately five to seven days after the onset of illness.[34] This is especially important when working with patients who are immunosuppressed. Also, if a person whom the practitioner lives with or has been in close contact with has a communicable disease, such as measles, mumps, chickenpox, shingles, hepatitis, mononucleosis, or TB, confer with the unit manager or employee health nurse regarding work status.

Summary

Touch therapists without prior health care experience often find the application of infection control standards to be one of the most difficult parts of learning to give massage in this milieu. It is not uncommon to have bouts of paranoia before settling into an ease and rhythm. As with any new skill, the learning period can be awkward, but eventually handwashing, gowning, masking, and gloving become second nature.

It is important for touch therapists to acknowledge every part of their learning journey, whether it is being in the presence of suffering, learning hospital dynamics, or getting to grips with gowning, masking, or gloving. It's a process. Mistakes will happen. Improvement will happen too.

Test yourself

Multiple choice: Circle all of the correct answers. There may be more than one.

1. A massage therapist should glove if the patient:

   A   Is taking oral steroids.
   B   Is receiving chemotherapy.
   C   Is under contact isolation precautions.
   D   Has a low platelet count.

2. Massage therapists should refrain from working with patients when they are experiencing the following:

   A   A runny nose due to hay fever.
   B   Day three of a cold.
   C   Conjunctivitis.
   D   An open cut on the hand.

3. Only soap and water should be used to clean the hands after working with patients infected with the following:

   A   MRSA.
   B   C. difficile.
   C   Norovirus.
   D   VRE.

4. Hands can be cleaned with a handrub in the following situations:

   A   When the skin is visibly clean.
   B   After giving a massage with lotion.
   C   After massaging a patient who has had diarrhea in the past 48 hours.
   D   After the therapist uses the toilet.

5. Which of the following are advisable with regard to lotion usage in the health care setting?

   A   Use single-serve, hospital lotion for patients who are immunosuppressed.

   B   Store bulk lotion containers on the shelf.

   C   If setting a lotion bottle on the floor, place a paper towel underneath it.

   D   When taking a massage bottle from patient to patient, clean the exterior between patients.

True or False: Answer true or false to each of the following statements. Rewrite each of the false statements to make it true.

1. If blood is not present, tears and perspiration are non-contagious body fluids.

2. Contact Precautions involve handwashing, gowning, masking, and gloving before entering the patient's room.

3. Fingernails should be kept short to minimize the presence of bacteria under the nails.

4. The hands should be cleaned before gloving.

5. Unused linen should be replaced onto the linen cart.

6. Infection Precautions are the protocols a health care worker implements in the presence of any potential body fluids.

7. A therapist should use an alcohol-based handrub to clean their hands after massaging a person with *C. difficile*.

8. When using personal protective equipment, practitioners should contact the dirty side of the equipment with the clean side.

9. One of the commonly missed areas when washing the hands is the web between the fingers.

10. Masks should be changed at the end of every shift.

11. The purpose of Reverse Isolation Precautions is to protect the patient from germs carried in by staff or visitors.

12. If a therapist is going to kneel on the floor to give part of the massage, place a towel under the knee in contact with the floor.

References

1. WHO. Health care-associated infections fact sheet. Available from: https://www.who.int/gpsc/country_work/gpsc_ccisc_fact_sheet_en.pdf

2. European Centre for Disease Prevention and Control. Infections in acute care hospitals in Europe – point prevalence survey. 2019. Available from: https://ecdc.europa.eu/en/health-care-associated-infections-acute-care-hospital

3. CDC. Current HAI progress report. 2018 National and state healthcare-associated infections progress report. 2019. Available from: https://www.cdc.gov/hai/data/portal/progress-report.html

4. Patient CareLink. Healthcare-acquired infections. Available from: https://patientcarelink.org/improving-patient-care/healthcare-acquired-infections-hais/

5. Interagency Coordination Group on Antimicrobial Resistance. No time to wait: securing the future from drug-resistant infections. Report to the Secretary-General of the United Nations. 2019. Available from: https://www.who.int/antimicrobial-resistance/interagency-coordination-group/IACG_final_report_EN.pdf?ua=1&utm_source=newsletter&utm_medium=email&utm_campaign=newsletter_axiosscience&stream=science

6. Global Health Security Agenda. 2019. Available from: https://www.ghsagenda.org

7. CDC. Infection control basics. 2016. Available from: https://www.cdc.gov/infectioncontrol/basics/index.html

8. Bjerke NB. Standard Precautions. 2002. Available from: https://www.infectioncontroltoday.com/hand-hygiene/standard-precautions

9. US Occupational Safety and Health Administration. Bloodborne pathogens and needlestick prevention. Available from: https://www.osha.gov/SLTC/bloodbornepathogens/

10. Komatsu H, Inui A, Sogo T, et al. Tears from children with chronic hepatitis B (HBV) infection are infectious vehicles of HBV transmission: experimental transmission of HBV by tears, using mice with chimeric human livers. J Infect Dis. 2012; 206(4):478–85.

11. Government of South Australia. Ways infectious diseases spread. 2019. Available from: https://www.sahealth.sa.gov.au/wps/wcm/connect/public+content/sa+health+internet/health+topics/health+conditions+prevention+and+treatment/infectious+diseases/ways+infectious+diseases+spread

12. WHO. WHO guidelines on hand hygiene in health care. First global patient safety challenge: clean care is safer care. 2009. Available from: https://apps.who.int/iris/bitstream/handle/10665/44102/9789241597906_eng.pdf?sequence=1

13. Global Handwashing Partnership. About handwashing: history. 2017. Available from: https://globalhandwashing.org/about-handwashing/history-of-handwashing/

13a. Kogani S, Alhmidi H, Tomas ME, Cadnum JL, Jencson A, Donskey CJ. Evaluation of hospital floors as a potential source of pathogen dissemination using a nonpathogenic virus as a surrogate marker. Infect Control Hosp Epidemiol. 2016; 37(11):1374–77.

14b. Galvin J, Almatroudi A, Vickery K, Deva A, Oliveira Lopes LK, de Melo Costa D, Hu H. Patient shoe covers: Transferring bacteria from the floor to surgical bedsheets. Am J of Infect Control. 2016; 44(11):1417–19.

15c. Mahida N, Boswell T. Non-slip socks: A potential reservoir for transmitting multidrug resistant organisms in hospitals. J Hosp Infect. 2016; 94(3):273–5.

16d. Deshpande A, Cadnum JL, Fertelli D, Sitzlar B, Thota P, Mana TS, Jencson A, Alhmidi H, Kogani S, Donskey C. Are hospital floors an underappreciated reservoir for transmission of health care-associated pathogens? Am J Infect Control. 2017; 45(3):336–8.

17. Harrogate and District NHS Foundation Trust. Community infection prevention and control guidance for general practice: hand hygiene. 2017. Available from: https://www.infectionpreventioncontrol.co.uk/content/uploads/2018/12/GP-07-Hand-hygiene-December-2017-Version-1.00.pdf

18. Harrogate and District NHS Foundation Trust. Standard Precautions (version 1.0). 2017. Available from: https://www.infectionpreventioncontrol.co.uk/content/uploads/2018/12/GP-20-Standard-precautions-December-2017-Version 1.00.pdf

19. CDC. Handwashing: clean hands save lives. How to wash your hands. 2020. Available from: https://www.cdc.gov/handwashing/show-me-the-science-handwashing.html

20. CDC. Antiobotic/antimicrobial resistance. Biggest threats and data. 2019. Available from: https://www.cdc.gov/drugresistance/biggest-threats.html

21. Jain S, Clezy K, McLaws ML. Glove: Use for safety or overuse? Am J Infect Control. 2017; 45(12):1407–10.

22. NHS England. "The gloves are off" campaign. 2018. Available from: https://www.england.nhs.uk/atlas_case_study/the-gloves-are-off-campaign/

23. Grice EA, Segre JA. The skin microbiome. Nat Rev Microbiol. 2011; 9(4):244–53.

24. Planned Parenthood. Oral and genital herpes. Available from: https://www.plannedparenthood.org/learn/stds-hiv-safer-sex/herpes

25. Government of Canada. Pathogen safety data sheets: infectious substances – Herpes simplex virus. 2011. Available from: https://www.canada.ca/en/public-health/services/laboratory-biosafety-biosecurity/pathogen-safety-data-sheets-risk-assessment/herpes-simplex-virus.html

26. CDC. Shingles (Herpes zoster). Transmission. 2019. Available from: https://www.cdc.gov/shingles/about/transmission.html

27. WHO. Glove use. Information leaflet. 2009. Available from: https://www.who.int/gpsc/5may/Glove_Use_Information_Leaflet.pdf

28. US Food and Drug Administration. N95 respirators and surgical masks (face masks). 2020. Available from: https://www.fda.gov/medical-devices/personal-protective-equipment-infection-control/n95-respirators-and-surgical-masks-face-masks

29. Kelsch N. Changing masks. 2010. Available from: https://www.rdhmag.com/infection-control/personal-protective-equipment/article/16407656/changing-masks

30. Harrogate and District NHS Foundation Trust. Standard Precautions (Version 1.0) — Appendix 1: Correct order for putting on and removing Personal Protective Equipment. 2017 Available from: https://www.infectionpreventioncontrol.co.uk/content/uploads/2018/12/GP-20 Standard precautions-December-2017-Version-1.00.pdf

31. CDC. Sequence for putting on personal protective equipment (PPE). Available from: https://www.cdc.gov/hai/pdfs/ppc/ppe-sequence.pdf

32. CDC. Infection control. Transmission-based precautions. 2016. Available from: https://www.cdc.gov/infectioncontrol/basics/transmission-based-precautions.html

33. CDC. Guideline for isolation precautions: preventing transmission of infectious agents in healthcare settings. 2007. Available from: https://www.cdc.gov/infectioncontrol/pdf/guidelines/isolation-guidelines-H.pdf

30a. Guo Z-D, Wang Z-Y, Zhang S-F, et al. Aerosol and surface distribution of severe acute respiratory syndrome Coronavirus 2 in hospital wards, Wuhan, China, 2020. 2020. Available from: https://wwwnc.cdc.gov/eid/article/26/7/20-0885_article

31. Drugs.com. Reverse isolation. 2020. Available from: https://www.drugs.com/cg/reverse-isolation.html

32. Graves L, Mullen L, Fouts J. Nursing Assistant Training Manual. Beaverton: Medical Express; 2002.

33. US National Library of Medicine. After an exposure to sharps or bodily fluid. 2017. Available from: https://medlineplus.gov/ency/patientinstructions/000442.htm

34. CDC. Influenza (flu). Guidance: use of masks to control influenza transmission. 2019 Available from: https://www.cdc.gov/flu/professionals/infectioncontrol/maskguidance.htm

Additional resources

Alliance for Massage Therapy Education. https://www.afmte.org/covid-19-related-recommendations-for-massage-therapy-and-bodywork-educators/

Association for Bodywork and Massage. COVID-19 Updates for the Massage Profession. Available from: https://www.abmp.com/covid-updates

CDC. Get the Facts about Coronavirus (COVID-19). 2020. Available from: https://www.cdc.gov/coronavirus/2019-ncov/index.html?CDC_AA_refVal=https%3A%2F%2Fwww.cdc.gov%2Fcoronavirus%2Findex.html

CDC. Handwashing: clean hands save lives. Available from: https://www.cdc.gov/handwashing/videos.html.

Federation of Holistic Therapies. FHT Statement on Coronavirus (COVID-19). Available from: https://www.fht.org.uk/news-item/fht-statement-on-coronavirus-covid-19

Hospital PPE - Infection Control: Donning and Doffing. Available from: https://www.youtube.com/watch?v=oxdaSeq4EVU.

NHS Education for Scotland: Standard Infection Control Precautions. Personal Protective Equipment. Available from: https://www.youtube.com/watch?v=S5p8vZ8zrWM.

NHS Guide to handwashing with soap and water. Available from: https://www.youtube.com/watch?v=bAwS0UslEDs.

OSHA. Guidance on Preparing Workplaces for COVID-19. Available from: https://www.osha.gov/Publications/OSHA3990.pdf

Werner R. http://ruthwerner.com/massage-therapy-and-covid-19/

WHO. Coronavirus disease (COVID-19) pandemic. Available from: https://www.cdc.gov/coronavirus/2019-ncov/index.html?CDC_AA_refVal=https%3A%2F%2Fwww.cdc.gov%2Fcoronavirus%2Findex.html

We are at our most powerful the moment we no longer need to be powerful.

Eric Micha'el Leventhal

At first glance, the high-tech machinery, side effects from treatment, and medical devices give the impression that massaging patients in a medical center is a complex undertaking. There is, however, a deceptive simplicity about giving bodywork in this setting. Once the information from the patient's chart and medical staff have been organized in the therapist's mind, the actual session is fairly straightforward. The more medically complex a person is, the simpler the massage session is.

In this chapter, a framework is presented that will form the foundation for much of *Hands in Health Care*. This organizational structure centers around three specific categories: **pressure** modifications, **site** considerations, and **positioning** adjustments. Most of the information about patients, such as side effects of medications, medical devices, procedures, or illness, can be placed into one of these three areas. Without a doubt, it is necessary to be knowledgeable about other parts of the patient's medical status, but the pressure, site, and position categories provide a basic structure for bringing order to the plethora of information that is given by the nurse, gathered from the medical chart, or shared by the patient. It can be used for quickly and thoroughly obtaining information about the patient's condition and then organizing it to create a safe massage plan. Figure 6.1 shows an example intake form which uses pressure, site, and positioning as part of creating a consultation form. This particular form is for an obstetrics patient.

OB/GYN Patient Information Form

PRESSURE CONSIDERATIONS ☐ Yes ☐ No

☐ DVT ☐ Nausea ☐ Phlebitis ☐ Varicose veins

☐ Bruising risk ☐ Recent surgery ☐ Edema ☐ Bedrest restrictions _____

SITE MODIFICATIONS ☐ Yes ☐ No

_____ Skin condition _____ Epidural

_____ Incision _____ Fetal monitor

_____ IV site _____ Severe varicosity

Other _____

POSITION ADJUSTMENTS ☐ Yes ☐ No

☐ Elevate head ☐ Lie flat ☐ No prone

☐ No L side-lying ☐ No R side-lying

☐ Elevate extremity ☐ No elevation of extremities

Other _____

FIGURE 6.1
Intake form organized around the pressure, site, position framework.

Chapter SIX

Massage therapists can apply this conceptual framework when working in any health care department, from obstetrics to oncology, general surgery, memory care, end of life, or rehabilitation. Extensive knowledge about each medical specialty is impossible for touch therapists as well as doctors and nurses; bodyworkers may be thoroughly familiar with a couple of specialties but have only superficial knowledge in others. With the pressure, site, and position framework as a focal point, they can move easily between areas of specialty without being completely conversant with each body of knowledge.

There is no one way to give massage to medically complex patients. A Swedish massage therapist will administer one type of session, a Shiatsu practitioner will give another, while someone trained in Craniosacral Therapy will perform still another. The purpose of the pressure, site, and position format is to give therapists from all disciplines a common frame of reference around which they can create a safe touch session that addresses the individual needs and desires of each patient.

Many of the adjustments that patients require are self-evident. For instance, all bodyworkers are aware of the dangers of massaging too near an incision or an open lesion. It is obvious that a person with breathing difficulties should not be positioned face down, or a person with a blood clot should not receive circulatory modalities. In many situations, common sense is enough to guide the massage process, but not in others. Specialized training is essential to understanding the needs of people who are medically complex. And, a specially designed system for organizing that information is helpful.

Pressure modifications

In 1917, British physician James Mennell headed the Massage Department at St. Thomas' Hospital in London. At that time, his focus was the rehabilitation of soldiers returning from the battlefields of World War 1. In the preface to his book, *Massage: Its Principles and Practice*, he writes: "I have undertaken the heavy task of writing a book in war-time, at the request of my publishers, with two main objects in view. The first is to try to point out, as far as I can, to the practising masseurs and masseuses, what I consider to be the rationale of massage treatment, and to endeavour to introduce into their technique more generally than is at present the case, the care and gentleness, which appear to me as the key to the riddle of the exact nature of the massage which will most speedily yield a successful result."[1]

More than 100 years ago, Mennell was trying to advance the notion of gentleness as the way that will "most speedily yield a successful result." This is the first and maybe most important adjustment when massaging patients in the health care setting. The case for gentler pressure is two-fold. First, deep or even moderate pressure may place demands on a body that is too sick to tolerate them, thereby directing energy away from the healing process. Ruth Werner, author of *A Massage Therapist's Guide to Pathology*, promotes the idea that: "Massage therapy challenges homeostasis. We create changes in the internal environment of our clients' bodies. Our first job, before we ever touch a client, is to determine whether that person is capable of adjusting to the changes massage precipitates."[2]

It must be remembered that people are in the hospital or other health care setting because they are acutely or chronically ill and require a level of care that cannot be given at home. Conditions such as low platelets, fragile areas of skin, neuropathy, edema, recent surgery, or bone metastases absolutely require the use of light pressure. Nearly all patients will have some factor that necessitates decreasing the usual amount of force. Table 6.1 categorizes a wide variety of health conditions and the appropriate massage pressure that is commonly needed.

The second reason for advocating the use of gentle pressure is in order to achieve comfort and relaxation: this is the main goal when working with people in a health care facility. In order to accomplish this, the attention of the therapist must shift away from the musculoskeletal system and toward the skin. It is here in the cutaneous nerves, through gentle touch, that the parasympathetic nervous system is activated. This is the system that causes thinking to be more coherent, breathing and heart rate to

TABLE 6.1 Pressure Scale for patients in health care settings

Pressure level		Indications for use
Level zero No physical contact with patient Hands held above affected areas Off the body energy techniques, e.g., Therapeutic Touch	0	Incisions IV sites Throat sore from NG tube Wounds
Level one Lotioning or energy technique Full-handed contact No pressure Places no demand on the body	1	Active dying Antepartum (severe blood clot risk) Ascites Bone metastases (severe) Bleeding or bruising risk (severe) Cachexia Cardiovascular event (severe, e.g. stroke, MI) Edematous extremity Extended bedrest (VTE risk) Fatigue (severe) Fever (noncontagious) Fragile skin and tissue (severe) Limb with PICC line Lymphedema (active) Nausea (severe) Neuropathy (severe) Neutropenia (ANC<500) Osteoporosis (severe) Respiratory distress (severe) Thrombocytopenia (<20,000 platelets per microL) Varices (veins that are bulging, ropey, twisted) VTE (recent Hx or Tx)
Level two Light, full-handed contact with superficial muscles Heavy lotioning No depth Places no demand on the body	2	Antepartum (moderate risk) Bone metastases (in limited sites) Fatigue (moderate) LE risk Nausea (mild) Neuropathy (moderate) Neutropenia (ANC>500–1500) Osteoporosis (moderate) Postoperative (general VTE risk) Postpartum (C-section & vaginal delivery) Respiratory distress (moderate) Thrombocytopenia (<50,000 platelets per microL; case by case assessment) Varices (discolored veins) VTE risk

continued

TABLE 6.1 Pressure Scale for patients in health care settings *continued*

Pressure level		Indications for use
Level three Slightly firm pressure to muscles, but still nurturing Typically used on a limited area No forceful depth No attempt to be ambitious Skin does not remain reddened after stroking	3	Fatigue (mild) Labor and delivery (back) Neuropathy (mild) Osteopenia (low risk of fracture) Outpatients (e.g. pain clinic, cardiac or orthopedic rehab)
Level four Moderate tissue displacement Firm but controlled pressure Focus on muscles	4	Most patients in a health care setting will require level 1 or 2 pressure. A few will require level 3. People who are healthy enough to receive level 4 are most likely to be healthier outpatients being seen for rehab.

The Pressure Scale is meant only as a general guideline. The circumstances of individual patients may allow or require slight variations in the amount of pressure used. However, it can't be overemphasized that too little pressure is better than too much.

Abbreviations: ANC, absolute neutrophil count; Hx, history; IV, intravenous; LE, lymphedema; MI, myocardial infarction; NG, nasogastric; Tx, therapy; VTE, venous thromboembolism.

The Pressure Scale was developed by and is used by the gracious permission of Tracy Walton. This pressure scale first appeared in Walton's course manual, *Oncology Massage Therapy/Caring for Clients with Cancer*. A later version appeared in Walton T, *Medical Conditions and Massage Therapy: A Decision Tree Approach*. Philadelphia: Wolters Kluwer Health/Lippincott Williams & Wilkins, 2011. ("Lotioning" pressures were first described by Gayle MacDonald and Dawn Nelson.)

slow, blood vessels to dilate, and digestion, elimination, and wound healing to improve. It is through sedation of the nervous system that rest and relaxation occur, not by the kneading or compression of muscles.

A vital component in initiating the parasympathetic response is trust and safety. Everyone, whether healthy or not, has a primitive area of the brain that is constantly asking, "Am I safe, or not safe?"[3] This part of the brain can't always distinguish between what is truly traumatic, such as an assault, and other events meant to be helpful. Many experiences during medical treatment or care can feel threatening and unsafe, although they are meant to be helpful. Imagine having constant blood draws, surgical procedures, being bound down by medical devices, pain, emotional uncertainty, or fear. Even something as seemingly as wonderful as having a baby can be a harrowing experience. Health care providers do their best to be sensitive when administering treatments, but there is an inherent intrusiveness that affects many people.

In addition to the strain of being in a health care setting, there can be somatic and emotional trauma from the cause of the hospitalization, such as a car accident, heart attack, or a fall. The disease, too, can bring on stress. Put yourself in the place of the person with limited breathing due to COPD, a cancer diagnosis, renal failure, or severe constipation due to pain medications. Touch therapy can be one of the services that contributes to a patient feeling safer.

Pressure is the hardest of the adjustments to gauge. Massage therapists generally are taught that firm or deep pressure is necessary to release stress or knotted muscles. However, they must learn to trust that forceful bodywork is not necessary to create a profound effect. Physical symptoms such as pain, nausea, fatigue, and insomnia can be alleviated with the use of gentle touch modalities, as can emotional discomforts such as isolation, hopelessness, or anxiety. Therapists can create deep presence without using deep pressure.

A patient's story 6.1 | **What works today may not work tomorrow**

As a person living with a port and being treated with bendamustine, my veins are so sore and painful that even level 1 pressure is too much for me. What works today may or may not work tomorrow. What gives pleasure one minute may create pain the next. This requires the therapist to be present and conscious every moment.

Meg Robsahm
Rochester, Minnesota

Therapist's journal 6.1
Who are you?

Most of us begin our careers thinking of ourselves as Massage Therapists. We have diplomas, licenses, or registrations that say so. At Oregon Health and Science University, our students have hospital ID badges telling people they are Massage Interns, but this label often obscures their deeper identity. One class in particular was having trouble adjusting the pressure they were using with patients who were particularly complex and vulnerable. One day I did an experiment with them. With eyes closed and sitting in a relaxed state, I asked them to be a Massage Therapist and notice what that felt like in their body. We did the same with four other identities: Touch Therapist, Complementary Therapist, Bodyworker, and Healer. Each of these identities felt different in their bodies: some softer, others more effortful; with some they felt more present, with other identities there was more sense of an agenda. The two identities that helped the class shift their ability to be softer and more present were Touch Therapist and Complementary Therapist.

Patient expectations can make it difficult to hold the line on pressure because, like healthy clients, they think the firmer the better – especially if the person has a history of receiving massage before being in a health care facility. Patients have been known to plead for deeper pressure, even during times when they have dangerously low platelet levels or have less than 20% heart function. While it is natural to try to respect the patient's wishes, in many health conditions, deeper pressure may cause harm to the patient or it can overburden body systems. Even if the patient is imploring the practitioner for more pressure, the therapist must stay within parameters of safety. Like physicians, bodyworkers are charged with the responsibility of "First Do No Harm."

There are many interpretations of "gentle pressure." Someone who is a sports massage therapist will have one idea, a person who practices Craniosacral Therapy will have another. Gentle bodywork may mean just resting the hands on the body, or it may entail systematically applying lotion, or using an open hand rather than thumbs to give a Shiatsu treatment.

The level of pressure will depend on a variety of influences, such as the patient's disease, treatment, age, length of illness, medications, and fitness level. Surmising the correct amount of effort and pressure is sometimes easy and straightforward. For example, a person with a platelet level below 20,000 per microliter (microL) of blood should be massaged *only* with the amount of pressure used to apply lotion to the skin. The patient whose legs are tight with edematous fluid because of chemotherapy or cardiac complications should also only be lightly lotioned in the lower extremities. However, the case of a 23-year-old patient with a spleen injury from a car accident is less clear-cut. A firmer pressure on some parts of his body might be well tolerated.

Patient vignette

Let's look at the case of Mrs C., an orthopedic patient. Underlined are four reasons why the pressure must be reduced to level 1 for her.

Mrs C., 72 years old, <u>underwent a left hip replacement 48 hours ago</u>. The surgery went smoothly, but Mrs C. needs to stay in hospital for longer than expected due to a <u>bleeding issue</u>. The hospitalist has ordered blood transfusions. She is on <u>morphine for pain</u> and <u>anticoagulant medication due to the risk of a blood clot</u>. Naturally, there is an incision and bruising at the left hip that extends down into the inner thigh. A peripheral IV catheter is in the right wrist, and she is wearing compression hose on her legs to diminish the possibility of a thrombus. Mrs C. is beginning to be ambulatory but still has a Foley catheter in place. The doctor has given permission for massage to the hands, head, and neck. Of paramount importance is to avoid pressure on any part of the body that would disturb the alignment of the replaced joint.

Site considerations

Medical devices, skin problems, intervention or injury sites, for example, will force therapists to avoid or at least be mindful of certain areas. Some locations, such as an area containing an incision, a weeping skin condition, or the site of a drain, should not be touched at all. Other areas may be touched but require an adjustment to the type of touch. An excellent example is diabetic neuropathy in the feet. Other examples are the site of a tumor, an epidural, or a skin condition called petechiae. Kneading or stroking the site of a tumor is inappropriate, but resting the hands lightly on it is not. Care needs to be taken near an epidural, but the area can be stroked up to a few inches away from the site. Petechiae, a hemorrhagic skin condition characterized by very small reddish-purple spots under the skin, does not need to be totally avoided. Pressure level 1 massage over the affected area is fine.

It is not uncommon for a patient to have a very limited area that can be massaged: one foot, a small area on the back, or just the hands. Focus on what is available to

Therapist's journal 6.2
Only the shoulder

A young man had fallen from a window five stories up. His injuries were severe, requiring him to be in the intensive care unit since the event happened (five weeks previously). His nurse asked if there was a massage therapist who could work with him. Because of my nursing background, my supervisor sent me. Despite 25 years in nursing, I was very nervous. The patient had been in a coma the entire time, had an open wound on the left hip that was stapled, a broken right foot, a lump on his right forearm the size of an egg, a catheter in his neck, compression devices on his legs, and a broken pelvis, to name just some of his injuries. The father of the young man thought that it would be good to massage him, but when I asked the nurse where I could touch him, she said the only place was his shoulder.

I didn't want to just start, so I whispered in his ear to tell him who I was, my name, and what I was going to do. On some level, I felt he could hear me. When I placed my hands on his shoulder, he took a big, long, slow, deep breath and I knew for sure I had reached him, even though he was unconscious. For half an hour I gently applied lotion to that small, uninjured area and then administered Therapeutic Touch to the remainder of the body for another half hour. At one point, the nurse came running in and asked me what I was doing, which made me nervous again. She said, "Whatever you are doing, keep doing it. His vital signs are normalizing." The father, who had rarely left his son's side for the five weeks, could see the relaxation in his son's body.

Mary Malinski RN, LMT
Portland, Oregon

be massaged rather than what can't be touched. Areas that can't be touched directly can be given indirect care through the use of a modality such as reflexology, Reiki, or Therapeutic Touch.

Patient vignette

Let's look at a cardiac patient, Mr R., 58 years old. Due to a coronary artery bypass graft (CABG) 72 hours ago, he has seven sites (underlined) that a therapist would need to be mindful of when working with his body.

Mr R has a <u>sternal incision</u> that is very painful and <u>a small incision on the right leg</u> where the saphenous vein was removed to graft onto the heart. <u>Drains were removed from the left side of his chest</u> at the end of post-op day 2. The patient has a peripheral IV catheter, also known as a <u>peripheral line, in the lower right arm</u>, compression hose on his legs to decrease edema and risk of blood clots, <u>two electrodes attached to the chest</u>, and his <u>throat is sore from the endotracheal tube</u>. Mr R. smoked for 35 years, which has diminished his pulmonary function. He is hemodynamically stable, which means the pressures in the heart and blood pressure are stable, but he has a low-grade fever. Mr R. is on a long list of medications: aspirin to prevent a blood clot; an antibiotic; oxycodone, and acetaminophen and hydrocodone (Vicodin) for pain; ketorolac (Toradol), an anti-inflammatory drug also used for pain; nitroglycerin for blood pressure; lovastatin (Mevacor) to control cholesterol; and nadolol to improve heart function. He is very fatigued. The nurses have him up twice a day for a short walk, and he takes his meals seated in a chair. Mr R.'s lower back is sore from lying in bed and his <u>shoulders hurt from being retracted to a 90° angle during surgery</u>. Changing positions is painful, but Mr R. is interested in having a massage. His doctor has given permission for massage to the back, neck, and feet.

Info Box 6.1 Common site considerations

Avoid directly touching sites of:
- Communicable diseases of the skin (e.g., herpes, shingles)
- Incisions (recent)
- Interventions (e.g., IV catheter, colostomy bag, epidural)
- Monitoring devices (e.g., cardiac, fetal)
- Severe pain
- Skin conditions that are weeping or painful (e.g., rash, radiation burn, fragility)

In situations where direct touch is contraindicated, there is anecdotal evidence that modalities such as Therapeutic Touch may be beneficial over the affected site. Practitioners not trained in one of these modalities can still give attention to restricted areas by holding their hands a couple of inches above the area for a few minutes.

Be mindful of the following areas. Gently resting the hands on the area or light stroking can be appropriate:
- Abdomen of a pregnant patient affected by preterm labor or obstetrical problem
- Bone and spinal metastases
- Extremities with or at risk for deep vein thrombosis (gentle holds are fine, but no pressure or stroking)
- Painful areas
- Phlebitis (resting the hands on the site is fine, but no pressure or stroking)
- Skin conditions (non-weeping, intact)
- Tumors (resting the hands on the site is fine, but no pressure or stroking)
- Varicosity, mild (all strokes should be toward the heart)
- Varicosity, severe (massage proximal to the varices)

Chapter SIX

Positioning adjustments

Depending on the area of the body that the patient desires to have massaged, the massage therapist will need to determine whether repositioning will enhance or compromise the patient's comfort. Things to consider include the patient's comfort in the current position, the patient's ability to tolerate a different position, the patient's energy level, and whether the process of repositioning will cause pain. It can be helpful to ask the patient: "Are you comfortable in this position, or would you like to try something different?"[4]

Each institution will, or should, have a policy regarding patient positioning by massage therapists. A therapist's status often will influence whether they are allowed to reposition patients: touch therapists who are members of staff may have more leeway than someone who is a volunteer.

Certain medical conditions require specialized training to safely position patients, for example joint replacements, amyotrophic lateral sclerosis (ALS)/motor neurone disease (MND), and stroke. Health care centers may prefer to have the nursing staff position patients who are unable to manage on their own. Other facilities may require bodyworkers to undergo instruction in how to perform transfers and position changes as part of their orientation to the hospital.

Generally, the nursing staff will allow the patient to determine which positions are comfortable, which is referred to as self-limiting. Most position adjustments involve the patient's inability to lie prone, which is often due to breathing difficulties, an incision, medical device such as a drain, urostomy bag, or an intravenous (IV) catheter. Those with respiratory or cardiac conditions may need to elevate the head to ease breathing difficulties. Orthopedic and stroke patients require a great deal of attention to positioning to maintain alignment of the affected area. If the patient is under

a strict and continuous position restriction, a sign will be posted on the wall above the head of the bed. For example, a person receiving chemotherapy directly to the liver will be required to lie on their back for a number of days with the head only being elevated at 30 degrees or less.

Whenever possible, allow patients to position themselves even though it is a slow, sometimes uncomfortable process. Therapists often feel bad when asking a patient to reposition. Nurses, however, encourage patients to make frequent position changes because it reduces the risk of pressure sore development, improves strength, and restores confidence in the body. The therapist should assist with repositioning such things as catheter lines or telemetry wires.

Therapist's journal 6.3
Too many pillows

A patient who had undergone a double mastectomy the previous day was recovering in her hospital room. I was eager to use my massage skills to help her relax, but about ten minutes into her 20-minute massage she still seemed uncomfortable. Why? I had missed a basic but vital detail: she had two giant, fluffy pillows behind her that were pushing her head so far forward that her chin was pointed to her chest. After the pillows were repositioned so she could relax her neck and shoulders, she relaxed into the massage and drifted off to sleep. Sometimes, the most important hospital-based massage skill is simple observation.

Christine Knapp CMT
Hospital-Based Massage Therapy student
Mayo Clinic, Rochester, Minnesota

Tip 6.1 Align the patient's hips with the fold in the bed

One of the most common sources of discomfort for a patient's back can be the semi-reclining position in a profiling bed. Patients should have their hips positioned at the angle where the bed folds, so that they can't slip downward leaving the mid-thoracic region at the fold. Patients may need help to be pulled up toward the head of the bed to correct their position (see Figure 6.10 regarding use of a draw sheet for this).

Patient vignette

Ms M., 82 years old, was in a rehab center for six weeks to recover from a knee replacement. Underlined are the positioning considerations for massage.

The affected right knee was supported by elevating the foot of the bed and placing pillows under the knee. Twice a day she had physical therapy that included joint manipulation and walking. For the first three weeks post-op, the staff advised her to sleep on her back. At about week 4 she progressed to side-lying, preferably on the right side, as this naturally created good alignment of the joint. Near the end of her stay, Ms M. was able to lie on her left side with support between the legs to maintain alignment. The patient was on several medications relevant to the joint replacement: tramadol for pain, celecoxib (Celebrex) for inflammation, and a muscle relaxant, methocarbamol (Robaxin). In addition, she took her regular medications for blood pressure and sleep.

Basic positions for receiving massage

Figures 6.2A–E show the positions commonly used for massaging hospital patients.

Info Box 6.2 Common indications for positioning adjustments

- Ascites
- Breathing difficulty
- Edema or lymphedema
- Fractures
- Heart conditions
- Incisions
- Joint replacements
- Medical devices
- Nausea or intestinal cramping
- Pain
- Pregnancy
- Tumors

- Figure 6.2A: Fowler's position, also known as semi-reclining or semi-seated. Patients may need to be in this position due to breathing issues, nausea, to reduce the pressure on a surgical incision, or because they want to socialize.

- Figure 6.2B: Side-lying. Notice the pillow under the top arm. When asked, patients will often say they don't need this, but on trying it, they find it very comfortable.

- Figure 6.2C: Supine. Sometimes a patient must lie completely flat because of their medical procedure.

- Figure 6.2D: Prone. Patients don't commonly lie prone in acute or long-term health care settings. If they want to try it, support under the torso often takes pressure off the neck.

- Figure 6.2E: Prone. Rolled hand towels under the axilla is another option for relieving pressure from the neck.

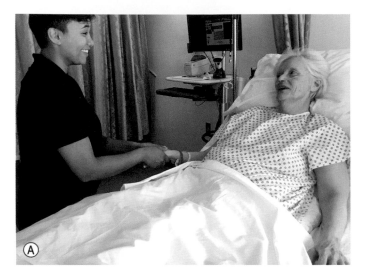

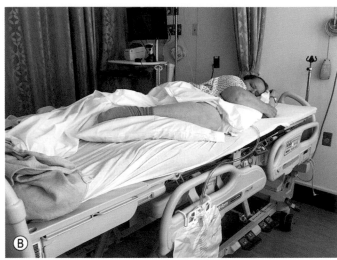

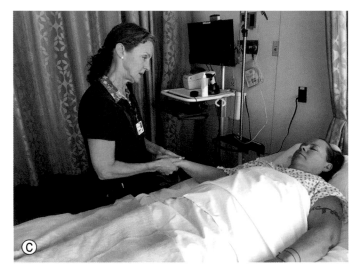

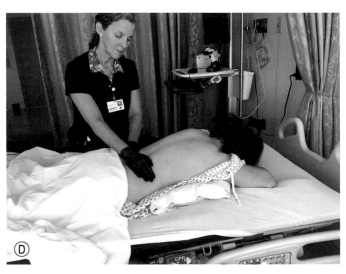

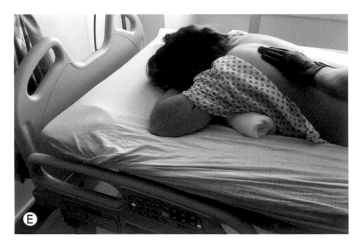

FIGURE 6.2
A Fowler's position. **B** Side-lying. **C** Supine. **D** & **E** Prone.

(Photos: A–D by Barbara Gideon; E by Carolyn Tague.)

Propping

Before the massage begins, it is well worth taking the time to make the patient more comfortable with the use of pillows, towels, and blankets, as this allows them to relax even further. Figures 6.3–6.9 show examples of how to use props that can be found in a health care facility. (*Author's note:* the lack of sufficient pillows is universal, but towels and blankets can often be substituted.)

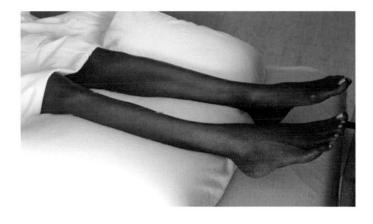

FIGURE 6.3
Support of the lower legs with the heels floating free.

(Photo by Candice White.)

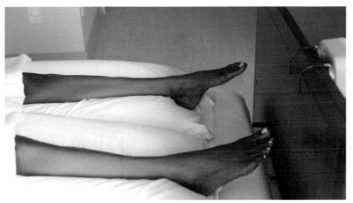

FIGURE 6.4
Support of the lower legs with the heels supported.

(Photo by Candice White.)

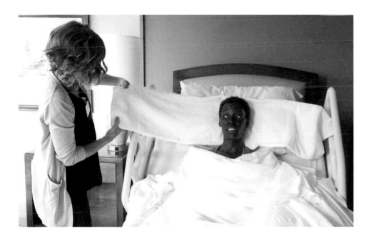

FIGURE 6.5
Fashioning head support from a towel.

(Photo by Candice White.)

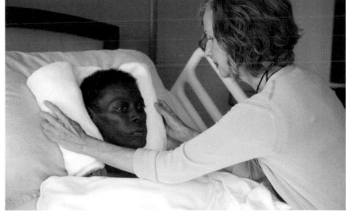

FIGURE 6.6
Head fully supported with a towel.

(Photo by Candice White.)

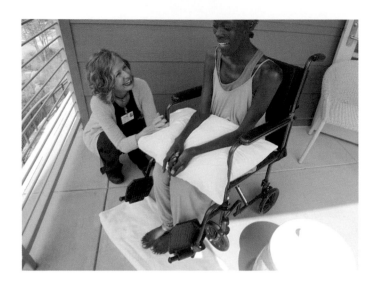

FIGURE 6.7
When seated, a pillow or two under the arms and a pillow or towel under the feet allow greater relaxation. A good laugh helps too!

(Photo by Candice White.)

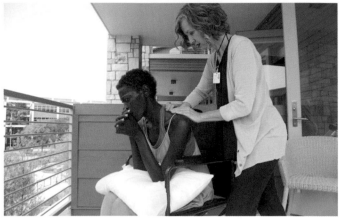

FIGURE 6.8
Reverent repose made comfortable by a pillow under the elbows.

(Photo by Candice White.)

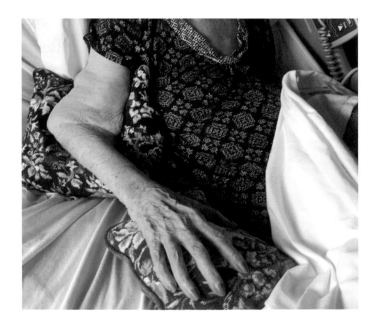

FIGURE 6.9
Props from home. Needlepoint pillows created in earlier days by the patient.

(Photo by Gayle MacDonald.)

Use of a draw sheet [4]

A draw sheet, sometimes called a "lift sheet," is often used in the inpatient environment to safely reposition a patient in bed. Draw sheets can be useful following surgery or other debilitating treatment, or any other time that patients are unable to move unaided.

The draw sheet is particularly useful in situations where the patient has slipped down toward the foot of the bed. When this happens, they are bent at the thoracic spine, which causes back discomfort. Helping the patient to shift back up toward the head of the bed will put their hips in the fold of the bed. It is a simple piece of positioning advice, but one that can bring great relief to the back. Two helpers, one standing on each side of the bed as pictured in Figure 6.10, can safely move most patients up toward the head of the bed. If the patient is very large, it may take additional helpers.

To move a patient up in bed, follow these steps:

1. Always tell the patient what you are about to do.
2. Use gravity to assist with repositioning by lowering the head of the bed. Patients with breathing issues may need reassurance that the bed will only need to be flat for a short time.

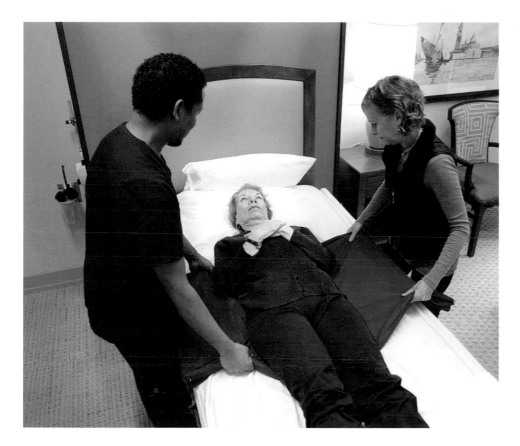

FIGURE 6.10
Using a draw sheet to move the patient up toward the head of the bed.

(Photo by David Spence.)

3. Have the patient fold their arms across the chest, or move the arms into this position if the patient is unable to do so. Be mindful of any tubing that needs to move with the patient.

4. If the head of the bed is against a wall, place an upright pillow between the wall and patient's head as a soft buffer.

5. The helpers, standing on opposite sides of the bed, should each grasp a corner of the draw sheet.

6. On the count of three, both helpers should slide the draw sheet and patient toward the head of the bed.

7. Raise the head of the bed as desired and reposition pillows as needed for the patient's comfort (see Figure 6.2A).

Repositioning from supine to side-lying position is possible for one experienced person to do, but it's easier for with people as pictured in Figure 6.11A. Follow these steps.

1. Tell the patient what you are about to do.

2. Remove pillows, if present, from under the knees.

3. Lower the head of the bed so that the bed is flat.

4. Uncross the patient's feet if they are crossed, so that the patient is lying flat.

5. Begin on the side of the bed where you want the patient's back to face.

6. Take the draw sheet in both hands, pull the patient toward you, so that the patient's body lies closer to one side of the bed (Figure 6.11A).

7. Reach across the patient and grab the draw sheet on the far side: this will be the side the patient will be facing. Pull the draw sheet so that the patient rolls toward you (Figure 6.11B).

8. Place pillows behind the patient's back for support.

9. Additional pillows can be placed between the legs and under the top arm for added support (see Figure 6.2B). The head of the bed can be raised slightly if desired by the patient.

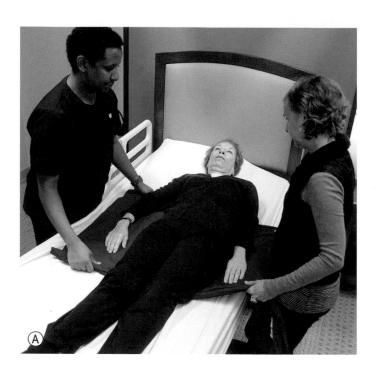
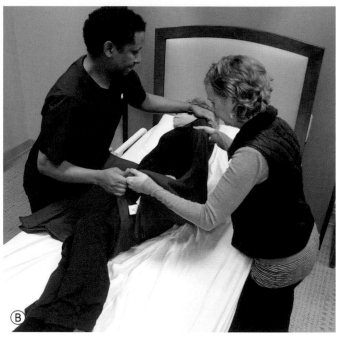

FIGURE 6.11
Rolling the patient from supine to side-lying. **A** Pull the patient toward one side of the bed. **B** Reach across the patient and pull the draw sheet so that patient the rolls onto their side.

(Photos by David Spence.)

Case history 6.1 — Exercise

Instructions: On a piece of paper mark three columns: pressure, site, and positioning. List two reasons for adjusting the pressure for Mr D., at least four sites to avoid, and the position he is most likely to be comfortable in.

Mr D. is recovering from radical neck surgery which took place 5 days ago. The 12-hour operation was for cancer in two sites along the left carotid artery. The surgeons replaced about 5 inches of the carotid artery with a Gortex stent and took a muscle from his stomach to replace a neck muscle. They also grafted some skin from the right thigh to cover the new neck muscle. A feeding tube is implanted in his stomach. Mr D. must relearn how to swallow because half of his esophagus is non-responsive. His left shoulder, neck, part of the larynx and tongue are numb because their nerves were cut during the surgery. He is experiencing headaches and back pain as a result of the surgery. The patient is on oxycodone for pain.

Summary

The pressure, site, and positioning framework can be applied to almost every part of a patient's situation: their disease or condition, side effects of medications, procedures or injuries, and as a tool to collect information. Like anything new, this framework, despite its simplicity, will feel a bit awkward to use at first. But in a very short time, it will become second nature and the massage practitioner will slot the patient's data into the framework as quickly as the doctor or nurse gives it. Touch therapists will feel confident as they expand their practice throughout the various health care units. Even though they may not have complete knowledge of a specialty, the pressure, site, and position framework gives therapists a springboard for effective questioning strategies and critical thinking, skills that are more valuable than the ability to memorize specialized medical details.

The following chapters will apply the pressure, site, and position framework in considering medical devices, medications, common reasons for admission, and common symptoms and conditions.

Test yourself

Multiple choice: Circle all of correct answers. There may be more than one.

1. Which of the following conditions indicate a high risk for a blood clot?

   A   Antepartum.
   B   Postsurgical.
   C   Psychiatric.
   D   Osteoporosis.

2. Being at high risk for a blood clot is an indication for:

   A   Reducing pressure.
   B   Avoiding touch in the affected area.
   C   Elevation of the head.
   D   Refusing to give massage until the person is no longer at risk.

3. Which of the following conditions require pressure modifications?

   A   Fatigue.
   B   Edema.
   C   Cesarean section.
   D   Congestive heart failure.

4. Which of the following conditions require positioning adjustments?

   A   Risk of easy bruising.
   B   Fracture.
   C   Breathing difficulty.
   D   Stroke.

5. Which of the following areas should not be touched directly?

   A   Weeping skin lesion.
   B   Incision site.
   C   Edema.
   D   Tumor site.

6. Which conditions require a reduction in the amount of pressure, either systemically or locally?

   A   Osteoporosis.
   B   Fragile skin.
   C   Herpes.
   D   Kidney failure.

7. Which conditions may require attention to the patient's positioning?

   A   Pregnancy.
   B   Tumor.
   C   Fatigue.
   D   Congestive heart failure.

8. Which condition is a site restriction that the therapist should avoid direct contact with?

A   Herpes.

B   Fever.

C   Varicose veins.

D   Neuropathy.

References

1. Mennell JB. Massage: Its Principles and Practice. London: J & A Churchill; 1917.

2. Werner R. Personal communication, 29 April 2010.

3. Adkins I. When the healing is through the body: understanding and supporting medical PTSD. Oncology Massage Healing Summit, 27 April 2018.

4. Spence C. Personal communication, 18 August 2019.

Every time we work with a client, we process an enormous amount of data, and we make decisions based on that information. What that looks like will vary depending on your unique skillset and approach to massage and bodywork, and your client's needs, priorities, and limitations. Most situations have many possible right answers; your job is to determine the course of action that fits your client's situation best.

Ruth Werner

The previous chapter outlined a framework of three categories that can assist bodyworkers in their session planning: *pressure modifications*, *site considerations*, and *positioning adjustments*. This chapter will continue to use of this framework, applying it to patient groups who commonly receive massage in health care settings. Later chapters will address in greater detail specific symptoms and side effects from illness, medications, medical devices, and procedures. The reader will need to combine the information in this chapter with that from subsequent chapters in order to create a complete clinical picture.

Each section of this chapter contains a feature called *Clinical considerations*. This feature suggests adjustments that may need to be made for the massage session. The reader should bear in mind that through the written medium, it is not possible to advise which modifications and to what level they should be made with regard to a particular patient. Many factors influence the performance of a massage session: the patient's clinical outlook is one thing, but so, too, are the preferences and beliefs of the staff, as well as the therapist's experience. Practitioners new to working in health care settings are usually more tentative, following the rules to a T. But as they settle in and have more experience, confidence is gained and therapists understand where they can push the envelope a bit more or need to hold back. For example, a new therapist might always keep to level 1 pressure for a patient whose platelet count is 30,000 per microliter (microL) of blood, whereas a seasoned therapist might use level 2 pressure on some patients with a platelet count of 30,000, depending on the patient's age, general health, tissue integrity, treatment regimen, and the cause of the platelet reduction.

This chapter is very substantial, but it cannot bear witness to all of the various patients who are admitted for medical and nursing care. It does, however, give the reader a starting place that hopefully allows them to ask the right questions of staff, patients, and sometimes the patient's family.

The following sections are presented alphabetically for ease of referencing.

Addiction, co-occurring conditions, and psychological disorders

Addiction treatment, sometimes referred to as behavioral health treatment, is often given in rehabilitation centers, but people being treated for drug dependence may also be cared for in a psychiatric hospital unit as in- or out-patients. People who enter treatment for substance abuse almost always have co-occurring conditions. Alcohol or drug abuse may be the primary reason for seeking rehabilitation, but there are usually a variety of other factors present, such as trauma, chronic pain, impulse control disorders, and mood disorders, such as anxiety or depression. These components co-mingle, making it difficult to separate out the primary cause of the addiction from the secondary ones.[1]

Patients in treatment for substance abuse or co-occurring conditions cover a wide spectrum. They may have a chemical imbalance, have become addicted to painkillers after surgery, or they may have been mentally or physically abused in childhood; or their suffering may be due to gender identification issues, PTSD from military service, or sexual assault, to name just a few causes. Regardless of the roots of addiction, there is generally a corresponding neurological change in the brain.

Touch therapies can make a profound contribution to the recovery process of these patients. In this setting, touch practitioners will work more closely with the

Chapter SEVEN

patient's care team, which will include doctors, nurses, psychologists, and other CAM therapists. There will be frequent communication about the bodywork sessions and the patient's response. Sometimes during a massage, memories stored in the tissues will surface and the patient will have an emotional response. It is tempting during these emotional times to step into the role of counselor, to encourage people to talk about their fears or grief, or to offer advice. However, it is imperative that practitioners avoid this pitfall and instead be active listeners rather than try to analyze; become skillful at just listening without interruption, providing a nonjudgmental space in which people can talk, and asking questions only to clarify meaning. Let the staff members who are trained to work in the emotional realm apply their specialty.

While recovering, patients will be prescribed a variety of medications. They may be on medication for allergic reactions, pain, sleep, nausea, sedation, anxiety, depression, psychosis, or muscle relaxation. Many of these drugs diminish a person's ability to give accurate feedback as well as causing other unwelcome side effects, such as pacing, leg shaking, tongue rolling, hand clenching, muscular rigidity, and a flat affect. Some people are eager to stop or cut down on their medications because of the dyskinetic effects, and also because some cause sluggishness or agitation. Touch therapies can calm these motor effects, and help during the process of tapering off or reducing medications.

Patients' diagnoses are complex and tangled, so there is no set way to deliver massage to them; however, there are tendencies within the subgroups. Those with a primary diagnosis of drug or alcohol addiction often request deep massage, while the person whose primary diagnosis is trauma-related typically needs a great deal of mindfulness, pacing, and focus on trust. The needs of people in treatment for mood disorders fluctuate from day to day, or even minute to minute. Each of these groups is addressed below in more detail.

Drug and alcohol recovery

People who have been abusing drugs and alcohol will need a number of days to detoxify. During that time, they may not want massage due to nausea, headaches,

breathing difficulty, and/or irritability. However, if they do want touch therapy during detox, the therapist should take a slow, gentle approach just as they would with someone receiving chemotherapy. As with chemotherapy patients, people detoxifying from drugs or alcohol can feel extremely unwell from massage that is too demanding. One patient and therapist found this out the hard way: thinking that a firm massage would help clear the drugs from his system more quickly, the patient requested a deep massage while in the midst of detox. A few hours later he paid the price with vomiting and various somatic pains.

Once the detoxification process is complete, these patients tend to want deep massage. However, on the whole, they are often disconnected from their bodies, so it is necessary to proceed with some level of caution. They may be unaware of how their bodies feel, including pain levels, and cannot give accurate feedback. One nurse massage therapist who specializes in addiction medicine tells about a patient who had had a hip fracture for some time but was so out of touch with his body that the pain didn't register. After a number of touch therapy treatments, he was able to feel his body again and the pain in it. This allowed him to communicate about the pain to the doctor and receive treatment for it.

These patients can have firm bodywork if it is appropriate for their general health, but the therapist needs to bear in mind the lack of physical awareness that long-time drug users experience. People who are detached from their bodies will sometimes allow invasive bodywork to be administered. Skilled, respectful touch will help these patients reconnect with their bodies.

Trauma

At the start of the therapeutic bodywork relationship, building trust is the only goal. This is true with all clients but especially for people with known trauma. And the doorway into trust is communication, especially prior to the session.

Often, the abuse or trauma is associated with touch, and relearning the experience of safe touch can be slow. One touch therapist tells the story of a woman whose tibias had been broken with the butt of a gun. At first she wouldn't allow her legs to be touched – even the idea of having them touched was intolerable. However, bit by bit, giving the patient complete control over the process, the therapist was able to extend the strokes from the feet up the legs. This client was eventually able to walk without a cane, her gait nearly normal.

Until patients have confidence in the massage experience, the bodyworker may need to honor various requests and limitations. People may need to keep their eyes open during the session so that they can see the therapist; others may not be able to lie prone on the massage table for fear of what is going on behind them. One man with PTSD was afraid to lie prone because he invariably fell asleep in that position – falling asleep triggered flashbacks, causing the man to thrash severely, and so he was afraid of falling off the table if he had an episode. Another man who received touch sessions in a regular chair would not let the therapist work behind him. The face cradle, too, may provoke a similar psychological discomfort, requiring the therapist to work on the client from supine and side-lying positions.

Many affected by trauma can be very sensitive and want gentler touch. And yet, surprisingly, there are others who want a firm pressure because they learned to cope with traumatic episodes by "leaving" their body. They may not have a sense of their physical body from years of this dissociative process, and a firmer pressure helps regain that awareness.

Choice and control are important to those recovering from trauma. Open-ended communication strategies can help in empowering patients: rather than asking, "Is that OK?" use a specific question such as, "Shall we include that area in the session this time?" Over time they may be able to tell the therapist exactly what they want in terms of pressure, music, temperature, and which areas to massage. Let the patient lead the process. And, very importantly, make no assumptions.

Mood disorders

Anxiety and depression are the most common mood disorders. People with these conditions fluctuate the most:

Therapist's journal 7.1
It takes time to feel safe

Our behavioral health patients receive some type of touch modality multiple times a week during their month-long stay. Since the second day after she arrived, I have been giving massage to a young woman who suffers from physical and sexual trauma. After two weeks, and many massages, her level of trust and awareness has grown enough for her to admit to me the she couldn't remember the first massage because she was so accustomed to "checking out" where her body was concerned. The other thing that she shared with me was that it helped to know exactly what I was going to do with the drape BEFORE I did it. Even though we tell our clients to let us know what will make them more comfortable, physically and emotionally, it took numerous sessions for her to feel safe enough to ask for what she needed.

Jacki Sellers LMT
Tucson, Arizona

---

one day their anxiety may be an 8 on a 1 to 10 scale and the next day it is a 3. Within a massage session their needs might change from wanting firm pressure to asking for gentle touch.

It can sometimes, with certain patients, be helpful to use a modality such as Therapeutic Touch, that works in the person's energy field rather than directly on the skin. In this way, the therapist doesn't have to enter into such close proximity with the patient, which, if done too quickly, can sometimes exacerbate the symptoms. A next step can be to massage only the hands, spending as many sessions with this area as needed, perhaps months, progressing next to the elbow and then eventually to the shoulder. The hands can be a good starting place when beginning to apply direct touch. As the hand opens, the heart opens, and then the whole body.

Clinical considerations: Addiction, co-occurring conditions and psychological disorders[2]

Pressure:

- Some patients will want a firm but gentle touch. However, the pressure should not be too light. Ultra-light touch may be misinterpreted, or the person may be too vulnerable for touch that is so intimate. Trust must be built before administering modalities that involve light touch, such as Reiki. Starting with Reiki above the body, using no contact, can be a good starting place for some patients.

- Other people in substance abuse rehabilitation want very deep massage, even those who have experienced psychological trauma. However, that is usually not the right starting place because they cannot give accurate feedback. A common denominator for these patients is the phenomenon of being *out of body*: the psychological term for that is dissociation. A more moderate beginning is advisable with this group of patients until they build more somatic awareness.

- Be mindful of pressure with people who have recently finished detoxification. They may think they are ready for deep massage, but the body, mind, and emotions are still finding their new normal.

- Avoid percussive strokes such as tapotement or techniques that involve prodding or digging, especially if patients have a trauma history. Gentle rocking may be appropriate.

- Be mindful that patients will be on a variety of medications, some of which decrease their ability to give accurate feedback.

Site:

- When giving touch therapy to patients who are affected by sexual trauma, consult and converse with the person every time you move to a new body part. This is different from asking for permission to move to a new body part, which is a therapist-centered approach. Instead, you might say, "Are you still interested in having massage to your neck or shall we skip that area?" Be aware of the areas of the body involved in the trauma. They may need to be avoided indefinitely or for a prolonged period. Often the buttocks, inner thigh, neck, or chest are areas that require mindfulness if the patient has experienced sexual abuse. Only massage these areas if the patient requests it.

Positioning:

- Positioning can be influenced by a variety of factors, most particularly trauma. Some patients cannot lie supine, but need a slight elevation because they can't breathe when they lie completely flat – the flat position reminds them of the trauma. Prone positioning can also feel unsafe because the patient cannot see what is behind them.

- Side-lying with plenty of pillows and bolsters is an option. It helps people feel cocooned.

Cancer treatment

Cancer is an umbrella term for some 100 separate diseases. The topic is so vast that entire books have been written on how to massage people with cancer. This section can only deal with generalities and point the reader toward other resources for specifics.

For many years, metastasis was the dominant issue with regard to massaging people with cancer. Scientific research now has shown that the initiation and spread of cancer is the result of an accumulation of genetic mutations and epigenetic changes, some of which are inherited, the bulk of which are acquired throughout a person's lifetime. There is no evidence that increasing the circulation through mechanical means causes cancer cells to form new tumors at distant sites. If this were the case, oncologists would ask their patients to refrain from exercising or being active in any way. Just the opposite is true, oncologists encourage cancer patients to remain active.

Metastasis is not the issue when creating a massage session plan for someone in treatment for cancer. The most relevant issues revolve around the side effects of treatment: chemotherapy, radiation, and surgery. It is true that the disease can cause side effects, but it is generally at the end of life that the disease process steps to the forefront. This section will address people receiving treatment as in- or outpatients in a medical setting. End of life care is beautifully addressed in Chapter 14, Sacred time: Touch at the end of life.

Many hospital massage service programs care for patients before, during, and after infusions, before or after a radiation treatment and surgery, or for treatment side effects, such as dehydration or electrolyte imbalance. Massage can also be given during a procedure, such as when a central IV catheter is attended to or during bone marrow biopsy. With the exception of their time receiving radiation, a person can have massage during any aspect of medical care.

Chemotherapy

There are a number of drug-related ways to treat cancer. Traditional chemotherapies work by killing cells that

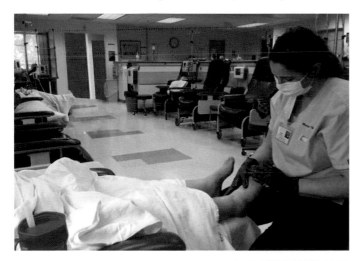

FIGURE 7.1
Chemotherapy – and foot massage – at the same time.

(Photo by Gayle MacDonald. Reprinted with permission from *Medicine Hands*, 3rd edition; Findhorn Press, 2014.)

grow quickly, such as cancer cells, but other cells get caught in the crosshairs of this type of treatment: these drugs are cytotoxic. Often they damage the bone marrow, which is responsible for the production of platelets, red blood cells, and white blood cells. This leads to suppression of the bone marrow resulting in bruising or bleeding risk, anemia, and immunosuppression. Other fast-growing cells, such as the skin and mucosal lining, are often affected, causing skin sensitivity or fragility, mucositis, diarrhea, and hand foot syndrome, for example. Specific chemotherapies are responsible for a multitude of other side effects, such as organ dysfunction, cognitive disorders, and neuropathy. Research on a reputable website, such as WebMD or Cancer Research UK, will further a therapist's knowledge of chemotherapy side effects. Chapter 10, Pharmaceutical factors: Adjustments for medications, should also be studied.

Two of the side effects that take center stage when working with hospitalized cancer patients are thrombocytopenia and neutropenia (some institutions use the term leukopenia, however, the two terms mean somewhat different things). Most often cytotoxic drugs are the cause of these two conditions. The neutropenic patient's immune system is compromised, leaving them vulnerable to infections. This can become a matter of life and death for some patients, rather than just the brief inconvenience of a cold or the flu. The massage therapist must take care to diligently apply Standard Precautions when working with this group.

Thrombocytopenic patients bruise easily; however, gentle touch therapy can be given during this time. Modalities that don't involve pressure, such as Reiki or Jin Shin Jyutsu®, are ideal. A light effleurage that basically lotions the skin also can be used. When massaging patients who bruise this easily, the practitioner should put their focus on the skin rather than the muscles. (Chapter 8 contains greater detail about thrombocytopenia and neutropenia.)

The debate around whether to glove for people who are receiving chemotherapy is ongoing. Most chemotherapies eliminate through the urine and feces, but there is evidence that some eliminate through the skin. There are hundreds of chemotherapies and few have been studied with regard to the metabolites that remain after the drugs have been broken down in the body. Case reports found in the literature implicate certain drugs leading to conditions in which the skin becomes irritated or inflamed. The authors of these studies suggest that the reactions indicate a possible connection between the concentration of antitumor drugs in sweat and tissue changes in the skin.[3–7] Doxorubicin (Doxil),[3] sorafenib (Nexavar), sunitinib (Sutent),[6] and imatinib (Gleevec)[7] are examples of oral drugs associated with various skin disorders that may be the result of metabolite accumulation in sweat glands. It is unrealistic for massage therapists, or even oncology nurses, to be up to the minute with the research on how chemotherapies metabolize. Because there are so many unknowns, a safe protocol is to glove if the patient has received any chemotherapy within the previous 72 hours.

It is important to be aware that cancer patients will be on a number of medications other than antitumor drugs. Steroids, antibiotics, sleep and pain medication, anxiolytics, and antiemetic drugs are commonly prescribed.

Targeted drug therapies take aim at a specific protein, gene, or tissue to control the cancer.[8] These drug-related treatments are the foundation of precision medicine, also known as personalized medicine. Precision medicine customizes cancer treatment based on a person's genetic makeup and tumor growth.[9] As the term implies, these drugs are more precise and usually cause fewer side effects than more traditional chemotherapy treatments.

Immunotherapy is a type of targeted therapy. One reason cancer cells flourish is because they are able to hide from the immune system, which is where immunotherapies come in. These treatments work in a variety of ways. Some target receptor sites on the cell surface to create or amplify an immune response. Other immunotherapies enhance existing anti-tumor responses. Certain immunotherapies mark cancer cells so it is easier for the immune system to find and destroy them. Vaccines are being used in a small proportion of patients. The vaccine can be made from the whole cancer cell, or from the DNA or certain proteins in the cancer cell, which helps the immune system recognize the diseased cells.[10,11]

Other targeted therapies work by aiming at a specific enzyme in the metastatic process. Gleevec, which is given for certain leukemias and gastrointestinal stromal cancer, is an example. Other targeted therapies, such as bevacizumab (Avastin) and lenalidomide (Revlimid), block the chemical signal that causes the development of new blood vessels that feed the tumor. These drugs are referred to as antiangiogenesis medications.

Targeted therapies sound benign, however, they can cause many of the same side effects as traditional chemotherapy. Flu-like symptoms are common, as well as fluid retention, heart palpitations, organ inflammation, skin problems, elevated liver enzymes, allergic reactions, fatigue, low blood cell counts, and high blood pressure.[12]

Clinical considerations: Chemotherapy

Pressure:

- Edema.
- Fatigue.
- Fever.
- Fragile veins or other tissue.
- Multiple medications, including pain medications.
- Nausea.
- Neuropathy (usually hands and feet).
- Neutropenia.
- Skin conditions and/or sensitivity.
- Thrombocytopenia.

Site:

- IV catheters.
- Skin conditions.
- Tumors.

Positioning:

- Central IV catheters (usually not prone).
- Nausea (minimize position changes).

Radiation

There are a number of types of radiation and methods of delivery, both externally and internally. The most common external method is external beam radiation. Typically, a patient will have between four to eight weeks of daily treatment, depending on the protocols followed in their country. Four-week regimens are common in the UK and Canada, while six to eight-week courses are frequently given in the USA. This form of treatment delivers high energy x-rays or gamma rays to a localized area from several angles, often three to five, but sometimes more. Compared to decades ago, modern radiotherapy minimizes the damage to surrounding healthy tissue.

The side effects of radiation can be similar to those of chemotherapy, such as fatigue, changes to blood counts, and damage to vital organs. However, unique to external beam radiation is its effect on the skin, fascia, and other tissues along the pathway of the beam. For example, the pathway of the radiation beam for prostate or colorectal cancer can affect the bladder, colon, and sexual functioning due to its inflammatory nature. A person treated for head and neck cancer with external beam radiation can have injury to the anatomical structures in that area, such as the tongue, teeth, cervical lymph nodes, fascia, blood vessels, larynx, and esophagus. Once the tissue is damaged, it tends not to regenerate normally.

Other methods of delivering radiation externally are tomotherapy, proton therapy, cyber knife, and gamma knife. With the appropriate adjustments, it is safe for the therapist to massage any of these patients – they are not radioactive.

It is common for a massage service to be created for people receiving radiotherapy on an outpatient basis. Typically, the medical staff prefer massage to be given after the person has completed their radiation session that day. Scheduling is very tight and once the patient is called to go back to the radiation suite, the staff need them to be there promptly rather than after an extra five minutes while the massage therapist finishes. Seated massage service is common, but some medical centers develop a program that offers both table or chair massage.

Brachytherapy is a way of delivering radiation internally using radioactive seeds, cones, or rods, depending on the area being treated. These patients will be radioactive for a certain number of days to weeks, but once the radioactive period has passed, it is safe to be with patients and give them bodywork.

Clinical considerations: Radiation – external beam

Pressure:

- Bone fragility in areas with history of radiation (late effect).
- Fatigue.
- Neutropenia.
- Skin sensitivity in area of treatment.
- Risk for lymphedema in treated quadrant (late effect).
- Thrombocytopenia.

Site:

- If the patient is receiving external beam radiation, do not use lotions or oils on the treated areas; recognize there will be entry and exit sites.
- Skin of treated area may be too sensitive to touch for 2–3 weeks afterwards. Also, be aware of the area opposite the treated site as it too may be affected.

Positioning:

- Sensitive skin in the field of treatment may affect positioning, especially on anterior body surfaces.
- The position required during radiotherapy may force the body into uncomfortable, static postures. Attention to these areas of the body may be very beneficial. For example, during radiation for breast cancer, patients must lie with the arm positioned over the head. The inflammation that accompanies the treatment shortens muscles and connective tissue in the chest and shoulders.

Surgery

Cancer patients will have surgery for a variety of reasons: removal of tumors is one of them; other common reasons are reconstruction, such as for breast cancer or head and neck cancers, pain management, placement of medical devices, or to prevent a calamitous problem, such as preventing the collapse of vertebrae due to spinal metastases. Further information can be found later in this chapter in the surgery section.

Many cancer patients have lymph nodes removed as part of the diagnostic process or the surgery. This, in combination with radiation therapy, puts them at risk for lymphedema. Because the massage given to the medically complex patient is basically comfort-oriented, the risk of a patient developing lymphedema from gentle strokes is negligible. People who have an active case of lymphedema can still have a touch session, but the safest course of action is to apply only light holds to the affected quadrant, unless a therapist is specifically trained in lymphatic techniques for lymphedema. Further information on lymphedema is given in Chapter 8.

Clinical considerations: Surgery

- Clinical considerations can be found in the surgery section at the end of this chapter.

Cardiovascular conditions

Cardiovascular diseases (CVDs) are disorders of the heart and blood vessels. Globally, they account for more deaths than any other cause.[13] Typically, cardiovascular diseases do not exist in isolation, and are commonly linked to obesity, diabetes, kidney and liver disease. This is a recurring theme throughout this chapter.

Common CVDs are coronary heart disease, most commonly caused by atherosclerosis, cardiomyopathy, congestive heart failure, cardiac arrhythmias, peripheral artery disease, and stroke. These conditions can lead to various outcomes, such as heart attack, poor cardiac output, blood clot risk, high blood pressure, and diminished peripheral circulation. Because strokes (cerebrovascular accidents) have a unique clinical profile, appropriate information is presented at the end of this section, with a separate list of Clinical considerations.

With the broad definition of massage being used in this text, some form of bodywork is appropriate for all types of cardiac patients. There are several factors common to all of them, each of which is an indication for a gentler touch. One is the use of anticoagulants, a group of medications that prevents platelets from adhering to one another and which may cause easy bruising if the dosage is high enough. Fatigue, edema, and comorbidities, such as kidney disease and diabetes, are other issues shared by many patients with heart problems. Typically, hospitalized heart disease patients also have certain positioning needs, such as the benefit of right side-lying, to decrease demand on cardiac output.

Severe conditions, such as heart attack, congestive heart failure, or heart surgery, require the bodywork practitioner to minimize cardiac output. A rough gauge of cardiac output can be made visually at the jugular vein. If there is any distension of this vessel, obtain doctor approval before embarking on massage that includes effleurage. Jugular vein distension occurs when the pressure inside the superior vena cava increases, causing the jugular vein to bulge. It is most visible on the right side of the patient's neck. A high central venous pressure is one of the signs of heart failure, a blockage, or other problems.[14]

Major lifestyle changes often must be made after a diagnosis of heart disease, and patients' resistance to these changes can be strong. Also, psychological issues, such as anxiety and depression, accompany serious cardiovascular concerns. Chapter 2, The frontier of knowledge: Exploring the research, presents a variety of studies showing that massage improves these variables for heart patients. Cardiac care often includes education activities such as guided imagery audiotapes for pre-surgical and post-surgical patients, and pairing massage with the tapes can be a powerful combination.

Arrhythmias

Arrhythmia is a condition in which the heart's electrical system goes awry. The damaged impulse can cause the heart to beat too fast, too slow, or erratically. This leads to the heart working inefficiently, with not enough blood being pumped to the lungs, brain, and other vital organs.

The most common arrhythmia is atrial fibrillation, which causes an irregular and fast heartbeat. Often the condition can be controlled with drugs that control the heart rate or convert the arrhythmia to a normal rhythm.[15,16] These patients will also be on anticoagulants to reduce the chance of a blood clot or stroke. Massage therapists will encounter many patients in geriatric settings affected by arrhythmia.

The touch therapist will encounter hospitalized arrhythmia patients when medications no longer can control the problem. Please see Chapter 9 for more details and information about massage adjustments for patients who have been treated in the heart catheterization lab.

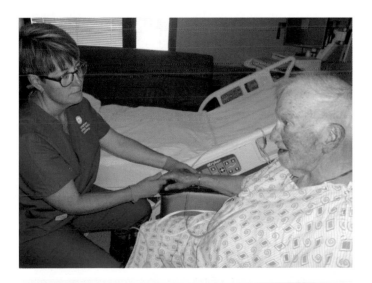

FIGURE 7.2
A cardiac patient receives hand massage sitting up rather than lying down due to breathing difficulties.

(Photo by Carolyn Jauco-Trott.)

Arteriosclerosis and atherosclerosis

Arteriosclerosis is the medical term for what is commonly called hardening of the arteries. When the arteries become thick and stiff from this condition, blood flow can be restricted to organs and tissues. Atherosclerosis is a specific type of arteriosclerosis. It refers to the build-up of plaque on the artery walls, which can restrict blood flow as well as lead to other problems, such as blood clots when plaque breaks off from the artery wall. The first line treatment for this is a group of medications called statins. Additionally, the person may be on an anticoagulant.

The complications of atherosclerosis can be very serious and depend on which arteries are blocked. If the narrowing is in coronary vessels, the outcome can be angina, a heart attack or congestive heart failure. The massage therapist might meet patients on the cardiac unit following a heart attack or coronary artery bypass graft (CABG) surgery (see Chapter 9 for more information.) If the stenosis is in the carotid artery, the risk is that the clot will break off and travel to the brain, causing a stroke. Peripheral artery disease can occur if the atherosclerosis develops in arteries that feed the arms and legs, causing circulation problems. Chronic kidney disease can occur if the narrowing is to the arteries leading to the kidneys, decreasing the body's ability to filter waste products.[17]

Congestive heart failure (CHF)

Congestive heart failure doesn't mean the heart has stopped pumping. Rather, it is the heart's inability to pump enough oxygenated blood. Eventually fluids can build up around the heart, in the lungs, abdomen, and lower extremities. There are many possible causes: hypertension, coronary heart disease, cardiomyopathy, chronic lung disease, anesthesia, surgery, pregnancy, drugs, diabetes, and obesity. To offset the side effects of diminished functioning, the heart rate increases, blood vessels constrict, and the heart enlarges, compensatory strategies that are themselves stressful to an already overworked heart.[18]

Poor oxygenation results in shortness of breath, fatigue, cyanosis, weakened immunity, anxiety, panic, and restlessness. These patients also are at increased risk for pneumonia. If they have been on prolonged bedrest, the touch therapist should be alert to the increased risk for pressure sores, thrombus, and pulmonary embolism.

Deep breathing is encouraged to avoid partial collapse of the lung, a condition known as atelectasis; massage to the respiratory muscles can support fuller breathing. In addition, it provides rest and alleviates psychological tension, fatigue, and insomnia. CHF patients don't sleep well at night due to restlessness and anxiety, a side effect of cerebral hypoxia.

The medical staff will manage the acute condition by reducing the heart's workload, administering oxygen, eliminating excess fluid accumulation, and increasing cardiac output with medications. Those with chronic congestive heart failure will commonly take diuretics to diminish excess fluid and various blood pressure and heart medications.[19]

Myocardial infarction (heart attack)

A myocardial infarction (MI) is commonly known as a heart attack. It occurs when a thrombus blocks one or more coronary arteries, depriving part of the heart muscle of oxygen. The area of the heart damaged when the oxygen supply is cut off is referred to as an infarct.

Treatment includes the administration of oxygen therapy and a multitude of drugs. Narcotics are given for pain; thrombolytics are used to dissolve the thrombus obstructing the coronary vessel; vasodilators, such as nitroglycerin, relax the coronary vascular system; beta-blockers are given to induce the heart to beat more slowly and with a more regular rhythm; calcium channel blockers decrease heart rate and blood pressure and dilate coronary vessels; and aspirin is prescribed as an anticoagulant.[20,21]

An important part of cardiac nursing care is to promote restfulness, which in turn will help the heart heal by lowering cardiac workload. *The Lippincott Nursing Manual* recommends: "back massage to promote relaxation, decrease muscle tension, and improve skin integrity."[22] Pain and anxiety reduction also could have been added to the above list. In addition to anxiety, a heart attack triggers a

host of other psychological reactions, such as depression, grief, and lowered self-esteem. These responses can hinder healing; anecdotal evidence indicates that massage may decrease some of these distressing feelings.

Clinical considerations: Cardiovascular conditions

Cardiac patients have many shared considerations. Where there is a clinical consideration specific to a certain group of heart care patients, an indication is given in parentheses.

Pressure:

- Blood clot risk.
- Bruising or bleeding risk due to thrombolytic and anticoagulant medications.
- Edema (CHF patients may also be affected by fluid in the lungs and body cavities).
- Fatigue.
- Fever (surgical patients most often).
- Light massage to the legs is often fine with staff approval.
- Minimize cardiac ouput. Maintain awareness of heart rate and distension of jugular vein.
- Pain medication.
- Possible cardiac and kidney complications.
- Psychological fragility.

Site:

- Blood clot risk (be mindful when massaging legs).
- Chest tubes (heart surgery).
- Electrodes on chest (MI and heart surgery).
- IV catheters.
- Leg incision (CABG surgery).
- Oxygen delivery device.
- Pacemaker or defibrillator site (usually under left clavicle).
- Sternal incision (open-heart surgery).

continued

Positioning:

- Elevate extremities if edematous. The feet should not be elevated above the heart to avoid stressing it through too much venous return.

- Flat position needed for a number of hours after an inguinal catheterization.

- Right side-lying, if the patient can tolerate, puts less strain on the heart.

- Patient should rise slowly from supine position.

- Semi-reclining position if the patient is short of breath.

- When rising from bed to a seated position, patient should sit with feet on the floor for a moment to minimize orthostatic hypotension.

Other:

- Certain patients may be on fluid intake restrictions. They may also be on diuretics and need to use the bathroom frequently. This can also lead to muscle cramps due to an imbalance in electrolytes.

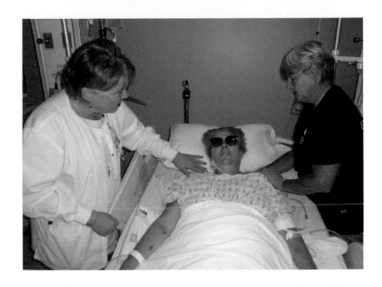

FIGURE 7.3
A stroke patient receiving massage in the ICU. (She is wearing sunglasses to protect her eyes from the light, which are sensitive due to headache.)

(Photo by Carolyn Jauco-Trott.)

Stroke

Stroke is the common term for a cerebrovascular accident. They are caused by internal brain vasculature problems, such as a blood clot, which is called an ischemic stroke. Another type of cerebrovascular accident is due to bleeding into the brain, which is known as a hemorrhagic stroke and is the result of a vessel wall that weakens to the point of breaking. A vessel can break because of an aneurysm, or as a result of a congenital malformation that reaches a point of breakage, referred to as an arteriovenous malformation (AVM). Transient ischemic attacks (TIAs) are considered "mini strokes" and rarely lead to hospitalization.[23,24]

The side effects of a stroke are dependent on where in the brain the occluded vessel is located. Usually weakness or partial paralysis, also known as hemiparesis, will occur on one side of the body. The affected side may have spasticity, diminished awareness of touch and proprioception, and lack of discrimination of size, shape, and texture. Mental processes may be affected and can manifest as changes in memory, judgment, concentration, and confusion. Impaired speech and vision, as well as incontinence, are also common. Following a stroke, patients are at risk for deep vein thrombosis, aspiration pneumonia, joint contractures, edema, fatigue, and other emotional states, such as hostility, uncooperativeness, and depression.

A cerebrovascular accident may be treated with thrombolytic drugs to dissolve the blood clot and anticoagulants to prevent formation of additional clots. Diuretics are given to reduce cerebral edema, and calcium channel blockers reduce blood pressure and help prevent spasm of the vessels in the brain. After the acute phase is over, medications may also be administered to reduce spastic paralysis and contracture.[25]

Rehabilitation is a core treatment. Physical therapy helps to reestablish range of motion, build strength, and regain motor control. Occupational therapy teaches the patient how to move and perform activities of daily living (ADLs). Manual therapists should work in conjunction with the rehabilitation experts and will commonly be a welcome addition to the health care team. While more specific research is needed, manual therapies may support the return to health of stroke patients by increasing circulation, limiting spasticity, diminishing joint contractures, and providing sensory stimulation, which in turn improves motor function.

Therapist's journal 7.2
Michael

Seven weeks ago, Michael, who is 60 years young, had a stroke that left him frustrated and depressed. It was his wife who briefed me on his condition. Michael had spent weeks in ICU due to complications post-intubation, and today he sat up in a chair for the first time since admission. His left side was compromised, he had swallowing problems, was being tube fed, had slurred speech, and had a urinary catheter. She was concerned that his chronically left-rotated head might be contributing to his swallowing difficulties and hoped that massage could help.

Michael's wife also told me that he was a passionate collector of rare guitars and had published a book documenting his major finds and transactions. Upon meeting Michael and recognizing our shared interest in guitars, I acknowledged his passion, which provoked a short interaction about instruments and music, during which time his wife proudly removed his book from a drawer to share with me. This sweet moment supported an easy transition to the subject of massage, which he was open to, and even requested me to treat specific areas. Although I couldn't fulfill his request for leg massage (due to our hospital policy), I assured him that shoulder, neck and feet massage were available.

As soon as I touched and gently held his upper left quadrant between my hands, he closed his eyes and let out a low sigh, his face softening. He continued to breathe easily with closed eyes as I massaged this area and his neck with slow, rhythmic and deliberate moves. As his body relaxed and settled in my hands, it was obvious that nothing forced or imposed was needed, or appropriate for that matter.

His wife sat quietly as I removed the compression device from his lower legs and continued the gentle rhythmic strokes to his feet. "This is the most relief he's had since we arrived 7 weeks ago," she said. Her face looked worn and anxious. "Can I give you a shoulder rub after I'm finished with Michael?" Her eyes looked a bit surprised as she nodded. "Yes. I can relax for a bit now that he looks so comfortable."

Michael slept soundly as I massaged his wife.

Kate Phelan CMT
San Francisco, California

Special attention to positioning is necessary when caring for stroke survivors. Because of a lack of motor control and strength, the person who has suffered a stroke may be unable to hold certain positions and may require special devices or supportive items to maintain body alignment and prevent contractures. The nursing staff will use footboards, night casts, splints, or braces to accomplish this. In addition to the client's limited abilities to self-reposition, extra attention is advised to help relieve pressure from the client's body pressing against the bed, wheelchair or even another body part. For example, when the patient is in side-lying position, a pillow placed between the knees and ankles will help to avoid the discomfort of one bony prominence pressing against another. While the able-bodied hospital patient could move their knee if it became uncomfortable, the person who is severely weakened or paralyzed cannot.

If spasticity is present, begin massage or stretches in the direction of flexion to the end range, but not beyond. Then, gently stretch in the direction of extension. Do not go beyond the limits of the tissues, but holding at end range is generally helpful. If contracture is found, do not attempt to stretch the soft tissue as the bone has over grown and is structurally limiting the range of motion.

Clinical considerations: Stroke

Pressure:

- Sensory impairment may affect a patient's ability to report potential micro-tears or other strains to tissue, so keep pressure to level 2 or below. Inch forward with clients once they are out of the acute phase and are recovering.
- Easy bruising due to thrombolytic or anticoagulant medications.
- Edema.
- Fatigue.
- Poor proprioceptive and touch awareness.
- Risk of further thrombus.
- Unstable joints on the affected side.

Site:

- Assess the skin for areas prone to developing pressure sores.

Positioning:

- Avoid side-lying on affected side for those with hemi-paralysis.
- Allow extra time for positioning.
- As noted elsewhere, if the patient is unable to reposition independently, request assistance from the patient's RN or caregiver.
- Do not allow the affected limb to hang or drop unsupported as muscle strength and control will be reduced or absent.
- Be careful not to use an affected limb to reposition or pull the patient into position.
- Supine and side-lying on the unaffected side are best.
- When the patient is side-lying, use pillows under the head, between the knees, under the top arm, and against the back (see Figure 6.2B). A pillow may be necessary behind the back to maintain the side-lying position.

- Position the affected limbs to avoid pressure on bony areas, such as the elbows, ankles, and knees.
- When the patient is in a seated position, elevate the affected arm and hand to prevent edema.
- Barring other factors, such as breathing difficulties, return the bed to a mostly flat position after the massage to prevent hip flexion contracture.

Other:

- The unaffected side can also benefit from massage to muscles that are compensating.
- With some stroke survivors, it may be important to speak slowly and patiently repeat questions as needed with an encouraging attitude. The communication tips in Info Box 7.2 will be useful for some stroke patients. For others without cognitive impairment, normal communication will be appreciated.
- Avoid doing things for patients that they can do themselves.
- When the massage session is over, return the overbed table, telephone, and TV remote to the unaffected side.

Diabetes

If this chapter were organized by frequency of diseases rather than alphabetically, diabetes, particularly type 2 diabetes, would be at the start. Diabetes is a chronic condition affecting the way the body processes blood sugar and is at the center of many modern-day illnesses, such as high blood pressure and heart, liver, and kidney diseases. Massage therapists will encounter this health situation more often than any other, especially within the medically complex populations seen in hospitals, nursing facilities, home health care, hospice, and rehabilitation centers. The World Health Organization reported the global level of diabetes in 2014 to be 8.5%.[26] In the United States, as of 2017, nearly 10% of adults have diabetes and another 34% are prediabetic.[27] Similar statistics are true in England.[28,29] In 5–19-year olds, according to UNICEF, nearly 20% of children were overweight in 2016, compared with 10% in 2000. No longer is this a problem in high and middle-income countries, it has also become a stark reality in lower income nations.[30] This is an issue because of the known links between obesity, diabetes, and heart, liver, and kidney diseases, as well as susceptibility to certain cancers, and endocrine, joint, and mental health problems. The obesity problem is a slowly ticking bomb that will explode in the future, overwhelming the health care system.

Diabetes can be the result of a variety of influences: pregnancy, medications, certain infections, heredity, lifestyle choices, or disease, such as cancer or hyperthyroidism. At first, the symptoms can be so mild that a person doesn't realize they are affected. Over time, diabetes worsens, even if a patient doesn't at first need medication to control the problem. Diabetes damages nerves, which mainly causes peripheral neuropathy.[31] It also damages blood vessels: deterioration of the larger blood vessels increases the risk of heart disease, hypertension, stroke, and aneurysm, while small blood vessel damage causes kidney and eye problems. People with diabetes develop atherosclerosis (arteriosclerosis) at a more aggressive rate. Not only is plaque laid down on the inside of blood vessels, but it can be deposited throughout the body. This leads to restricted blood flow to organs and tissues.[32] Poor circulation also gives rise to edema in the limbs, as well as diminished wound healing and fragile skin. In the advanced stages of diabetes, the connective tissues can be very fragile and easily injured. Ulcerations and gangrene are a possibility and can eventually lead to amputation, most often in the extremities.[31]

Generally, diabetes is managed on an outpatient basis with diet, exercise, and medication, including insulin injections, and oral diabetes medications, such as metformin. If a patient is hospitalized, it is due to a severe episode of destabilization. Secondary complications, such as renal or cardiovascular disease, are the other common reasons a person with diabetes is hospitalized.[33]

The medical history of a person who has had the disease for a long time can be complicated and may require a number of massage adjustments. Massage should not be demanding on the body and thereby contributing to a disruption of the homeostatic equilibrium. In his book, *Massage Therapy and Medications,* Randall Persad warns against increasing the metabolic demands on the body or the workload of the heart for those with advanced diabetes. Shorter sessions, perhaps 20 minutes, are advisable at the beginning to gauge the person's response to the massage.[34] Using gentle modalities may be best during periods of severe destabilization.

Patients with uncontrolled diabetes are more susceptible to infection, and once they have an infection, it is slow to resolve. The tissue in areas that have received repeated insulin injections tends to become fibrotic. It may have poor color and sensation, and like a scar, it can cause tugging on nearby structures, reduce range of motion, and create edema distal to the area. Massage or stretching to these sites should be performed with care.

A patient's story 7.1   It's never too late to try something new

I was in the hospital overnight because of a kidney problem. To my amazement, a foot massage was offered to me by a student massage therapist. I was hesitant and only agreed to try it because my daughter wanted me to. I'm 75 years old and had never had a massage. Plus, I was uncomfortable about having my feet massaged – the big toe on my right foot was removed 3 weeks before, a side effect of diabetes. The student said that she could just massage my hands and the unaffected foot. So I gave it a try. I liked it so much that I even let the therapist touch the foot that had had the amputation. I had no idea it could feel so good. It's never too late to try new things.

D.R. Portland, Oregon

Clinical considerations: Diabetes

Pressure:

- Cardiovascular and renal disease.
- Easily destabilized.
- Easy bruising.
- Edema.
- Fatigue.
- Fragile skin or connective tissue.
- Lack of sensation locally or systemically.
- Old injection sites.

Site:

- Insulin pump and continuous glucose monitoring sites.
- Fragile skin.
- Old injection sites.
- Slow-healing wounds.
- Ulcerations.

Positioning:

- Edema.
- Ulcerations.
- Amputations.

Other:

- Become knowledgeable about the signs and symptoms of low blood sugar shown in Info Box 7.1.

Info Box 7.1 Signs and symptoms of low blood sugar[35]

- Irregular heart beat
- Fatigue
- Pale skin
- Shakiness
- Anxiety
- Sweating
- Hunger
- Irritability

Geriatrics

Geriatrics is the medical field that specializes in health care for aging adults. More than any other group, massage practitioners will meet older people in every aspect of health care. They will see them in hospitals, rehabilitation centers, care homes, and assisted living and nursing facilities. The reader might then think that this should be the most sizable section in this chapter. However, in a way, Chapters 7–10 are primarily about older adults. So, just a few specific hints will be given here about this very large section of the global population.

One hint is not to underestimate aging people. They are perceived as being delicate and frail, requiring massage pressure to be greatly reduced. It is true that adjustments should be made because of thin skin, diseases, joint replacements, or failing memories, but older people can rail against the overly tentative treatment they often receive from massage therapists. There may be areas of the body where an older person could safely receive a more firm touch, such as the upper trapezius muscles or feet.

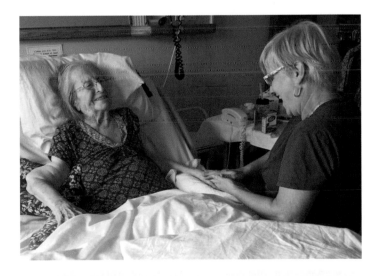

FIGURE 7.4
A patient loving her weekly massages for the touch and laughter.

(Photo by Gayle MacDonald.)

An older person will readily appreciate the benefits of massage. If they have mobility issues due to arthritis, there may be a feeling of tension in their body, which massage ameliorates. Touch therapies support relaxation, increase energy, improve shortness of breath, and joint mobility. There is also the emotional benefit that everyone experiences from kind, compassionate touch. It is not uncommon for older adults to be isolated, which can lead to depression. Perhaps their spouse has died and their children live far away. Hearing loss and vision changes can add to the isolation. Never make assumptions about older adults and how they will react to an offer of massage. They are often at the front of the line.

Clinical considerations: Geriatrics

Pressure:

- Bruising/bleeding risk, which can be due to blood thinners, thin skin, or diabetes.
- Thin, fragile skin.
- Osteoporosis.

Site:

- Skin conditions, such as torn or scabbed-over areas, especially over the shins and forearms.
- Medical equipment and aids, e.g., oxygen delivery systems.

Positioning:

- Fall precautions. Offer support/assistance with dressing/undressing if needed. This can be related to brain changes as the person ages, low blood pressure, neurological problems, muscular weakness, and medications.
- Be certain to allow the patient plenty of time to get into and out of the massage position.
- Arthritic changes may affect mobility.
- May require extra use of pillows or bolstering.
- A seated position may be the best option for people with poor mobility or breathing issues.

Other:

- Older adults are commonly admitted to the hospital for three reasons: dehydration, falls, and misuse or over-prescription of medications. Both dehydration and medication problems can present with mental confusion.

Infections

Infections are the result of a combination of factors, bacterial or fungal exposure and lowered immunity for the most part. Hospitals, rehab centers, and nursing facilities are prime environments for their development. Below, the focus is on four common infections: pneumonia, cellulitis, septicemia, and urinary tract infections. Chapter 5 gives the reader a broader view of infections as they relate to protective practices.

Pneumonia

Pneumonia is a very common reason for hospital admittance and is a leading cause of infection-related deaths. It is not a single disease but can be one of more than 50 different diseases, each of which inflames the lungs. Bacteria, viruses, or fungi are common causes. The various pneumonias are divided into four main categories: 1) community-acquired, which are triggered by micro-organisms found in the community, such as pneumococci or influenza; 2) hospital-acquired; 3) health care-acquired, which occur in people who live in long-term care facilities or receive care in outpatient clinics, such as a hemodialysis clinic; and 4) aspiration pneumonia, caused by aspirating foreign matter. Pneumonia is often secondary to another condition, such as immunosuppression, chronic obstructive pulmonary disease (COPD), or cardiac failure. It results in fluid around and in the lungs, which accounts for breathing difficulty, coughing, and chest pain. People admitted to the hospital for pneumonia usually have a fever and fatigue and sometimes mental confusion, nausea, vomiting and diarrhea.[36,37]

Clinical considerations: Pneumonia

Pressure:

- During the most acute phase, especially when the patient is febrile and fatigued, bodywork should consist of level 1 stroking and/or holding techniques.

Site:

- Oxygen delivery device.
- IV catheters.

Positioning:

- Change of position is good to prevent pooling of secretions in lungs.
- The patient will need to maintain an upright or semi-reclining position due to cough and dyspnea.

Other:

- Deeper breathing is helpful.
- If the patient is hypoxic, mental status may be affected.

Cellulitis

Cellulitis is a common bacterial infection that can be serious, potentially spreading throughout the body. The infection frequently appears on the lower legs, but can present on the face, arms, chest, and other areas. It tends to occur when a break in the skin allows bacteria, most often *Streptococcus* or *Staphylococcus*, to enter. The classic symptoms are heat, tenderness or pain, redness, and swelling. The red area of skin affected by the infection tends to spread, which is worrisome.

There are many risk factors for cellulitis. It can be caused by injuries, such as a fracture, burn, or scrape; or a weakened immune system, such as in older people, those being treated for cancer, diabetes, or HIV/AIDS. The risk increases with that of lymphedema, and for people who are overweight.[38] Touch practitioners will encounter people with cellulitis in every type of venue. In fact, they may be the ones who notice the symptoms first and report it to the nursing staff. A person with diagnosed or suspected cellulitis could have a touch session with holds only: traditional massage should be discontinued until the patient finishes the course of antibiotics and has been given the all-clear by staff.

Septicemia

According to the 2015 Healthcare Cost and Utilization Project data, septicemia was the most common reason in the United States for hospitalization except for labor and delivery.[39] Septicemia, commonly called *blood poisoning*, most often occurs in people who have low immunity, such as the elderly, those with chronic conditions, or patients taking immunosuppressing drugs. It often occurs due to a bacterial infection entering the bloodstream as a result of pneumonia, a urinary tract infection (UTI), a scratch received while working in the garden, a surgical incision, an IV line or urinary catheter, cellulitis from lymphedema, or a severe burn. Fungal-induced septicemia, such as from *Candida auris*, is also on the rise in health care facilities.[40]

Septicemia can develop into sepsis, which can be life-threatening. The pathophysiology of sepsis is extremely complicated. The body reacts with a severe inflammatory response that causes fever or hypothermia, increased heart rate and breathing, mental confusion, and either a high or low white blood cell count. Coagulation problems occur that may cause either easy bleeding or the formation of blood clots that reduce the flow of blood to limbs and internal organs. In the worst-case scenario, the blood pressure drops, leading to poor circulation to the organs and thus multiple organ failure.[41]

Urinary tract infection (UTI)

Urinary tract infections are caused by the presence of pathogenic bacteria in the urinary tract. People might be hospitalized because of a UTI, or it may develop in the health care facility secondary to another condition, such as an indwelling urinary catheter or as a result of treatment for kidney stones. Common symptoms are the frequent and urgent need to urinate, pain or discomfort just above the pubic bone, abdominal tenderness, fever, nausea, and vomiting.[42] Urinary tract infections are one of the most common reasons for hospital admittance in the elderly.[43] Commonly, elderly patients with a UTI undergo a change in their mental status because of the infection.

The treatment for a UTI is generally with antibiotics. When a person is diagnosed with only a UTI, the clinical considerations for the massage are more straightforward. Massage for individuals in whom the UTI is secondary to other factors, such as aging or kidney disease, will be more complex and require the therapist to study other sections of this book.

Clinical considerations: Infections

Pressure:

- Until a person is well stabilized and has completed the course of antibiotics, the therapist should use only gentle holds.

- Once the medical or nursing staff have given approval, massage should be confined to a slow level 1 pressure (lotioning).

Site:

- Touch therapy should be avoided in areas containing localized infection, such as cellulitis.

Intensive care unit (ICU)

Providing massage therapy in the ICU is simple in terms of the actual hands-on intervention. The environment, however, is unique in the amount of information there is to be gathered from fellow practitioners, from the activity on the unit, in the patient's room, and during interactions with the patient. Patients in the ICU are, by definition, too medically unstable to be cared for on another unit in the hospital. Their health status may be so unstable that it may change during a massage session.

A variety of skills are required in order to provide massage therapy in the ICU: concise communication, moment-to-moment awareness, and real-time critical thinking. Therapists need to understand the essentials of the body's systems and the ways in which it is affected when one or more vital organs are compromised. A medically complex patient is unable to maintain homeostasis on their own, so any challenge to the body's attempt to achieve stability can result in grave consequences.

Session planning for massage in the ICU is focused on supporting the body in the already difficult work it is doing to heal or to die. Therapists must learn as much as they can about what has brought a patient to the state of injury or disease that necessitates intensive care. The touch session should not cause the body to shunt resources away from its basic function – the goal is to add to the patient's reserves, not deplete them in any way.

Massage practitioners will need to formulate key questions to discern a patient's health status. The questions will vary depending on the patient, and other members of the health care team are usually happy to collaborate in this process. However, they don't typically know what is useful for a massage therapist to know, so it is the massage practitioner's responsibility to ask specific questions to ascertain the required information.

Providing safe massage in the ICU requires an understanding of a patient's skin integrity, bone fragility, infection status, input and output of fluids, stage and severity of disease, and goals of care. Massage therapy can often result in subtle changes in vital signs like blood pressure, breathing and oxygen saturation. In a healthy person, these imperceptible changes are no cause for worry, but for a patient who has pulmonary, cardiac, or neurological issues, such slight differences can be serious. A massage therapist needs to check with the patient's nurse about the possibility of these changes occurring during the massage. In this way they can understand the safe ranges for the patient and be on the lookout for anything that would necessitate a shift in focus, intensity, or pace of the massage or that may require a nurse's attention.

In addition to the patient, it is vital to understand who else is in the room. If there are concerns or issues related to family dynamics, part of providing good care is maintaining an awareness of these issues in communicating with the various visitors. It's very easy to accidentally divulge protected health information if the relationships between the patient and their visitors are not understood. For example, it may seem obvious to the therapist, based on their conversations with the health care team, that a patient is in an end-of-life process, but it should not be assumed that a patient's loved ones share that understanding. A well-meaning reassurance or sharing of something you understand as fact can result in great confusion and unnecessary suffering.

Therapist's journal 7.3
He knew me from my touch

After major heart surgery, one of our cardiac intensive care patients had to be placed in a medically induced coma in order to heal. Before they put him under, his nurse asked him if he wanted gentle massage while he was in a coma because of his extreme shoulder and neck tension. He answered in the affirmative. Twice I massaged him while he was in a coma and the third time after he was awake. When I started to massage him the third time, he commented that he knew me from my touch and it had been so soothing when he was "under."

Del Delashmutt LMT
Portland, Oregon

Many patients in the ICU are not able to communicate verbally, either because they are medically sedated, or due to brain or other injuries. Some of these patients can blink their eyes or squeeze a hand in answer to simple, slowly-asked questions. However, most practitioners are not accustomed to asking simple yes/no questions. Therapists tend to say things such as, "How can I make you more comfortable?" or "Do you need another pillow or should I move the one you have?" These are hard questions to answer with a blink or a squeeze. Learning to ask one, simple question at a time when working with

these patients is key to understanding their needs and to creating trust and comfort with massage therapy – likely an uncommon experience in the ICU.

When patients are not able to communicate at all, touch practitioners need to slow the process even more. It is hard to know if a person who cannot communicate wants to be touched. Training and experience will help to cultivate the skill of tuning in to the subtle signals that will give massage therapists a sense of whether touch is welcome and how to modify the session.

It is not easy to interpret these signs – it requires patience and keen perception. Commonly the patient's heart rate or breathing may accelerate when you first come into contact with their body. If these stay elevated after you have been in contact for a few minutes, this could be a sign that your touch is too stimulating for a patient. A patient's brow may furrow or maybe their legs or arms move slightly or their eyelids flutter. One helpful practice is to stand outside the patient's room but where the patient can be clearly seen, and simply observe for 60 seconds or so. This gives the therapist an opportunity beforehand to note some of the patient's signs before contact, which gives a baseline from which to gauge the possible signals.

It's important to maintain physical contact with the patient. Each time the practitioner takes their hands off the patient and then places them in another location, the patient's nervous system can be slightly jarred. Contact should be full and confident without sinking into the tissue as you might with a more robust patient. It's important to have complete, full-handed contact, even when using a gentler pressure. However, massage strokes that are deep or long are potentially unsafe for the ICU patient: small, gentle, circular effleurage or compressions, still holds, or thumb circles are commonly employed strokes. A tentative, feathery touch can be irritating to the nervous system. It can be helpful to use a patient's breathing, even when it's very slow or even a little unpredictable, as a guide for pacing.

Finally, the ICU can be a place of great confusion and sadness for families as well as patients. Families feel helpless as they watch their loved one in a critically ill or injured state. They want the pain and suffering to be lessened and will often immediately reject massage as "one more thing they don't need" or they might ask the therapist to work with the patient even though the practitioner is getting clear signals from the patient that massage is not wanted. The patient must always be the priority and the center of the interaction. It can be difficult to maintain that focus when family members are crying or upset or when they are saying, "They can't feel it anyway," or "They can't hear you. You don't have to introduce yourself," or "They've always loved massage in the past."

Kidney disease

Because kidney disease is a silent killer, most people don't realize how common it is. The World Health Organization states that it is: "possible that, each year, at least as many deaths are attributable to kidney disease as to cancer, diabetes, or respiratory diseases."[44]

The job of the kidneys is to filter waste and excess water from the blood and excrete them in urine, produce red blood cells, secrete hormones that build bone, control blood acidity, and keep electrolytes balanced. If the filters, which are known as nephrons, are damaged, kidney function is reduced. The two most common causes of this damage are hypertension and diabetes. The previous section on diabetes details how the kidneys can become damaged. When the kidneys don't filter wastes and manage the extra water build-up, other health problems can occur.[45] Kidney diseases are categorized as chronic kidney disease, acute kidney injury, and end stage renal disease.

Chronic kidney disease

The number of people worldwide who have chronic kidney disease (CKD) is rising. The reason for the rise in this condition is three-fold: an escalation in diabetes due to greater obesity levels, an increase in hypertension cases, and an aging global population. Studies show that 10–13% of the global adult population has chronic kidney disease,[46] which is consistent with European and UK numbers.[47,48] However, the CDC estimate is even higher for adults in the USA at 15%.[49]

People often don't realize they have CKD at first as there are no symptoms, which is why it is referred to as the silent killer. By the time the condition is discovered, a significant amount of a patient's kidney function has been destroyed. As CKD worsens over time, other health problems can occur: anemia; low calcium and high phosphorus levels which cause osteoporosis; high potassium levels which cause an abnormal heart beat; nausea and loss of appetite; fluid retention; a weakened immune system; insomnia, and depression.[50]

There is no research to guide massage therapists in their work with patients who have chronic kidney disease. Common sense, anecdotal experience/evidence, and an understanding of the function of the kidneys along with the impact of CKD's co-morbidities must steer the way when a therapist is making clinical decisions. For example, if the person has swollen ankles, it is a sign that the kidneys are not functioning well and therefore the massage session plan should be made less demanding.

The decision-making process for patients in the next two categories, acute kidney injury and end stage renal disease, is much easier and clearer because of their complexity.

Acute kidney injury

Acute kidney injury (AKI), sometimes called acute kidney (or renal) failure, happens when the kidneys are suddenly damaged within a few hours or days. Although AKI can happen to anyone, those with diabetes, hypertension, or of advanced age are at higher risk. AKI is often a hospital-acquired complication due to surgery or an acute illness, such as a heart condition, liver failure, or sepsis. It can also be triggered by severe bleeding, shock, severe burns, dehydration, or toxic drugs.

People with acute kidney injury will not pass enough urine, will experience severe fatigue, swelling in the lower extremities, shortness of breath, confusion, nausea, chest pain or pressure, and in severe cases may have seizures or fall into a coma. An incidence of AKI increases the risk of developing CKD, stroke, and other cardiovascular events. Treatment is with temporary hemodialysis, medications, and the administration of fluids; however, death is also a real possibility.[51]

Despite the severity of this condition, touch therapy can be given, but, clearly, massage therapy must be in the level 1 range or gentle holds given with the intention of comfort.

End-stage renal disease

Once damage occurs to the kidneys, it cannot be reversed. Both chronic kidney disease and acute kidney injury can advance into end-stage renal disease. One happens progressively over years and the other develops very quickly, but both lead to the same end point, dangerous levels of fluid, electrolytes, and the build-up of wastes in the body. This leads to symptoms such as hypertension, shortness of breath, fatigue, nausea and vomiting, sleep difficulties, muscle cramps and twitches, and rapid heartbeat. In addition, the skin of renal patients is dry and more susceptible to breakdown due to itching and poor skin integrity from edema. The mental status of some patients in kidney failure can be highly impaired because of high levels of toxicity.[52]

For patients to survive, dialysis or kidney transplantation is needed. Hemodialysis is the most common way to cleanse the blood. A smaller group of patients are treated with peritoneal dialysis. People who qualify for kidney transplantation will be on dialysis until a new kidney is found. (More information about dialysis can be found in Chapter 9.) Dialysis will allow a person to have a functional life, but is not a permanent solution.[52]

Clearly, massage needs be less demanding for most people with kidney disease. For those in end-stage kidney disease, it needs to at level 1 or 2, bearing in mind that the kidneys are not filtering the waste products in the blood, leaving more toxins in the body of these patients.

Clinical considerations: Kidney disease

Pressure:

- Cardiovascular complications, e.g. stroke risk, shortness of breath.

- Co-existing conditions, e.g., diabetes, hypertension.
- Edema.
- Fatigue.
- Homeostatic disequilibrium.
- Abnormal toxin levels.

Site:

- Shunt site if patient is receiving hemodialysis. Stay well away from this.
- Skin fragility.
- Tenderness from kidney surgery.

Positioning:

- Tenderness from kidney surgery, past or recent. Allow the patient to guide this process. Most likely they will prefer supine at first. Some people find side-lying uncomfortable.
- Shortness of breath in advanced cases.

Liver disease

The liver performs over 500 different functions. It is part of the digestive system, metabolizes drugs, detoxifies other wastes, and creates proteins for a variety of functions related to immune function, blood plasma, and coagulation, to name but a few.[53] This very important organ can be damaged by excessive alcohol use, over-the-counter medications, viruses, liver cancer, autoimmune diseases, and the accumulation of fat in the liver. Diseases of the liver are a serious issue, with incidences on the rise globally in line with increasing obesity levels. The UK, Europe, Asia, Africa, and the USA all report an increase in liver disease.[54]

Fatty liver disease

In some areas of the world the increase in liver disease is due to higher levels of obesity, diabetes, and alcohol consumption, all of which cause an accumulation of fat inside the liver cells.[55,56]

Nonalcoholic fatty liver disease (NAFLD) has become common in the developed world. In Europe, the rate is slightly lower than 25%.[57] The NHS reports that approximately 30% of Britons have early stage NAFLD,[58] and in the USA, 25–30% of adults have NAFLD.[59] NAFLD is usually not problematic unless the liver becomes inflamed, which happens in about 20% of cases. This condition, referred to as nonalcoholic steatohepatitis (NASH), can lead to fibrosis and cirrhosis of the liver. Alcohol-related fatty liver disease can lead to hepatitis and cirrhosis.[56]

Hepatitis

In other parts of the world, liver disease is largely due to viral hepatitis. The World Health Organization reports that: "deaths from HIV, tuberculosis, and malaria are declining while mortality caused by viral hepatitis is on the rise."[54] The viruses that cause significant liver disease are hepatitis B (HBV) and C (HCV). These viruses lead to inflammation of the liver, which can cause scarring, diminishing its ability to function. HBV and HCV are not transmitted by casual contact. While they can be communicated via semen or vaginal secretions, their primary route of infection is via blood from tainted transfusions, use of a contaminated needle, or from an accidental needle stick injury while performing a medical procedure on an HBV or HCV patient. Contact with contaminated blood can also enter another person's bloodstream through an open wound, cut, or scratch.[60,61]

According to the British Liver Trust, Hepatitis B is 50–100 times more infectious than HIV.[60] The HBV virus is able to survive outside the body for at least a week: this means that objects used by the patient such as razors, toothbrushes, or blood stains on linen can convey the virus.[60] Hepatitis C can remain on a surface at room temperature for up to three weeks.[61] The implications of this information would seem obvious to bodyworkers, reinforcing the observance of Standard Precautions. A series of vaccinations for hepatitis B is available, although touch practitioners are not at risk of blood-borne contact in the same way as nursing staff or phlebotomists. No vaccine yet exists for hepatitis C, but highly effective treatments are available.

Two other common hepatitis viruses are type A (HAV) and E (HEV). Both are transmitted through the fecal-oral route, which is usually by way of contaminated water and food, but can also happen via oral to anal contact during sexual activity or from failing to handwash after changing a baby's diaper. Hepatitis A can survive for months outside of the body, including in freezing temperatures. Fortunately, most people recover from the virus without any long-term effects. It is very unlikely that a massage practitioner would be exposed to HAV or HEV within the scope of their health care duties.[62,63]

The symptoms for each type of virus are similar and include fatigue, fever, headache, nausea, vomiting, and jaundice. Patients with hepatitis B and C also may display skin disruptions, light sensitivity, edematous areas of skin, myalgias, arthritis, and vasculitis, the inflammation of which causes thickening, narrowing, and scarring of the blood vessels.[60,61] The inflammation caused by HBV and HCV can also develop into cirrhosis, the medical term describing the end stage scarring of the liver.

Cirrhosis and end stage liver disease

Cirrhotic scarring diminishes the liver's functioning. No matter the reason for developing cirrhosis, a person with it is susceptible to a variety of comorbidities, such as type 2 diabetes, cardiovascular disease, chronic kidney disease, chronic obstructive pulmonary disease, and liver cancer. Patients with advanced cirrhosis and end stage liver disease will develop a variety of complications. Ascites is common (see the ascites section in Chapter 8.) Swelling can also occur in the legs. Bile salts can deposit on the skin, causing intense itching. GI problems such as nausea, diarrhea, and constipation are common, as well as significant weight loss. There is a build-up of toxins, such as ammonia, causing concentration and memory problems and irritability. Platelet levels can drop due to coagulopathy, putting the person at risk for bleeding and bruising, and electrolytes can become unbalanced, causing muscle cramping.[64]

Clinical considerations: Liver disease
Pressure:

- Fatigue.
- Swelling in legs and abdomen.
- Bleeding and bruising risk.
- Fever.
- Myalgia.
- Nausea.

continued

Positioning:

- Nausea.
- Swelling in the legs and abdomen.

Neurological disorders

Neurological challenges range from conditions such as drop foot to traumatic brain injury (TBI). Any compromise or dysfunction in the central or peripheral nervous system can lead to a vast range of disabilities or challenges. The neurological conditions practitioners are likely to see in medical center environments include spinal cord injury (SCI), traumatic brain injury (TBI), and diseases including Alzheimer's, Lewy body dementia or other brain pathologies. Patients with recent injury may have a long hospital stay. Once the patient is stable, they may be discharged to a nursing facility, or rehabilitation center. Modified bodywork is appropriate in any of these medical settings and may truly be a significant support for patients in the healing process.

Traumatic brain injury (TBI)

Traumatic brain injury refers to events that cause brain injury from an outside impact as may happen in a fall, vehicle collision, or a direct hit from an object. The specific mechanisms of injury are classified as: direct impact, rapid acceleration and deceleration, penetrating injury, or blast waves. Damage caused by these events may include contusion or hematoma (bruising, temporary internal bleeding, swelling), and concussion: "a type of traumatic brain injury caused by a bump, blow, or jolt to the head or by a hit to the body that causes the head and brain to move rapidly back and forth. This sudden movement can cause the brain to bounce around or twist in the skull, creating chemical changes in the brain and sometimes stretching and damaging brain cells."[65] Defuse axonal injury is twisting of the brain tissue that can cause axons to shear or break. This often includes bleeding in the brain or brain lining. Many secondary mechanisms of injury may follow, including free radical injury to cells, electrolyte imbalances, inflammatory response, secondary ischemia, and infection.[23,24,65]

People living with TBI experience a wide range of changes to lifestyle and abilities. If the injury was to the front of the head (frontal cortex), it is likely the person has some level of personality changes. Depending on the extent of injury, activities of daily living (ADLs), speech, comprehension, motor coordination, or social skills may be affected. Remember that a patient's health status is not fixed: there will be changes over time – sometimes improvements, sometimes decompensation.

Clinical considerations: Traumatic brain injury

Pressure:

- If the patient has limited ability to give clear feedback and input, start with level 2 pressure and inch forward. Slow lotioning or level 1 may also provide benefit. Avoid over-stimulating the client and look for somatic indicators of discomfort or irritation.

Site:

- Avoid circulatory techniques to head during acute injury phase to limit any possible increase of inflammation to the brain. Gentle holds with limited duration may be helpful.

Positioning:

- For significantly impaired patients, caregiver assistance may be required. Be mindful of good communication, even if speech or comprehension is limited (see Info Box 7.2, Communicating with the person who is neurologically impaired).

- Avoid draping that may be too tight or restricting; allow for easy movement of all limbs to avoid sensation of constriction or binding as it may be misunderstood and/or agitating for the client.

Other:

- Uninhibited behaviors are common in persons with history of TBI and can range from overly affectionate to easily frustrated or angered. These are the result of compromised processing in the brain and should not be taken personally.

Spinal cord injury (SCI)

Spinal cord injuries are categorized as *complete* or *incomplete*. For those with a complete injury, it means that nerve damage is obstructing all signals coming from the brain to the body below the injury. An incomplete injury, on the other hand, causes varying degrees of motor function loss distal to the damaged area. Typically, sensation is partially preserved in dermatomes below the area of injury to a greater extent than motor function.[66] Initially, after the injury, there is a phase referred to as spinal cord shock, in which the person may experience cardiovascular symptoms, such as dilation of the peripheral blood vessels, dangerously low blood pressure, a slow heart rate, and the risk of hypothermia. Other serious complications often associated with SCI are respiratory infections, DVT/VTE/PE risk, pain, pressure sores, urinary and bowel motility issues, and of course, reduced abilities to perform many activities of daily living.[67]

Besides providing the usual benefits, massage has specific uses for people with spinal cord injury. A study that examined massage and guided imagery for pain and fatigue showed that both interventions given weekly over a five-week period reduced both pain and fatigue.[68] Over time, massage techniques and careful stretching may help relieve painful postural distortions. Commonly, people with SCI have overuse problems in their hands, wrists, elbows, and shoulders.

Clinical considerations: Spinal cord injury[66,67,69,70]

Pressure:

- Limit pressure to level 2 or below for sensory-impaired areas (generally below the level of injury).
- Level 1 pressure is indicated for keeping skin healthy.
- For acute injury and during early rehabilitation, keep pressure to level 2 or below in non-affected areas as well. Over-stimulation can be an issue for patients with limited internal controls, therefore firmer pressures are contraindicated during this phase of healing.
- Continued risk for DVT.

Site:

- Avoid medical devices and be aware of catheters, feeding tubes, and ostomy bags.
- Notify patient and/or health care provider if pressure sores are suspected.
- If muscle is spastic, stretch into the direction of contraction first, then use caution to stretch and extend muscle in opposite direction, just short of its limitation.
- If muscle is flaccid, gentle holds or energy work is indicated.
- Calcium deposits can form bone fragments in the soft tissue, causing inflammation and thus pain at the site.

Positioning:

- Caregiver assistance will be required for any transfers or repositioning unless patient is able to self-position.
- Providing touch therapy while patient is in a wheelchair is a viable option.
- Be watchful for limbs leaning into rails or wheelchair parts that may lead to pressure sores or bruising. Add a rolled towel for comfort and pressure relief. Notify caregivers of any tissue damage observed. Even skin reddening can be a symptom of a pressure sore beginning. Early detection and correction can save days or weeks of wound healing procedures.

Other:

- The duration of sessions with SCI clients may be appropriately longer than sessions with other medically complex clients. In addition to gentle touch that is not "medical", companionship, conversation and general social interaction can be powerful medicine. SCI patients are often more socially isolated and mistaken for being cognitively impaired, which is not generally the case.
- Follow the lead of the client, but be open to including conversation as part of the session.

continued

- Avoid doing things for patients that they can do themselves.
- When the massage session is over, be extra mindful to return the bedside table, telephone, and TV remote to the original location.

Other neurological diseases

There are many neurological diseases, but rarely will they require hospital admission. As diseases progress however, practitioners may find clients and patients with neurological conditions, such as dementia, Parkinson's disease, multiple sclerosis (MS), and amyotrophic lateral

---

Info Box 7.2 Communicating with the person who is neurologically impaired

Any time the brain is affected by a medical condition, the patient may be easily confused, forgetful, discouraged, hostile, uncooperative, withdrawn, depressed, or emotionally unsteady. Communication often becomes difficult. The following suggestions will ease the communication process with those who have suffered a stroke, have dementia, or have brain damage.[71,72]

Non-verbal communication:
- Assume an equal or lower physical position when with the person.
- Connect with the person while communicating. Make eye contact, call them by name, or hold their hand while talking.
- Use gestures and facial demonstrations along with words.
- Keep distractions to a minimum. Provide a quiet environment to induce restfulness.
- If the person is restless and won't sit still, play soft music or familiar music (perhaps from their younger years if elderly). Sing along if possible for even greater connection.
- Never force physical contact if the person is not open to receiving it.
- If the person seems to become more agitated with physical contact, take your hands away and "hold" the person with your focused attention and presence. If the person continues to be agitated, calmly say that you are not going to continue the massage/touch them. Ask a carer or member of health care staff that the person relates with to assist in calming them.

Verbal communication:
- Get the person's attention before speaking.
- Face the person, making eye contact if possible.
- Be patient. Allow the person plenty of time to speak and respond. It is difficult for patients to translate what is being said and then form a response if they feel pressured. Don't talk for the patient unless absolutely necessary.
- Speak slowly, clearly, calmly, and with normal volume.
- Speak to the patient as you would any reasoning adult. Avoid baby talk. Call people and objects by their proper name.
- Don't talk to the person as if they aren't there.
- Keep it simple. Use short sentences. "Yes" and "No" questions are helpful for stroke and dementia patients, depending on their status.
- Present one idea at a time.
- Avoid changing the subject abruptly.
- Use the same wording consistently when asking questions or giving instructions.
- If the person is having trouble communicating, provide gentle encouragement and comfort, letting them know it is OK.
- Until speech returns, encourage communication through gestures, writing, or drawing if able.
- If patients have had a stroke, face them on the unaffected side.
- From time to time, restate what the patient has said.
- Don't act as if you understand when you don't.
- Elicit responses through statements such as, "Nod your head if you understand."
- Don't be abstract. The patient is often in a concrete frame of mind and takes everything literally. When you say you'll be back in a minute, the patient may understand it to mean "one" minute.
- Avoid criticizing, correcting, or arguing.
- Avoid using slang, nonspecific, or abstract words.
- Offer choices, especially if the person might be resistive. If someone is reluctant to try massage, offer them a choice between having their neck or feet massaged.
- Take a break if you are frustrated.

sclerosis (ALS; also known as Lou Gehrig's disease or motor neurone disease), in skilled nursing, rehabilitation, and memory care facilities. Dementia, MS, Parkinson's, and ALS are discussed below as they are common conditions likely to be found in medical center settings.

Dementia

Dementia is a generic term used to describe nonreversible declines in mental function, encompassing Alzheimer's disease, Lewy body disease, vascular dementia, and others.[73,74] These are conditions that practitioners will encounter in many types of long-term care residences. Each client is unique and may present very differently at each session. As they would with any patient, the therapist will need to ascertain health specifics, such as medical devices, medication side effects, and musculoskeletal issues. However, the unique aspect of working with people who have dementia, is the type of communication and presence required. The communication suggestions given in Info Box 7.2 for engaging with people who have traumatic brain injury or stroke are also useful for people with any type of dementia.

Multiple sclerosis (MS)

Multiple sclerosis causes damage to myelin sheaths, the protective sleeves that surround the nerves of the central nervous system.[75] The immune system attacks the myelin sheaths, causing destruction and scarring of nerves, thus the term sclerosis. The sclerotic action influences the way messages are sent or received, creating a variety of side effects that occur along a spectrum. Some people have motor weakness, others experience neuropathic pain, and some have musculoskeletal pain or spastic muscles. The symptoms often occur in cycles, disappearing after an episode only to recur later on. This is thought to happen because the myelin sheath is damaged, repaired, and then damaged again in a cyclical fashion.

About 1 in 7 MS patients experience Lhermitte's sign, a sudden sensation like an electric shock that travels down the back of the neck and spine, sometimes radiating out into the arms and legs.[76] Constipation is common for 70% of those with MS.[77] In addition, urinary incontinence can be caused when nerve signals to the bladder are blocked or delayed by the MS lesions.[78]

Stress is not the cause of MS, but it very likely exacerbates symptoms. This is where bodywork can play a role, by inducing relaxation[69] and reducing fatigue.[79,80] Bodywork may also ameliorate pain[69,80,81] and improve muscle tone and joints affected by spasticity. Pressure is important when focusing on muscle rigidity. Too little pressure can be irritating or difficult to sense, while deep pressure can cause inflammation and pain. Abdominal massage may also support bowel health for those who experience constipation.[69]

Clinical considerations: Multiple sclerosis

Pressure:

- Fatigue.
- Medication side effects.
- Spasticity.
- Painful areas.
- Use full-hand contact with moderate firmness, starting with a level 2–3 pressure. Inch forward over time.

Site:

- Neuropathic pain.
- Painful areas caused by spasticity.

Positioning:

- Take time to support areas affected by spasticity.

Other:

- When stretching spastic areas, including joints, use a cautious approach. Inch forward.

Parkinson's disease (PD)

Parkinson's disease is the result of reduced dopamine levels in the brain, the neurotransmitter that regulates coordinated muscle movement, behavior, cognitive function, and a sense of well-being. Typically, the side effects are tremor, muscle rigidity, poor balance, and a general slowness of movement, known as bradykinesia. A shuffling gait, difficulty changing positions, difficulty swallowing, and a blank facial expression are some of the common features of PD.[69]

The above symptoms can also be associated with parkinsonism, which is distinct from PD. Parkinsonism can be the result of some medications, particularly those given for psychiatric disorders; head trauma, such as happens to boxers; exposure to toxins; brain lesions; and liver failure.[82]

People living with Parkinson's or parkinsonism will often have a tremor that comes and goes. Hands, head, and feet and legs may occasionally or regularly move in uncontrolled ways. Patients often feel the need to apologize and explain their uncontrolled movements. Normalizing this side effect and literally going with the tremor flow is reassuring and comforting. Practitioners who show no fear, but rather understanding and gentle care, are truly appreciated.

Clinical considerations: Parkinson's disease

Pressure:

- Approach painful and rigid muscles and joints with gentleness.
- Fatigue.
- Focus on relaxation as a potential measure for relieving stress. Stress can exacerbate symptoms.
- Provide gentle abdominal massage for constipation.

Positioning:

- Allow the positioning process to be an integral part of the session. Allot extra time for it.
- Poor balance may necessitate assistance when undressing and dressing, as well as positioning and transferring on and off the bed or to a chair.
- Postural changes, such as stooping, may require extra support under the head when supine, or side-lying rather than prone.

- Use semi-reclining position if the person has swallowing difficulty.

Other:

- For people with a tremor, hold more firmly with one hand to help stabilize the limb but keep flexible in your own body to move with the waves of the client.
- Practitioners should keep their head a comfortable distance away from client's limbs that move uncontrollably. Sometimes a stimulated leg or arm will fly up without warning.
- Personality changes and limited affect, especially facial expression, are common. Do not make assumptions about the client's experience based on what is visible externally. Be sure to ask how they are feeling after the session. Words and hand gestures are likely more accurate.
- Apply the communication principles listed in Info Box 7.2.

Amyotrophic lateral sclerosis (ALS)/motor neurone disease (MND)

In some parts of the world this disease is referred to as amyotrophic lateral sclerosis (ALS), in others it is known as motor neurone disease (MND). This is a condition that affects nerve cells in the brain and the spinal cord needed to stimulate motor neurones. The progressive degeneration of the motor neurones causes muscles to become weak and wasted, eventually leading to paralysis. People may lose the ability to speak, eat, move, and breathe. The weakness, paralysis, and immobility can lead to musculoskeletal pain, therefore, keeping all joints in the body flexible through range of motion exercises is an important pain-prevention action.[83]

ALS is a relentless disease without remission. Typically, it advances over a course of three to five years, although, with technological advances, people are living longer. As ALS progresses, a lot of equipment may be involved, such as sophisticated wheelchairs, suctioning equipment, a BiPAP, and communication devices. Therapists will need help from family and/or other professional caregivers to become familiar with this equipment and its impact on the session. Communication especially is important to figure out because these patients can and should be very involved in developing their own care plans and letting the therapist know what is helpful. Despite needing the aid of communication devices, the personality of these patients comes through. Their minds continue to be sharp and they are eager to remain engaged with others.[84]

Clinical considerations: ALS/MND[84]

Pressure:

- Moderately firm pressure, with full-hand contact is best. Start with level 2–3 in most areas of the body. In some areas, the patient will prefer level 1.
- Bruising risk due to blood thinning medications.
- Edema is common in legs and feet.
- Fatigue.

Site:

- Mindfulness is needed of areas that have become flaccid or rigid.
- Once respiratory muscles are affected, intercostal, scalene, and pectoralis work can soften and open those muscles.
- Skin breakdown is a big risk due to long-term immobility.
- Some patients will have a feeding tube, tracheostomy to support their breathing, and a few may have a Portacath through which they receive IV medication.

Positioning:

- There will come a point at which the patient is not ambulatory and will spend much of the time in their wheelchair. This is a great place for them to receive massage. Many chairs can be set at any angle from upright to fully reclined. If the patient can tolerate it, the headrest can be taken out for better access to the head. Or, the head can be accessed by standing to one side of the chair and slipping a hand between the head rest and the curve of the neck.
- Flaccid or rigid areas will need extra support that conforms to the patient's comfort.
- Positioning also needs to consider breathing and difficulty swallowing saliva; many patients in advanced stages need frequent suctioning because they can't manage their secretions.

Other:

- Using lotion or wax is good for the patient's skin, which often is dry. When using one of these products with a person in a wheelchair, be very careful to not get it on the chair. Use towels to protect arm and foot rests. Oil is not a good choice in this situation.
- Once ambulation is lost, much of the session will be given over the patient's clothes. Lotion or wax can be applied to lower extremities by rolling up sleeves and pant legs.
- The movement of strokes is preferred because it is more easily sensed on the skin, rather than holds. The nerves that supply sensation to the skin are still fully functional.
- Muscle cramping is common.
- Warm compresses can be helpful.
- Music played through earphones during the massage can give a break from the noise of the BiPAP machine.
- Caregiver fatigue is a huge issue with ALS patients, since they require total care over a long period of time. Families/caregivers need a lot of support.

Obstetrics

Obstetrics (OB) is the branch of medicine that is concerned with pregnancy and childbirth. For eons, massage has been used to support mothers through the birthing experience. Until recently, women mostly delivered their babies vaginally. However, the use of cesarean section (C-section) has increased dramatically to the point that the World Health Organization and other institutions are calling for an examination of the practice.[85] The rate globally has nearly doubled between 2000 and 2015.[86] Rather than being used for specific medical purposes, C-sections are now often used for scheduling convenience, to reduce the possibility of lawsuits, or for patient preference, all non-medical reasons.

The overuse of C-sections is causing worldwide concern because they are associated with a number of risks, such as an increased likelihood of admission to the NICU, breastfeeding complications, childhood asthma and obesity, and postpartum depression.[87] On the other hand, vaginal delivery benefits the infant's immune system and prepares the lungs by emptying them of fluid, thus decreasing the chance of respiratory distress.[88] To help reduce the number of C-sections in the USA, the American College of Obstetrics and Gynecology and the American College of Nurse Midwives encourages women be provided with continuous labor support and non-pharmacological methods for pain management.[89] According to *The Lancet*: "Approaches such as labour companionship and midwife-led care have been associated with higher proportions of physiological births, safer outcomes, and lower health-care costs relative to control groups without these interventions, and with positive maternal experiences, in high-income countries."[90]

This trend is highlighted here because massage therapy may be one component that supports women to deliver their babies in the traditional way when medically possible.

Antenatal

The term antenatal, or antepartum, means before birth. There are a handful of precautions that must be observed when offering massage to pregnant patients regardless of whether they are enjoying a healthy pregnancy or have a high-risk condition. During pregnancy, a woman is five times more likely to develop a thrombus. The frequency of clot development is similar in all three trimesters,

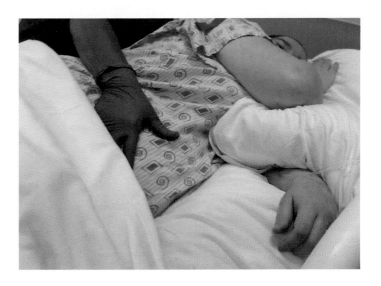

FIGURE 7.5

A pregnant patient in left side-lying position with support under the head, top arm, abdomen, and legs.

(Photo by Cathrine Weaver.)

including up to six weeks postnatal. This is because the body increases its clotting capacity, which is nature's way of protecting mothers from excessive bleeding during miscarriage and childbirth. By weeks 25–29 of gestation, venous flow has reduced by 50%, which lasts until six weeks after birth. Most commonly the left lower leg is the site of VTE.[91] It is imperative, therefore, that massage to the legs should be superficial and never deep.[92]

The recommended position during pregnancy is "SOS"– *sleep on side*, preferably the left side. Side-lying on the left will increase the amount of blood and nutrients that reach the placenta and baby. When supine, the patient should be in a semi-reclining position, also referred to as Fowler's position. Lying flat can result in the mother's abdomen resting on the intestines and major blood vessels, particularly the aorta and vena cava. This can cause low maternal blood pressure and decreased circulation to mother and baby, a condition known as supine hypotensive syndrome.

High-risk pregnancy

A number of complications can force early hospitalization during pregnancy. If contractions start too early in the pregnancy, referred to as preterm labor, a woman may be hospitalized on bedrest until the contractions are stopped or the fetus reaches a viable age. Hypertensive disorders, such as severe pre-eclampsia; placenta previa, a condition in which the placenta implants in the lower part of the uterus; and abruptio placentae, the premature separation of the placenta from the uterus, are other disorders that can require hospitalization.

Nowadays, fewer patients with high-risk pregnancies are placed on absolute bedrest. They are encouraged to walk, especially those who are at high risk of thrombus. Although less common than in the past, it is important to ask about mobility restrictions because practitioners can never assume a patient's restrictions or limitation. Patients with preeclampsia or those whose contractions have started early may be on a high dose of magnesium sulfate to relax the contracting muscles, which affects all of the muscles, including the eyes. The woman may be limp and disoriented. High dose magnesium sulfate also causes low blood pressure, an indication to elevate the head slightly. It is best to give the touch therapy session to these patients in situ, rather than moving them.

A high-risk pregnancy places greater demands on the prospective mother's heart, lungs, vascular and lymphatic systems, kidneys, and liver than a healthy pregnancy. This is an indication for extra gentle, nurturing, supportive massage. In addition, the mother is anxious about the health of her unborn baby and is not inclined toward any activity that would pose a threat to the pregnancy, such as vigorous massage. However, if she has been on bedrest for a prolonged period of time, the patient's back will be sore, and she will be bored, restless, and feel sluggish from inactivity. Some careful bodywork will be welcomed.

Labor and delivery

The use of epidurals in obstetrics has never been more popular. Once a patient receives an epidural, she will be restricted to bed. Prior to this she may be walking around the unit, sitting on an exercise ball, in the bathtub or shower. Once the device has been placed, the mother-to-be and the nurse are usually under the impression that no other pain management is necessary or useful.

An epidural, however, only diminishes the pain sensations. Many laboring women are still uncomfortable and anxious, feelings that massage can address. Massage may help stimulate labor, allow the patient to rest, and decrease pain. (Be sure to study the massage research presented in Chapter 2.)

During early labor (1–3 cm dilation), full-body massage that includes long strokes down the back, legs, and arms will feel good. (Practitioners need to glove if they are in contact with the lower back or legs or if the bedding is soiled with body fluids.) The light, downward direction of the strokes encourages a sense of openness, outwardness, and calmness. Therapists can also perform firm circles to the sacrum with the palm of the hand, apply acupressure along the spine, and pay special attention to the labor-stimulation points. It is during labor that these points are most potent. Contrary to popular belief, they are not particularly effective when administered to the woman not yet in labor.[93]

Giving massage during active labor (4–7 cm dilation) the therapist must be adaptable while at the same time maintaining focused concentration. While there are fewer precautions to implement than with medically complex patients, the needs and emotions of women preparing to deliver a baby change frequently, making it an intense experience for everyone in the room. One moment the laboring woman may be enjoying the sensations of massage, while in the next it becomes intolerable. During contractions, she may not want any touch or just *still* touch.

Women aren't always sure what they want in the midst of labor. The touch therapist may have to lead them by saying: "I am going to rub your feet for two contractions. You tell me how it feels." Communicate in shorter phrases rather than long sentences. This will allow the laboring woman to stay connected to that deep, primal place that birthing can lead to – during labor, the cortex shuts off, allowing the lower brain to take over.[94]

If she is tolerating massage between contractions, effleurage to the inner thighs will help relieve fatigue and trembling of the legs. If the legs cramp, extend and stretch them after contractions. Pressure to the sacrum and massage to the buttocks feels good to some women during this phase of labor; to other women, simple massage to the feet, shoulders, jaw, and scalp may be more relaxing.

Depending on the wishes of the patient and the hospital staff, the massage therapist may or may not be allowed to stay in the room during the transitional phase (8–10 cm dilation) and delivery. If the bodyworker is able to remain, their role will be to provide reassurance to the laboring woman, to encourage breathing, to help her assume whatever position is comfortable, to hold her hand, or to support the legs.

The massage literature contains a wealth of material on pregnancy massage that the reader is encouraged to study. These books list many ideas to ease the discomfort related to labor, such as the use of birthing balls, certain positions, or walking. The hospital massage therapist usually is not free to suggest the use of these directly to the patient; instructions for positioning and walking must come from the midwife. A massage therapist acting in the role of doula or a massage therapist who has a long-standing rapport with the labor and delivery staff may be more influential in this area.

There is also an array of relaxation skills that can be helpful during labor. However, often the hospital massage therapist is meeting the mother-to-be for the first time and has not had a chance to develop a rapport with her. New skills such as focusing or breathing techniques are difficult, although not impossible, to learn in the middle of such an intense experience.

Postnatal

Following delivery, women who give birth vaginally can be massaged with few precautions in the upper body. Their muscles are sore and fatigued from the exertion of delivery and respond well to slightly firmer bodywork. Most are not inclined to lie prone, but the midwife usually leaves the decision to the patient. Attention to the neck, shoulders, arms, and hands will be welcomed. The pelvic bones and attachments will be unstable; therefore, deep compression that displaces the musculature or mobilizing techniques to the area should be avoided. Patients who have had an epidural may have a headache. Massage to the head and neck can be effective

in relieving the discomfort. The legs should only be given gentle attention as a thrombus is still a strong possibility, especially if the delivery has been via C-section. The risk of developing a blood clot continues for the first six weeks following delivery, then gradually decreases.[91]

Therapist's journal 7.4
Jumping, screaming toddlers

I walked into a room on the OB floor where a mom was having a hard time breastfeeding her newborn. Two toddlers were jumping around, screaming, using hospital blankets as capes. Dad sat in a chair arguing with the kids to please calm down so mom and baby could bond and relax and the baby could be fed. The mom and dad both seemed frustrated and exhausted. The children were having a blast.

I greeted the new mother and asked if she would be interested in a foot massage. Her face lit up. The first five minutes of the session, baby and mom were restless. But, as mom settled, so did the baby. Mom appeared to fall asleep and the toddlers' screams had ceased. They sat quietly, wrapped in their cape blankets, smiling, and watching me give their mom a massage. I peeked over at dad who was fast asleep, snoring. After completing the massage, I moved quietly so as not to wake anyone. Mom peeked at me, smiled, and whispered, "Thank you, this is true bliss."

Heather E. Stauffer LMT
Royal Oak, Michigan

Clinical considerations: Obstetrics

Pressure:

- Anxiety about health of unborn baby (high-risk pregnancy).
- Blood clot risk, especially C-section (avoid firm pressure to the legs).
- Edema (particularly the legs).

continued

- Firmer pressure to upper body is generally fine postnatally.
- High-risk pregnancy causes demands on vital organs.
- Ligaments become overstretched, resulting in joint instability.
- Pain medication, especially for C-section.
- Varicosities (if severe, massage only proximal to the site).

Site:

- Abdomen (some patients will want no touch, some only gentle holds, and others will be happy with effleurage).
- C-section incision.
- Epidural site (gentle massage within a few inches of the site is OK).
- IV catheter.

Positioning:

- Semireclining or left side-lying is best antenatally. Offer to place a pillow under the abdomen for support when side-lying. Some find this comfortable, others don't (see Figure 7.5).
- Self-limiting post-natally.
- C-section patients most likely to stay semi-reclining.

Organ transplantation

What was once a novel treatment for organ failure has become almost commonplace. The most commonly transplanted organ is the kidney, followed by liver, heart, and lungs. In the modern world of transplantation, even pancreas and intestines are sometimes transplanted. Because of the increase of kidney and liver disease, the need for organ transplantation has increased while the pool of available donors has decreased.[95,96]

Pre-transplant

Organ transplantation is characterized by waiting. People not in crucial need of a new organ wait at home for word that an organ matching their tissue type and body size is available. Those who are medically unstable wait in the hospital, where they can receive the medications and care necessary to sustain their life. Sometimes the wait is weeks; sometimes, as with a heart, it can be many months; and sometimes an organ does not become available.

Many of the side effects requiring adjustments to the massage session are similar for kidney, liver, and heart failure: fatigue, shortness of breath, edema, ascites, nausea, and difficulty concentrating. The person in liver failure will experience specific side effects, such as a build-up of ammonia, one of the toxins metabolized by a healthy liver, causing poor mental functioning, confusion, and irritability.[97] Platelet levels also drop due to coagulopathy, putting the person at risk for bleeding. People in liver failure may be on diuretics, lactulose to counteract the ammonia build-up, antibiotics to suppress enteric bacteria, antiemetics, and pain medication.[98]

The person needing a new heart can be sustained for a certain period of time on medications or a ventricular assist device (VAD), but not indefinitely. A VAD is a mechanical pump implanted into the chest to help pump blood from the heart's ventricles. Sometimes this is a temporary bridge until a new heart is found or, for people who don't qualify for heart transplantation, it is used to prolong their life and improve its quality.

Therapist's journal 7.5
Joe

Joe had been on an LVAD for about 7 years. In the beginning it had allowed him to play pool, poker, and go fishing with his friends. As long as he could do these things, life was good. Eventually, however, the device was in need of repair, but it was so old that it couldn't be fixed. Unfortunately, a new device couldn't be placed because, prior to receiving the LVAD, Joe had had four other heart surgeries, which had created significant scar tissue. He also had developed multiple co-morbidities, such as diabetes and damage from the anti-rejection drugs. This meant he would most likely not survive a heart transplant.

continued

As time progressed, Joe began to have more and more frequent hospitalizations – more time in the hospital, less at home. It became obvious that the LVAD would fail; the doctors estimated in about three months. Rather than let that happen, Joe took control and chose a day to turn it off.

I had massaged Joe on and off for two years during his frequent trips to the hospital. He had a lot of enthusiasm for his massages and tried to make people jealous that he was getting massage, telling them he was in a spa. The day of his last massage, I was unaware of Joe's decision to turn off his LVAD. He was as chipper as ever. The room was full of friends and family, but that really wasn't unusual. There was, however, a heaviness in the atmosphere. When I finished, Joe and other people in the room hugged me. I said to Joe, "See you next week my friend." He replied back, "You bet you will!"

As usual, I left his room and went out into the hall; it was then that the social worker told me what was going to happen that afternoon. I cried while she held me.

Later that day, with family and friends in the room, Joe turned off the failing LVAD. The staff weren't sure what would happen because no one had ever done it. Would his heart keep going without the device? But once he turned it off, Joe only lived for another ten minutes.

Some of my hospital memories are hard to relive. But the experience with Joe warms my heart and lifts my soul. It is a blessing to remember our time together.

Del Delashmutt LMT
Portland, Oregon

Post-transplant

Potential complications from transplantation surgery are significant and can include infection, blood clots or bleeding, a heart attack or stroke, and rejection of the new organ.[99–101] Despite this, gentle touch therapy can begin soon after surgery. Foot massage is a common starting place.

After an organ transplant, almost all patients will be on immunosuppressive drugs, such as tacrolimus or cyclosporine, for the remainder of their lives.[102] These drugs help prevent the body's immune system from seeing the new organ as foreign and rejecting it. Most long-term complications are related to the immunosuppressants, the major risk being infection. Patients will also be on a long list of other drugs at the beginning, such as antifungals, antibiotics, corticosteroids, pain medication, diuretics, blood pressure medication, statins, laxatives, and anxiolytics. Touch therapists needs to remain mindful of the number of medications an organ transplant patient may be on as well as of the accumulation of side effects. For example, some of the anti-rejection medications can cause kidney toxicity, high blood pressure, diabetes, and electrolyte imbalances; others can cause diarrhea, cramping, nausea, and vomiting. Steroids can result in fluid retention, increased appetite and weight gain, stomach irritation, mood swings, insomnia, poor wound healing, and acne. These are just some of the side effects. Over time the transplant team will taper the dosages as well as the number of medications.[103] (See Chapter 10 for greater detail.)

Clinical considerations: Organ transplantation

Pressure:

- Blood clot risk.
- Concern about organ rejection.
- Multiple side effects of medication regimen.
- Fatigue.
- Incision sites.
- Pain medication.

Site:

- Drains.
- IV catheters.
- Incisional sites:
  - Kidney: In prior years, incisions for kidney surgery were made into the back or laterally. Nowadays, the incision for a transplant is made into the lower abdomen. The new kidney is placed inside this area. The surgeon connects the artery and vein of the new kidney

continued

to the artery and vein of the pelvis. Unless the original kidney is causing a medical problem, it is left in place.

° Liver: Will be in upper right quadrant.

Positioning:

• Mostly semi-reclining while hospitalized.

• Liver and kidney transplant patients may be able to be positioned side-lying on the unaffected side.

Other:

• Immunosuppression.

• Infection risk.

Orthopedic

The massage therapist who works with orthopedic patients will encounter a world of medical hardware such as pins, screws, rods, plates, and apparatus used to stabilize the body such as slings, halos, and traction devices. The types of patients vary. There are those having elective surgery for joint replacements, most often knee and hip; elderly people, especially women, who have broken their hip in a fall; and victims of trauma, often due to motor vehicle accidents. Commonly, these patients will be transferred to a rehabilitation or long-term care center to complete their healing process.

Positioning is a primary concern with orthopedic patients. If the hospital staff allow patients to make position changes in the bed, maintaining skeletal alignment is imperative. For example, the person who has had a hip replacement eventually will be able to assume a side-lying position on the unaffected hip, but it is important to place a pillow between the entire length of the legs so that neutral alignment is preserved, thereby placing no stress on the newly replaced joint. The person who has had a knee replacement can have the knees bolstered while receiving massage in supine position. Afterward, however, the knee should be repositioned so that it is flat and does not remain in flexion. Following back surgery, spinal alignment is important. Positions or movements that cause the spine to torque or twist should be avoided.

Bruising is a common occurrence with orthopedic patients. It can happen near the surgical site or be the result of trauma. Once the discoloration has become yellow-green, gentle massage can be administered in the bruised area if the patient is agreeable. Elderly orthopedic patients are likely to have osteoporosis. Be mindful of this when massaging the non-injured parts of the body. Many of these patients will be on high doses of pain medication, which inhibits their ability to provide feedback to the massage therapist. Additionally, they may be on anticoagulants, another indication for gentle massage because of the possibility of easy bruising.

Despite the medical equipment that must be worked around and the many precautions, systematic touch is very beneficial for this group. It may promote circulation in the affected areas, provides pain relief, and can assist the work of the rehabilitation staff working to increase range of motion, rebuild strength, and control edema. Massage practitioners should work closely under the direction of the physical therapy staff to integrate range-of-motion or other movement exercises into the massage session.

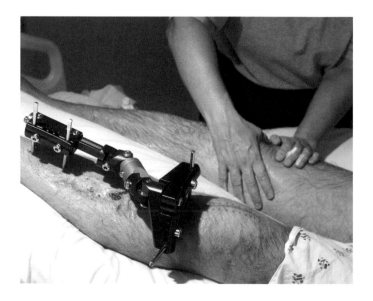

FIGURE 7.6

A patient with an external orthopedic fixator receives massage.

(Photo by Don Hamilton.)

Clinical considerations: Orthopedic

Pressure:

- Edema often occurs in the affected limb. (See Chapter 8 for edema protocol.)
- Pain medications.
- Anticoagulants.
- Veins of the lower extremities and pelvis are highly susceptible to a blood clot after a fracture or surgery in the lower regions.
- Avoid pressure on any part of the body that would disturb the alignment of a replaced joint, surgical site, or fractured limb.

Site:

- The involved area may be affected by muscle spasm, which is the body's attempt to stabilize the area. Massage in the vicinity of the surgical site should be very gentle and in no way destabilizing.
- Avoid getting lotion or oil on the skin in the vicinity of casts or external orthopedic fixation devices.
- Take notice of the skin around the edge of casts for signs of irritation.
- Be aware of signs that circulation is being cut off by a cast: cold, numb, tingling sensation, or blue or pale fingernails or toenails in the affected extremity.
- With the approval of the health care team, it may be acceptable to reach under the cast of certain patients and massage the accessible skin.

Positioning:

- Elevate the affected limb above the level of the heart.
- Ensure that bedding and clothing are wrinkle-free. This helps prevent irritation to the skin for those who are severely immobilized.
- If the patient has a cast, avoid resting it on hard surfaces or sharp edges that may dent or flatten the cast, which may then cause pressure sores.

- If the hip has been replaced, maintain alignment of the new hip. When the patient is side-lying, place a pillow under the head, top arm, and especially between the entire length of the legs so that the new joint remains in a neutral position. The nursing staff may want to help the patient reposition to ensure that the process is performed properly.
- Following knee replacement, avoid leaving the knee in flexion after the massage. Elevate the leg on pillows to control swelling.

Other:

- Anxiety and depression can occur if a significant part of the patient's body is in a cast. The person is subjected to immobility in a confining space, dependence on others, and loss of control. Massage may take the edge off these emotions.
- The decrease in activity combined with pain medications may cause constipation. If the foot or hand is accessible, attention to the bowel reflexology zones may be beneficial (see Tip 8.1).

Stem cell transplantation

Hematopoietic stem cell transplantation (HSCT) is best known for its role in treating certain cancers, particularly bone marrow-related, such as leukemias, lymphomas, and multiple myeloma. Some nonmalignant diseases also respond well to HSCT from a donor, such as aplastic anemia, myelodysplastic syndrome, and myelofibrosis, all diseases in which the bone marrow is defective. This treatment has also been successful with some autoimmune diseases, most particularly lupus, MS, and systemic sclerosis and in some people affected by sickle cell anemia and thalassemia.[104]

HSCT should not be confused with stem cell therapies. These are more recent techniques that are offered to regenerate areas affected by age-related inflammation and pain, such as the knees, spine, neck, and shoulders. Stem cell therapy for joint regeneration harvests stem cells from one part of the patient's body and injects them into the damaged part, with the aim that the cells differentiate into cartilage cells and repair the joint. These stem cells are of a different type than the ones used in hematology oncology.[105]

HSCT collects blood stem cells, which are immature or primitive blood cells that grow into red or white blood cells, and platelets. HSCT rebuilds a patient's bone marrow after high-dose chemotherapy and total body irradiation (TBI) have been used to destroy the defective bone marrow. This increases the possibility of curing the patient's disease. In the past, these high doses of chemotherapy and total body irradiation were often fatal because the patient's immune system was decimated for 5–6 weeks. The implementation of HSCTs rescues the immune system.

There are two main types of transplantation, autologous and allogeneic. The type used is dependent on the disease and its level of advancement, patient's age, and donor availability. If a person is producing enough healthy bone marrow cells, they can donate their own stem cells before treatment. This is referred to as autologous transplant. An allogeneic transplant involves the cells of a donor whose tissue matches that of the patient as closely as possible, such as a sibling. However, sometimes the donor is unrelated, and is referred to as a *matched unrelated donor* (MUD).[106]

HSCT recipients are admitted to the hospital up to 7 days before the transplant to undergo what is known as a "conditioning regimen." This protocol involves high-dose chemotherapy, and sometimes total body irradiation, or both. It is for the purpose of killing remaining cancer cells, suppressing the immune system to prevent rejection of the new cells, and creating space in the bone marrow for the cells to engraft. The days before transplantation are referred to as Day –7, Day –6, Day –5, etc.

HSCT is not a surgical procedure like an organ transplant. It takes place in the patient's room and is similar to a blood transfusion. The stem cells are contained in a blood products bag that is hung on an IV pole and infused into the patient's central IV catheter. The day of the transplant is referred to as Day 0 and is often treated like a birthday.

There is no medical reason that gentle touch modalities cannot be administered during stem cell infusion. However, patients are sometimes so anxious that they are not receptive to the idea. Also, the nursing staff are particularly attentive during this time in case patients have a reaction to the preservative the cells are stored in. Allogeneic HSCT recipients in particular may experience side effects similar to those from a blood transfusion: shortness of breath, chills, fever, rash, chest pain, and hypotension.

Engraftment, which takes 2–4 weeks, is the process of the stem cells traveling to the bone marrow and producing new blood cells.[107] Until this occurs, patients are severely neutropenic and thrombocytopenic. The white blood cell count usually drops to 0.1 (the normal range is 4.5–10), and platelets can plummet to less than 10 (150–450 is the normal range). (For explanations of platelet and white blood cell counts, see Chapter 8 "Bruising and bleeding" and "Immunosuppression", respectively.) This is a dangerous time because the immune system is greatly compromised, and the patient is at risk for spontaneous bleeding into the brain or retina. The risk of bleeding is so severe that patients may not be allowed to brush their teeth in case the gums bleed.

A number of other side effects occur. The kidneys and liver may go into failure, and the heart and lungs become toxic, which are potentially fatal complications. People frequently have fevers, tremors from cyclosporine, and mouth and esophageal sores from mucositis, making eating and talking difficult to impossible.[108] The skin of the hands and feet can peel off down to the dermal layer, and the fatigue is fierce and unyielding. No words can truly describe how hellish a hematopoietic stem cell transplantation can be, particularly an allogeneic one.

Patients who have allogeneic transplants almost always suffer from some degree of graft-versus-host disease (GVHD).[108] The new stem cells (the graft) see the body (the host) as an enemy and attack it, creating a severe inflammatory process. GVHD can affect the skin, gastrointestinal (GI) tract, and liver, resulting in skin rashes or discoloration, nausea, vomiting and diarrhea, an inability to absorb nutrients, and liver dysfunction. Even massage lotion will not absorb into the skin of some people with GVHD. Over time, the inflammatory process can cause the skin and connective tissue to develop a sclerotic condition. Patients often think deep massage will "break up" and alleviate the condition, which is completely untrue.

Hematopoietic stem cell transplantation is often an isolating experience for patients due to the need to protect them from infectious agents during immunosuppression. (Fresh food and flowers are not even allowed due to the bacteria and fungi that are on them.) Emotional problems can arise during this time. Further contributing to mood shifts are drug reactions or the patient's lack of preparation for the physical and emotional intensity of the treatment. Anxiety, depression, and panic are common.

Massage is highly beneficial during this time but must be performed with great mindfulness and care. Nurses are very protective of these patients for two reasons. The first is thrombocytopenia, which puts people at severe risk of bleeding or bruising – a bruise for one of these patients is potentially a serious event. The touch therapist must use only the amount of pressure required to spread the lotion or apply noninvasive modalities such as Reiki. Amazingly, patients with low platelets are just like many massage clients – they want more pressure. However, no matter how much the patient tries to talk the therapist into it, the practitioner absolutely must use only gentle pressure! Besides the risk for bruising and bleeding, a number of other complications demand the use of light pressure, such as organ toxicity, fatigue, and nausea. The other reason nurses are vigilant of their stem cell transplant patients is severe neutropenia, which means people are at significant risk of opportunistic infections. Strict adherence to Standard Precautions is a must.

Patients are discharged when the blood counts have returned to certain levels, generally 15–30 days after transplantation. However, they must remain within 20–30 minutes travelling distance from the hospital for an extended period of time, usually 80–100 days. A medical crisis can develop quickly for stem cell recipients, and they must be able to get to the hospital rapidly if an emergency occurs.

Practitioners are perhaps reading this section with wide eyes, wondering if they dare massage people affected by such grave complications. The answer is yes. Massage is one of the few pleasant sensations patients experience, especially during hospitalization. Massage gives them something to look forward to during the long days of semi-isolation. It can temporarily reduce anxiety, pain, fatigue, nausea, and

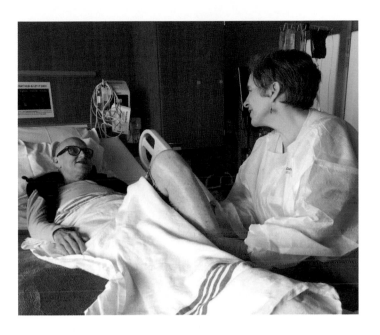

FIGURE 7.7
HSCT patient feedback. "You are a prayer to me."

(Photo by Gayle MacDonald.)

even neutropenic fevers. One person even told her therapist that massage gave her the will to live.

Clinical considerations: HCST

Pressure:

- Neutropenia (severe.)
- Thrombocytopenia (severe).
- Fatigue (severe).
- Organ toxicity.
- Skin sensitivity.

Site:

- Central IV catheter.
- Skin conditions, e.g., mucositis, rashes.

Positioning:

- Self-limiting.

Chapter SEVEN

When I was first diagnosed with AML, it surprised me and my young family. I was tired all the time, which I thought was just part of being a mom, wife, and teacher. But I knew that something wasn't right.

I was admitted to the hospital to begin chemotherapy. When it came time to bring the kids to the hospital and tell them that I would be there for a while, we were very thoughtful in the way we wanted to share this news. I took off the hospital gown and put on my regular clothes. "You look like a normal person," my nurse said. I never put on a hospital gown again! I wanted to stay a normal person.

When the kids arrived in my hospital room, I showed them my bed. I sat with the girls, aged 6 and 8, and we pushed all the buttons, making it go up and down, feet up, feet down, head up, head down. What a toy, they thought it was great! Then I said, "Watch this!", and I pushed the nurse call button and a sweet voice came on, "May I help you?" I replied, "Please could you bring me three ice waters with straws." The girls looked at me with wide eyes and questioned, "Mom! You have a maid?!" This made me smile and I told them, "Yes, I do! And I have a nice young man that brings me breakfast in bed with cloth napkins, a fun-loving lady with a glorious smile that sweeps my room and wipes everything down, another young lady comes in and makes my bed while I am showering, a woman brings me art supplies every Wednesday, AND I get a massage twice a week!"

In talking with my girls that day, I was seeing through the eyes of children. I saw all the amazing people taking care of me, making me feel like a queen at a spa and giving me hope in what could have been a really dark time of chemotherapy and a bone marrow transplant. From that day on, I looked at my time in the hospital as a selah moment. Selah is a Hebrew word meaning a time to pause and reflect and truly find what has value in my life: God and other people. I am here to love others and forgive. Period. I felt very loved in the hospital.

When I think about the massage therapists that came twice a week, it was something I looked forward to. They would listen while gently massaging my arms and legs. My body was working so hard to process the chemo and rid itself of cancer. Their gentleness with me showed that they understood my process. I could just be me, not needing to put on a strong face for them. They reminded me that I was still here on this earth and that my body was still alive.

D.H. Portland, Oregon

Surgery

Surgery is an injurious event to the body, as well as to the entire being. Systematic touch can be instrumental in piecing together the whole person and in releasing the trauma. When receiving massage, whether it is after gynecological surgery, a coronary bypass, or the removal of a tumor, postsurgical patients require some common adjustments. An increased risk of blood clots is one of the primary considerations. When blood vessels are injured, as they are during an incision, platelets adhere to one another to form a plug that staunches the flow of blood. These cells can clump together in the body and come to rest on the interior of blood vessel walls, forming a thrombus. Heavy massage could dislodge a clot, thereby creating a pulmonary embolism. Patients who have had surgery to an area with an abundant supply of blood vessels are at greater risk for a blood clot. The abdomen and chest cavity are good examples, as opposed to the tonsils or hands.

Massage can occur as soon as the patient returns from the recovery room and the nurse has settled the patient into their room. For some patients, massage can ameliorate pain, decrease anxiety, and provide faster recovery from anesthesia. Nausea is a common side effect of anesthesia: general massage or specific attention to the acupressure nausea points has been shown to be helpful. The application of a non-circulatory modality such as Reiki or Jin Shin Jyutsu® is very soothing. Of course, the incision site cannot yet be massaged, but patients report decreased incisional pain from the application of an off-the-body modality such as Therapeutic Touch over the surgical site.

During this time, patients will be on pain medication and unable to give accurate feedback. Anticoagulants may make patients susceptible to bruising. Antibiotics are also commonly given. The practitioner doesn't usually need to make any adjustments because of them, but it underscores the need for robust usage of Standard Precautions as a protective action for the patient. Preventing health care-acquired infections is a high priority, which is why patients are now discharged from hospital as quickly as possible.

Medical devices may present the bodyworker with many areas that must be avoided. Surgical patients often have sequential compression devices on their legs to prevent the formation of a blood clot, a Foley catheter inserted into the bladder, an IV catheter in at least one wrist, and possibly a drain at the surgical site. Gloving is more often necessary with this group of patients due to the drainage of body fluids, which not only will be around the treated area but also may seep into the gown and bedding. Staying alert to this is important. If in doubt about whether to glove, err on the side of caution and glove.

Clinical considerations: Surgery

Pressure:

- Blood clot risk.
- Edema.
- Fatigue.
- Incision.

Site:

- Incision.
- Medical devices (e.g., IV catheters, epidural, drains, ostomy bag).

Positioning:

- Generally, massage will occur in the position the therapist finds the patient.
- Patient may not want to reposition due to pain or disorientation.
- Side-lying may be tolerated on the unaffected side.

Case history 7.1 Exercise

Instructions: On a piece of paper, make three columns: pressure, site, and position. List the conditions that would require pressure reduction, those that could be a site restriction, and the ones needing positioning adjustment.

Mr Williams is 68 years old and was admitted to the hospital with diabetic-related side effects. A scratch on his left foot developed into a serious infection after he waded in dirty water. Despite heavy doses of antibiotics, the infection could not be controlled, which is not uncommon with diabetes. The doctor was in favor of amputating the foot and the entire lower leg, but Mr Williams insisted on a more conservative approach, removal of only half the foot.

The procedure was performed 2 days ago. The surgical site requires elevation and is dressed with a compression bandage. There is some seepage in the area. The right foot is affected by neuropathy. The patient has a Foley catheter in the bladder and a urine collection bag attached to the side of the bed. Pain medication, insulin, and antibiotics are being given through an IV catheter inserted in his left wrist.

Other long-term side effects from diabetes include poor eyesight, causing Mr Williams to be very dependent on his wife; 3 years ago he had coronary bypass surgery; and his skin is fragile.

Chapter SEVEN

Summary

This text can only provide a thumbnail sketch of each patient group. The reader is referred to pathology texts, online medical dictionaries, nursing manuals, and websites to more deeply study the diseases and conditions. This textbook cannot replace those texts but is a complement to them.

One of the main purposes of *Hands in Health Care* is the creation of an intellectual infrastructure that will lead new and experienced therapists to develop critical thinking skills. The ability to ask the right questions and to connect the dots between knowledge and practice is more desirable than memorization of a vast quantity of information. The pressure, site, and position framework combined with the knowledge of some basic concepts is the skeleton around which intake skills and questioning strategies can be built. Touch therapists who can combine critical thinking with the practice of Standard Precautions, develop the ability to perform gentle massage, relate to patients, and act in concert with the other health care professionals will be on their way to mastering massage in the medical setting.

Acknowledgments

The authors wish to thank the following people for their contributions: Jacki Sellers for the section on addictions, co-existing conditions, and psychology disorders; Lauren "Cal" Cates and Kerry Jordan for the intensive care section; and Karen Armstrong for additions to the obstetrics section.

Test yourself

Multiple choice: Circle all of the correct answers. There may be more than one.

1. Which of the following conditions are typically associated with peripheral neuropathy?

   A   Congestive heart failure.
   B   Diabetes.
   C   Substance abuse.
   D   Cirrhosis.

2. Which of the following may contribute to immuno-suppression?

   A   Cancer treatment.
   B   Diabetes.
   C   Aging.
   D   Surgery.

3. Touch therapy is contraindicated for:

   A   End stage kidney disease.
   B   Stroke.
   C   Arrhythmia.
   D   Septicemia.

4. One important clinical consideration when massaging a post-operative patient is:

   A   Skin sensitivity.
   B   Peripheral neuropathy.
   C   Anemia.
   D   Blood clot risk.

5. Fatigue is one of the side effects of:

   A   Diabetes.
   B   Liver disease.
   C   Congestive heart failure.
   D   Edema.

6. Edema often accompanies:

   A   Renal failure.
   B   Liver disease.
   C   Pregnancy.
   D   Urinary tract infection.

7. Which of the following has an interrelationship with obesity and diabetes?

   A   Certain cancers.
   B   Mental health problems.
   C   Endocrine problems.
   D   Liver disease.

8. When communicating with people affected by dementia or a brain injury:

   A   Keep distractions to a minimum.
   B   Allow the person plenty of time to respond.
   C   Speak softly.
   D   Use short sentences.

9. Which of the following patients are at increased risk of blood clot development?

   A   C-section.
   B   Post-operative.
   C   Antenatal.
   D   Organ transplant.

10. Obstetric patients:

   A   Are at risk of developing a blood clot for a week after childbirth.
   B   Are recommended to sleep on the right side.
   C   Are at risk of developing a blood clot weeks to months before delivery. Increasing the clotting ability is nature's way of protecting mothers from excessive bleeding during childbirth.
   D   Should have superficial massage to the legs before and after delivery.

11. Blood clot risk is first and foremost a _____ precaution:

   A   Positioning.
   B   Time.
   C   Pressure.
   D   Site.

12. Which of the following can be true about massaging people recovering from substance abuse or trauma?

   A   Start with deep pressure so that the patient is able to feel the contact.
   B   Patients often can't give accurate feedback about massage pressure.
   C   They are commonly out of touch with their body.
   D   Patients in detoxification should have gentler pressure.

13. Hematopoietic stem cell transplantation:

   A   Is used in conjunction with high dose chemotherapy, which decimates the patient's bone marrow.
   B   From an unrelated donor can result in graft-versus-host disease.
   C   Rescues the patient's immune system and ability to create red blood cells and platelets.
   D   Typically engrafts in 2–4 weeks.

14. _____ is a primary concern with orthopedic patients:

   A   Communication.
   B   Positioning.
   C   Length of session.
   D   IV catheters.

15. Older people can be a fall risk because of:

   A   Bruising risk.
   B   Skin conditions.
   C   Medications.
   D   Neurological problems.

References

1. American Addiction Centers. Co-occurring disorders & dual diagnosis treatment guide. 2020. Available from: https://americanaddictioncenters.org/co-occurring-disorders

2. Sellers J. Personal communication, 5 June 2019.

3. Jacobi U, Waibler E, Schulze P, et al. Release of doxorubicin in sweat: first step to induce the palmar-plantar erythrodysesthesia syndrome? Ann Oncol. 2005; 16(7):1210–1.

4. Horn TD. Antineoplastic chemotherapy, sweat, and the skin. Arch Dermatol. 1997; 133:905–6.

5. Apisarnthanarax N, Duvic M. Chapter 144: Dermatologic complications of cancer chemotherapy. Holland-Frei Cancer Medicine, 5th edition. Hamilton: BC Decker; 2000.

6. Lee WJ, Lee JL, Chang SE, et al. Cutaneous adverse effects in patients treated with the multitargeted kinase inhibitors sorafenib and sunitinib. Br J Dermatol. 2009; 161(5):1045–51.

7. Dib EG, Ifthikharuddin JJ, Scott GA, Partilo SR. Neutrophilic eccrine hidradenitis induced by imatinib mesylate (Gleevec) therapy. Leuk Res. 2005; 29(2);233–4.

8. American Society of Clinical Oncology. Understanding targeted therapies. 2019. Available from: https://www.cancer.net/navigating-cancer-care/how-cancer-treated/personalized-and-targeted-therapies/understanding-targeted-therapy

9. American Society of Clinical Oncology. What is personalized medicine? 2020. Available from: https://www.cancer.net/navigating-cancer-care/how-cancer-treated/personalized-and-targeted-therapies/what-personalized-cancer-medicine

10. National Institutes of Health. National Cancer Institute. Immunotherapy to treat cancer. 2019. Available from: https://www.cancer.gov/about-cancer/treatment/types/immunotherapy#4

11. Cancer Research UK. Vaccines to treat cancer. 2017. Available from: https://www.cancerresearchuk.org/about-cancer/cancer-in-general/treatment/immunotherapy/types/vaccines-to-treat-cancer

12. MD Anderson Cancer Center. Targeted therapy (precision medicine). 2019. Available from: https://www.mdanderson.org/treatment-options/targeted-therapy/html

13. World Health Organization. Cardiovascular diseases (CVDs). 2017. Available from: http://who.int/news-room/fact-sheets/detail/cardiovascular-diseases-(cvds)

14. Medical News Today. What to know about jugular vein distension (JVD). 2017. https://www.medicalnewstoday.com/articles/320320.php

15. American Heart Association. About arrhythmia. 2016. Available from: https://www.heart.org/en/health-topics/arrhythmia/about-arrhythmia

16. Cleveland Clinic. Arrhythmia treatments. 2019. Available from: https://my.clevelandclinic.org/health/treatments/16751-arrhythmia-treatments

17. Mayo Clinic. Arteriosclerosis/atherosclerosis. 2018. Available from: https://www.mayoclinic.org/diseases-conditions/arteriosclerosis-atherosclerosis/symptoms-causes/syc-20350569

18. Mayo Clinic. Heart failure: symptoms and causes. 2017. https://www.mayoclinic.org/diseases-conditions/heart-failure/symptoms-causes/syc-20373142

19. Mayo Clinic. Heart failure: diagnosis and treatment. 2017. Available from: https://www.mayoclinic.org/diseases-conditions/heart-failure/diagnosis-treatment/drc-20373148

20. Mayo Clinic. Heart attack: diagnosis and treatment. 2018. Available from: https://www.mayoclinic.org/diseases-conditions/heart-attack/diagnosis-treatment/drc-20373112

21. Cleveland Clinic. Heart Attack (Myocardial Infarction). 2019. Available from: https://my.clevelandclinic.org/health/diseases/16818-heart-attack-myocardial-infarction

22. Nettina S. The Lippincott Manual of Nursing Practice. Philadelphia: Lippincott Williams & Wilkins; 2001.

23. Caplan LR. Patient information: stroke symptoms and diagnosis (beyond the basics). 2019. Available from: https://www.uptodate.com/contents/stroke-symptoms-and-diagnosis-beyond-the-basics

24. The Aneurysm and AVM Foundation. About brain aneurysm. 2019. Available from: https://taafonline.org/conditions/aneurysm/about

25. Mayo Clinic. Stroke. 2020. Available from: https://www.mayoclinic.org/diseases-conditions/stroke/diagnosis-treatment/drc-20350119

26. World Health Organization. Diabetes. 2018. Available from: https://www.who.int/news-room/fact-sheets/detail/diabetes

27. CDC. National diabetes statistics report. 2018. Available from: https://www.cdc.gov/diabetes/data/statistics/statistics-report.html

28. Mainous AG, Tanner RJ, Baker R, et al. Prevalence of prediabetes in England from 2003 to 2011: population-based, cross-sectional study. 2014. Available from: https://bmjopen.bmj.com/content/4/6/e005002

29. Diabetes UK. Us, diabetes, and a lot of facts and stats. 2019. Available from: https://www.diabetes.org.uk/resources-s3/2019-02/1362B_Facts%20and%20stats%20Update%20Jan%202019_LOW%20RES_EXTERNAL.pdf

30. UNICEF. The state of the world's children: children, food, and nutrition. 2019. Available from: https://www.unicef.org/media/60806/file/SOWC-2019.pdf

31. Mayo Clinic. Diabetes. 2018. Available from: https://www.mayoclinic.org/diseases-conditions/diabetes/symptoms-causes/syc-20371444

32. Mayo Clinic. Arteriosclerosis/atherosclerosis. 2018. Available from: https://www.mayoclinic.org/diseases-conditions/arteriosclerosis-atherosclerosis/symptoms-causes/syc-20350569

33. Bailie C. Personal communication, 17 April 2019.

34. Persad R. Massage Therapy and Medications. Toronto: Curties-Overzet Publications; 2001.

35. Mayo Clinic. Hypoglycemia. 2018. Available from: https://www.mayoclinic.org/diseases-conditions/hypoglycemia/symptoms-causes/syc-20373685

36. Mayo Clinic. Pneumonia. 2018. Available from: https://www.mayoclinic.org/diseases-conditions/pneumonia/symptoms-causes/syc-20354204

37. Weurth BA, Bonnewell JP, Wiemken TL, Arnold FW. Trends in pneumonia mortality rates and hospitalizations by organism, United States 2002–2011. 2016. Available from: https://wwwnc.cdc.gov/eid/article/22/9/15-0680_article

38. Mayo Clinic. Cellulitis. 2018. Available from: https://www.mayoclinic.org/diseases-conditions/cellulitis/symptoms-causes/syc-20370762?p=1

39. HCUP Fast Stats. Most common diagnoses for inpatient stays. 2019. Available from: https://www.hcup-us.ahrq.gov/faststats/NationalDiagnosesServlet

40. CDC. *Candida auris*. 2018. Available from: https://www.cdc.gov/fungal/candida-auris/c-auris-drug-resistant.html

41. WebMD. What is sepsis? 2017. Available from: https://www.webmd.com/a-to-z-guides/qa/what-is-sepsis

42. CDC. Urinary tract infection. 2019. Available from: https://www.cdc.gov/antibiotic-use/community/for-patients/common-illnesses/uti.html

43. AARP. Most common causes of hospital admissions for older adults. 2012. Available from: https://www.aarp.org/health/doctors-hospitals/info-03-2012/hospital-admissions-older-adults.html

44. Luyckx VA, Tonelli M, Stanifer JW. Bulletin of the World Health Organization. The global burden of kidney disease and the sustainable development goals. 2018. Available from: https://www.who.int/bulletin/volumes/96/6/17-206441/cn/

45. National Kidney Foundation. How Your Kidneys Work. Available from: https://www.kidncy.org/kidneydisease/howkidneyswrk

46. Bikhov B. Chronic kidney disease: impact on the global burden of mortality and morbidity. Available from: https://www.thelancet.com/campaigns/kidney/updates/chronic-kidney-disease-impact-on-global-burden-of-mortality-and-morbidity

47. Stel VS, Bruck K, Fraser S, et al. International difference in chronic kidney disease prevalence: a key public health and epidemiologic research issue. Neph Dialysis Transplant. 2017; 32(supl_2):ii29-ii35. Available from: https://academic.oup.com/ndt/article/32/suppl_2/ii129/2999740

48. Kidney Care UK. Facts and Stats. 2019. Available from: https://www.kidneycareuk.org/news-and-campaigns/facts-and-stats/

49. National Kidney Foundation. Chronic Kidney Disease Fact Sheet. 2019. Available from: https://nkf.egnyte.com/dl/h2PeqRLmEB/

50. Mayo Clinic. Chronic Kidney Disease. 2019. Available from: https://www.mayoclinic.org/diseases-conditions/chronic-kidney-disease/symptoms-causes/syc-20354521

51. American Kidney Fund. Acute kidney injury. Available from: http://www.kidneyfund.org/kidney-disease/kidney-problems/acute-kidney-injury.html

52. Mayo Clinic. End-stage renal disease. 2019. Available from: https://www.mayoclinic.org/diseases-conditions/end-stage-renal-disease/symptoms-causes/syc-20354532

53. Johns Hopkins Medicine. Liver: anatomy and functions. Available from: https://www.hopkinsmedicine.org/health/conditions-and-diseases/liver-anatomy-and-functions

54. WHO. Global hepatitis report, 2017. 2017. Available from: https://www.who.int/hepatitis/publications/global-hepatitis-report2017/en/

55. American Liver Foundation. Alcohol-related liver disease. 2017. Available from: https://liverfoundation.org/for-patients/about-the-liver/diseases-of-the-liver/alcohol-related-liver-disease/#information-for-the-newly-diagnosed

56. WebMD. Fatty Liver Disease. 2019. Available from: https://www.webmd.com/hepatitis/fatty-liver-disease#1

57. Pimpin L, Cortez-Pinto H, Negro F, et al., EASL HEPA-HEALTH Steering Committee. Burden of liver disease in Europe: epidemiology and analysis of risk factors to identify prevention policies. J Hepatology. 2018. Available from: https://www.journal-of-hepatology.eu/article/S0168-8278(18)32057-9/fulltext

58. NHS. Non-alcoholic fatty liver disease (NAFLD). 2018. Available from: https://www.nhs.uk/conditions/non-alcoholic-fatty-liver-disease/

59. Tommolino E. Medscape. Fatty Liver: Epidemiology. 2018. Available from: https://emedicine.medscape.com/article/175472-overview#a4

60. British Liver Trust. Hepatitis B. Available from: https://britishlivertrust.org.uk/information-and-support/living-with-a-liver-condition/liver-conditions/hepatitis-b/

61. British Liver Trust. Hepatitis C. Available from: https://britishlivertrust.org.uk/information-and-support/living-with-a-liver-condition/liver-conditions/hepatitis-c/

62. British Liver Trust. Hepatitis A. Available from: https://britishlivertrust.org.uk/information-and-support/living-with-a-liver-condition/liver-conditions/hepatitis-a/

63. British Liver Trust. Hepatitis E. Available from: https://britishlivertrust.org.uk/information-and-support/living-with-a-liver-condition/liver-conditions/hepatitis-e/

64. Mayo Clinic. Cirrhosis. 2018. Available from: https://www.mayoclinic.org/diseases-conditions/cirrhosis/symptoms-causes/syc-20351487

65. CDC. What is a concussion? 2019. Available from: https://www.cdc.gov/headsup/basics/concussion_whatis.html

66. Christopher & Dana Reeve Foundation. What is a complete vs incomplete injury? Available from: https://www.christopherreeve.org/living-with-paralysis/newly-paralyzed/how-is-an-sci-defined-and-what-is-a-complete-vs-incomplete-injury

67. Werner R. Working with clients who have spinal cord injuries. Massage Today. 2009. Available from: https://www.massagetoday.com/articles/10465/Working-with-Clients-Who-Have-Spinal-Cord-Injuries

68. Lovas J, Tran Y, Middleton J, et al. Managing pain and fatigue in people with spinal cord injury: a randomized controlled trial feasibility study examining the efficacy of massage therapy. Spinal Cord. 2017; 55(2);162–6.

69. Walton T. Medical Conditions and Massage Therapy: A Decision Tree Approach. Baltimore: Lippincott Williams & Wilkins; 2011.

70. Hansebout R, Kachur E. Acute traumatic spinal cord injury. 2019. Available from: https://www.uptodate.com/contents/acute-traumatic-spinal-cord-injury

71. Mayo Clinic. Alzheimer's and dementia: tips for better communication. 2019. Available from: https://www.mayoclinic.org/healthy-lifestyle/caregivers/in-depth/alzheimers/art-20047540

72. Jackson G. Personal communication, 15 September 2019.

73. Alzheimer's Association. What is Alzheimer's Disease? 2019. Available from: https://www.alz.org/alzheimers-dementia/what-is-alzheimers

74. Tague C. Massage Therapy for People Living with Neurological Challenges: Student Workbook. San Francisco: Tague Consulting; 2019.

75. WebMD. What is multiple sclerosis? 2019. Available from: https://www.webmd.com/multiple-sclerosis/what-is-multiple-sclerosis#1

76. Multiple Sclerosis Trust. Lhermittes sign. 2018. Available from: https://www.mstrust.org.uk/a-z/lhermittes-sign

77. Multiple Sclerosis Association of America. Bowel problems. 2016. Available from: https://mymsaa.org/ms-information/symptoms/bowel-problems/

78. Multiple Sclerosis Association of America. Bladder dysfunction. 2018. Available from: https://mymsaa.org/ms-information/symptoms/bladder-dysfunction/

79. Arab M, Radfar A, Madadizadeh N, et al. The effect of massage therapy on fatigue of patients with multiple sclerosis. J of Adv Pharma Ed & Research. 2019; 9(S2):44–9.

80. Backus D, Manella C, Bender A, Sweatman M. Impact of massage therapy on fatigue, pain, and spasticity in people with multiple sclerosis: a pilot study. Int J Ther Massage Bodywork. 2016; 9(4):4–13.

81. Hughes CM, Smyth S, Lowe-Strong AS. Reflexology for the treatment of pain in people with multiple sclerosis: a double-blind randomized sham-controlled clinical trial. Multiple Sclerosis. 2009; 15(11):1329–38.

82. Mayo Clinic. Parkinsonism: causes and coping strategies. 2019. Available from: https://www.mayoclinic.org/diseases-conditions/parkinsons-disease/expert-answers/parkinsonism/faq-20058490

83. MND Association. Basic facts about MND. 2019. Available from: https://www.mndassociation.org/about-mnd/what-is-mnd/basic-facts-about-mnd/

84. Spence C. Personal communication, 3 November 2019.

85. World Health Organization. WHO statement on caesarean section rates. 2015. Available from: https://www.who.int/reproductivehealth/publications/maternal_perinatal_health/cs-statement/en/

86. Boerma T, Ronsmans C, Melesse DY, et al. Global epidemiology of use of and disparities in caesarean sections. 2018. Available from: https://www.thelancet.com/journals/lancet/article/PIIS0140-6736(18)31928-7/fulltext

87. WHO Europe. Experts address alarming increase in caesarean sections at meeting in Tbilisi, Georgia. 2018. Available from: http://www.euro.who.int/en/countries/georgia/news/news/2018/12/experts-address-alarming-increase-in-caesarean-sections-at-meeting-in-tbilisi,-georgia

88. Cleveland Clinic. Why you should carefully weigh c-section against vaginal birth. 2017. Available from: https://health.clevelandclinic.org/why-you-should-carefully-weigh-c-section-against-a-vaginal-birth/

89. American College of Obstetrics and Gynecology. Approaches to limit intervention during labor and birth. 2017. Available from: https://www.acog.org/Clinical-Guidance-and-Publications/Committee-Opinions/Committee-on-Obstetric-Practice/Approaches-to-Limit-Intervention-During-Labor-and-Birth

90. Betrán AP, Temmerman M, Kingdon C, et al. Interventions to reduce unnecessary caesarean sections in healthy women and babies. 2018. Available from: https://www.thelancet.com/journals/lancet/article/PIIS0140-6736(18)31927-5/fulltext

91. Davis P, Knuttinen MG. Deep vein thrombosis in pregnancy: incidence, pathogenesis and endovascular management. Cardiovasc Diagn Ther. 2017; 7(Suppl 3):S309–S319.

92. WebMD. Pregnancy masssage. 2019. Available from: https://www.webmd.com/baby/pregnancy-and-massage#2

93. Osborne-Sheets C. Personal communication, 21 November 2003.

94. Gray C. Personal communication, 17 March 2001.

95. United Network for Organ Sharing. Transplant. 2019. Available from: https://unos.org/transplant/?gclid=Cj0KC-QjwjrvpBRC0ARIsAFrFuV_2uvBj-XZoVa6tcrCumfY3hGG-HZywvwQur3bsdbl2rexxgGkBmADsaAvJZEALw_wcB

96. European Commission. Journalist workshop on organ donation and transplantation. Recent facts and figures. 2014. Available from: https://ec.europa.eu/health//sites/health/files/blood_tissues_organs/docs/ev_20141126_factsfigures_en.pdf

97. WebMD. What is an ammonia test? 2019. Available from: https://www.webmd.com/a-to-z-guides/ammonia-test#1

98. Medscape. Liver transplantation treatment and management. 2019. Available from: https://emedicine.medscape.com/article/431783-treatment

99. Mayo Clinic. Kidney transplant. 2019. Available from: https://www.mayoclinic.org/tests-procedures/kidney-transplant/about/pac-20384777

100. Mayo Clinic. Liver transplant. 2019. Available from: https://www.mayoclinic.org/tests-procedures/liver-transplant/about/pac-20384842

101. Johns Hopkins Medicine. Heart transplant. Available from: https://www.hopkinsmedicine.org/health/treatment-tests-and-therapies/heart-transplant

102. United Network of Sharing. Post-transplant medications. Available from: https://transplantliving.org/after-the-transplant/preventing-rejection/post-transplant-medications/

103. MedlinePlus. Kidney transplant. 2019. Available from: https://medlineplus.gov/ency/article/003005.htm

104. Lucarelli G, Isgro A, Sodani P, Gaziev J. Hematopoietic stem cell transplantation in thalessemia and sickle cell anemia. Cold Spring Harb Perspect Med. 2012; 2(5):a011825.

105. WebMD. Stem cells for knees: promising treatment or hoax? 2017. Available from: https://www.webmd.com/osteoarthritis/news/20170407/stem-cells-for-knees-promising-treatment-or-hoax#2

106. MD Anderson Cancer Center. Stem cell transplants. Available from: https://www.mdanderson.org/treatment-options/stem-cell-transplantation.html

107. National Cancer Institute. NCI dictionary of cancer terms. Stem cell engraftment. Available from: https://www.cancer.gov/publications/dictionaries/cancer-terms/def/stem-cell-engraftment

108. American Society of Clinical Oncologists. Side effects of a bone marrow transplant (stem cell transplant). 2018. Available from: https://www.cancer.net/navigating-cancer-care/how-cancer-treated/bone-marrowstem-cell-transplantation/side-effects-bone-marrow-transplant-stem-cell-transplant

Additional resources

In Care of Dad. 40 things a stroke survivor might need. Available from: http://www.incareofdad.com/article-detail/140/40-things-a-stroke-survivor-may-need.html

MacDonald G. Medicine Hands: Massage Therapy for People with Cancer. Findhorn: Findhorn Press; 2014.

Maddox S. Paralysis Resource Guide (3rd edition). New Jersey: Christopher & Dana Reeve Foundation; 2013.

Motz J. Hands of Life. New York: Bantam Doubleday Dell Publishing Group; 2000.

Muscular Dystrophy Association. Everyday Life with ALS: A Practical Guide. Available from: https://www.mda.org/sites/default/files/publications/Everyday_Life_with_ALS_P-532.pdf

Naparstek B. Audio recordings to support all types of patient groups and health conditions. Available from: www.healthjourneys.com

Nelson D. From the Heart Through the Hands: The Power of Touch in Caregiving. Findhorn: Findhorn Press; 2006.

Osborne C. Pre- and Peri-natal Massage Therapy (2nd edition). Baltimore: Lippincott Williams & Wilkins; 2012.

Rossato-Bennett M. Alive inside (film). 2014. Available from: http://www.aliveinside.us

Sanford M. Walking: A Memoir of Trauma and Transcendence. USA: Rodale; 2006.

Shapiro A. Healing Into Possibility: The Transformational Lessons of a Stroke. Navoto: New World Library; 2009.

Stillerman E. Mother Massage. New York: Delta Trade Paperback; 2006.

Taylor J. My Stroke of Insight: A Brain Scientist's Personal Journey. New York: Penguin Group; 2006.

Taylor J. "My Stroke of Insight" TEDTalk. 2008. Available from: https://www.ted.com/talks/jill_bolte_taylor_my_stroke_of_insight/up-next

Van der Kolk B. the Body Knows the Score: Brain, Mind, and Body in the Healing of Trauma. New York: Viking; 2014.

Yates S. Pregnancy and Childbirth: A Holistic Approach to Massage and Bodywork. Edinburgh: Churchill Livingstone; 2010.

The symptom…is a request for support; not support for simply getting rid of, or fixing it; but support for bearing it, for suffering it as an experience of life.

Dianne M. Connelly,
All Sickness is Homesickness

Massage therapists are trained to take their cues from the body's musculature. Are the muscles firm or flabby? Are joints supple or limited? Is the posture in alignment or out? These indications are helpful for musculoskeletal bodywork. However, for medically complex patients, symptoms, such as edema, fatigue, and bruising, are the signposts that give the massage therapist guidance: they reflect the deeper processes happening within the person.

The purpose of this chapter is to present more detailed information about symptoms that are common to a variety of diseases and conditions. While a symptom may appear the same in all patients, the underlying cause can be very different, and, therefore, require different adjustments to the massage session. For example, a touch practitioner could encounter edema in five patients. With one patient, it may be a byproduct of congestive heart failure (CHF); with another, pregnancy may be the cause. Prednisone use, extended bedrest, a blood clot, and many other situations can also cause edema. In four of the above scenarios, light massage could be safely given; in the fifth, any type of stroking motion would be contraindicated. By becoming more familiar with various symptoms and their causes, bodywork practitioners will have a deeper understanding of massage precautions.

Ascites

Ascites is the build-up of excess fluid between the two layers of the peritoneum, a membrane that lines the abdomen.[1] The abdomen swells, becoming large and distended, resembling pregnancy. The most frequent cause of ascites is advanced liver disease and cirrhosis, but other nonmalignant conditions, such as renal disease, COPD,

CHF, and TB, can cause ascites. Ascites also develops when certain advanced cancers spread to the peritoneum or the liver, typically ovarian, colon, stomach, endometrial, pancreatic, breast, or lung cancer. This is referred to as malignant ascites and the outlook for this type is poor. However, those with ascites due to a chronic condition, such as liver disease, CHF, and COPD, have a more optimistic prognosis and can manage their disease over a long period of time.[2]

The pathophysiology behind this condition is not completely understood. One theory is that hypertension within the hepatic portal vein creates an imbalanced pressure gradient between the fluid in the hepatic vessel and the abdominal cavity. The fluid flows from a place of high pressure, the hepatic vessel, to a place of lower pressure, the abdominal cavity. Additionally, the diseased liver produces less albumin, a protein that keeps fluid in the bloodstream so that it doesn't leak out of the vessels into surrounding tissue.[2]

Depending on the cause of ascites, treatment by the medical team may include reduced sodium intake, reduced fluids, and/or diuretics. When these approaches fail or are deemed inappropriate, ascites may be managed by paracentesis, a bedside procedure in which fluid is removed through a needle under local anesthesia. The volume of fluid may be quite large, five liters or more, which typically provides immediate relief of symptoms. If the cause of ascites is ongoing, such as occurs with end-stage liver disease or advanced cancer, the fluid will return, requiring repeat paracentesis. Surgical placement of a shunt is sometimes used to manage chronic ascites.

Patients whose abdomens are distended from ascites can experience discomfort or pain, loss of appetite, indigestion, nausea, vomiting, shortness of breath, and edema of the lower extremities. The extra liters of fluid impact simple daily activities such as breathing, sitting, and walking, which further compounds the patient's suffering.

There is no scientific evidence about how to proceed when massaging patients affected by ascites. The clinical experience of many practitioners has shown that it is safe to perform gentle, comfort-oriented strokes or touch to these patients. The root cause of the swelling will impact the massage session plan. A patient with malignant ascites or end-stage liver disease will be more medically complex and less stable than someone with chronic congestive heart failure or chronic liver disease. The latter groups of patients will, most likely, be able to have massage therapy that is slightly more demanding.

Clinical considerations: Ascites

Pressure:

- Level 1 strokes or holds to lower and upper extremities and posterior trunk.

Site:

- Some patients will not tolerate touch to the abdomen. If they do, apply level 1 abdominal effleurage (in a clockwise direction), or abdominal holds may be comforting to some patients.
- Be mindful of skin integrity.
- Avoid areas where recent paracentesis was performed.

Positioning:

- Usually a Fowler's (semi-recumbent) position, works best to ease shortness of breath. The angle of the head of the bed will depend on the patient. Let them be the guide to their own comfort.
- Traditional side-lying in a flat position is usually not tolerated due to breathing difficulties. However, for a short time, many patients find side-lying from a Fowler's position allows them to breathe adequately while giving the therapist access to their back for massage. Also, it takes the pressure off the sacrum for a short while.

Other:

- A shorter session is often indicated.

Bruising and bleeding

People bruise easily for a variety of reasons. Diabetics bruise easily because their disease causes blood vessels to become fragile. Poor oxygenation, such as occurs with CHF or COPD, can cause tissues to become fragile and therefore more susceptible to trauma. Advanced age also can cause patients to bruise more easily as a result of fragile tissues.

A bruise can be painful and unsightly, which is sufficient reason for massage therapists to take care when working with those whose tissues are fragile. However, bruising can be a sign of thrombocytopenia, a condition with more serious implications. In thrombocytopenia, there are insufficient platelets, the clotting component of blood. When the number of platelets is low, bruising can occur easily and clotting time is slow. More dangerous than bruising, however, is the risk for bleeding. A normal platelet count is between 150,000 and 450,000 per cubic microliter of blood, expressed as $150–450 \times 10^3$/microL. (The zeros are dropped off to make the numbers more manageable.) If a person's platelet count is below normal, they are considered thrombocytopenic.[3]

A number of medications, most notably anticoagulants, such as aspirin, heparin, and warfarin (Coumadin), and many antitumor drugs, cause physiological changes that affect the coagulation of platelets. Specific diseases cause the platelet level to be low due to decreased production. Leukemias, multiple myeloma, and some lymphomas are examples, as well as liver diseases. HELLP syndrome, a severe complication of pregnancy-induced hypertension, causes low platelets, and platelets can also be destroyed as a result of an infection such as *Escherichia coli* (E. coli), trauma to the body, or medications.[3,4]

While a platelet count of 150,000/microL is below the norm and technically qualifies as thrombocytopenia, it is not a particularly dangerous level. Unless there are other influencing factors, patients can be given the usual bodywork that any hospitalized person receives. However, when levels drop to 50,000/microL, usually expressed by health care staff as 50, special attention must be paid to the amount of pressure. It should not exceed anything more than heavy lotioning or a level 2 pressure. There may, however, be some patients whose platelet count is 50, but who have other influencing factors that call for level 1 pressure. Age, comorbidities, and previous health status would be examples of influencing factors. Take for instance a 25-year-old and a 65-year-old patient being treated for lymphoma with chemotherapy, both with a platelet count of 50. The 25-year-old has no previous health problems, while the older patient has a history of diabetes and kidney dysfunction. It would be best to use level 1 massage strokes with the older person because of their previous longstanding health conditions. However, the 25-year-old person who has no comorbidities could receive level 2 pressure, since they will likely have much better tissue integrity that is less at risk for bruising than the 65-year-old. Many therapists want black and white guidelines, however, there are often gray zones in which they must apply their clinical thinking abilities.

A platelet count of below 20,000/microL, or 20, will necessitate a very gentle level 1 touch, focusing just on the skin. Lotion with good glide should be used to avoid any drag or friction on the skin. A count below 20 puts the patient in danger of bleeding, the most serious of which are brain and retinal bleeds. Without sufficient platelets, any bleeding whether internal or external, no matter how miniscule, is difficult to stop. Occasionally, the platelet level is so low that patients aren't allowed to brush their teeth for fear of causing the gums to bleed. Patients who receive high-dose chemotherapy, such as stem cell transplant patients, are most at risk for this level of thrombocytopenia: counts below 10 are not unusual in this group.

When massaging patients who bruise easily, the practitioner should put their focus on the skin rather than the muscles. Applying lotion in a systematic way with a very gentle effleurage stroke is safe, as are techniques that do not employ pressure or stroking, such as craniosacral therapies or Polarity Therapy. However, patients with seriously low platelet counts often will be hesitant to accept touch therapies, and their doctors and nurses will be reluctant to approve them for fear the touch will be too heavy and cause bleeding. Most hospital staff are unfamiliar with the broad range of bodywork modalities. Their knowledge may come from the experience of receiving massage as a healthy person or from information seen in the popular media where massage is given in a more vigorous manner. The touch practitioner can help foster approval by using such phrases as "gentle massage" or "light touch" and briefly demonstrating on the doctor's or nurse's back (having of course asked for their permission.) Referring to the massage as "lotioning" is also helpful and truly describes what will occur with these patients.

Hospitals have varying policies about the massage of thrombocytopenic patients. Some set the threshold at 20, forbidding all touch therapy if a patient is below that level. Other institutions have a policy of only gentle holds when the platelet level is below 20, while some allow holds or level 1 pressure at 20. A few hospitals have higher thresholds, such as 50, only allowing massage if the patients are above that level. The therapist is bound to observe the policies of each health care facility regardless of suggestions in this book.

Therapist's journal 8.1
The messy aftermath

Yesterday I provided massage for a 59-year-old patient with multiple myeloma who has thoroughly stolen my heart. He started a "Go Hat Me" campaign rather than a "Go Fund Me" page and now has a collection of several hundred hilarious hats, which he changes out frequently throughout the day. He had a terrifying nosebleed that lasted for over an hour, during which I massaged his feet and conversed with him in an effort to quell his understandable anxiety. All the while, the medical team kept packing his nostril with gauze that repeatedly became saturated with blood within seconds. We keep black towels at the unit for such situations, but this all happened too quickly to grab the right towels.

Once the staff had the bleeding under control, they departed and the patient and I were left alone in the room. The bed was soaked with blood. He was nodding off, all the while clutching his cell phone in his

continued

blood-covered hands. He'd attempted to text a friend to come be with him, but was not able to operate the phone. I asked if I could help him dial the number, but he declined. Then I asked what else I could for him and he said (this makes me cry to write) could I help "clean up a bit" while the nursing staff were attending to another patient. I put on gloves and gathered all the bloody gauze in a biohazard bag. I put all the bloody towels in the dirty hospital linen bag. I did not move him, afraid the bleeding would start again. The bloody fitted sheet and draw sheet I couldn't remove, so I laid clean pillowcases on top to cover the blood until the CNA was able to change his bedding.

Because we've just moved onto a new unit, it's been all hands on deck while we figure out staffing for the new floor. Everyone has been working really hard, stretching to cover patients, family, phones, and housekeeping. Sometimes I find myself doing things that are way outside my job description. It's often reality versus the ideal.

This experience was all pretty intense for a soft, serenity-loving therapist. There was nothing in my background to prepare me for this event, or the messy aftermath of blood-soaked linens. Our staff talk about patients whose deaths are due to "bleeding out," but I thought that was just a term used on "Grey's Anatomy" for dramatic effect.

Cindy Spence MPH, LMT
Dallas, Texas

Clinical considerations: Bruising and bleeding

Pressure:

- Light pressure, generally level 1 or 2.
- When massaging thrombocytopenic patients, use a lotion with good glide to avoid friction to the tissues. If a good product is not available, apply touch over the sheets. Sheets have surprisingly good glide.

Site:

- Be mindful of areas that are bruised.

Constipation

Readers might be surprised at how serious and painful constipation can be. Narcotics are the chief culprit due to a slowing of peristaltic activity in the colon, but other drugs, such as chemotherapies, also contribute. Decreased activity and fluid intake can play a part in bowel problems, as do certain diseases, such as stroke, MS, and Parkinson's disease.[5]

Constipation can range from mild to impacted, the latter requiring medical intervention. Massage is not effective in cases of impaction. However, in mild to moderate cases, there is a great deal of anecdotal evidence supporting the success of using various touch modalities, such as Shiatsu, Polarity Therapy, Reiki, or Swedish massage. It is necessary to look to anecdotal evidence because the research is sparse and inconclusive. A few studies have applicable information that can be integrated into practice. A study of people with opioid-induced constipation were given a 15-minute abdominal massage training video and asked to perform the technique twice a day for four weeks. Compared to the control group, the abdominal massage group had a decrease in the severity of constipation, the feeling of incomplete bowel emptying, and other improvements.[6] A study done by the MS Trust trained an experimental group in abdominal massage and encouraged them to carry out massage once a day for six seeks. There was improvement in the bowel problems but it didn't reach statistical significance, which may be due to the design of the study protocol.[7]

Patients are accustomed to being asked by nurses about their bowel movements. Massage therapists, too, should feel at ease in speaking to patients about their bowel health. Today's massage therapist working in health care not only gives comfort and nurturance but also plays a part in managing specific symptoms. Constipation is a condition in which practitioners have a great many tools to accomplish this: acupressure points, reflexology zones, and Swedish massage to the abdomen. Figure 8.1 illustrates the direction and sequence in which to apply Swedish massage techniques to the abdomen. When doing reflexology on the foot, the same sequence should be applied.

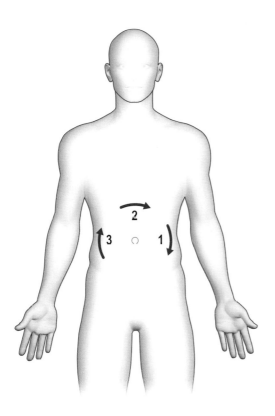

FIGURE 8.1
Massaging the abdomen. The arrows are numbered to correspond with the order of strokes. Begin with #1, the descending colon, proceed next to #2, the transverse colon, and then #3, the ascending colon, ending with long, continuous strokes in a clockwise direction.

Clinical considerations: Constipation

Pressure:

- Patients can be in mild to severe discomfort because of constipation, which can distress their entire body. Even if constipation is their only complaint, gentler pressure will be required over the entire body.

Site:

- If the patient can't tolerate direct touch to the abdomen, indirect techniques, such as reflexology, Shiatsu meridians, or acupressure, may be helpful.

Positioning:

- Self-limiting.

Tip 8.1 Common acupressure points for constipation

Stomach 25 and 36, liver 2, large intestine 4 and 11, conception vessel 6, 10, and 12, pericardium 6, spleen 6.[8]

Dyspnea (shortness of breath)

Dyspnea, the feeling of being short of breath, is the result of a many conditions: COPD is a common one, and others include heart diseases, such a CHF or cardiomyopathy, lung cancer, anxiety disorders, obesity, pulmonary embolism, and pulmonary hypertension. The adjustments needed for the massage session will vary depending on the root cause.[9] For example, dyspnea due to anxiety will have different implications than that of in someone with heart disease. Although the following sections may give the impression that there are clear boundaries between types of respiratory patients, in reality, there is a great deal of overlapping between groups. Pulmonary hypertension is an example: this condition can lead to COPD in some, while in others it causes heart failure.[10]

Chronic obstructive pulmonary disease (COPD)

Three conditions commonly cause COPD: asthma, chronic bronchitis, and emphysema. All three disorders cause airways to narrow, preventing the lungs from

157

performing efficiently. Airflow into and out of the lungs requires more time, slowing the exchange of oxygen and carbon dioxide. The end result is labored breathing. Over a period of time, poor lung functioning causes the heart to overwork, the potential consequence being right-sided heart failure. Management of the disease is through medications such as bronchodilators, corticosteroids, cough suppressants, and decongestants.

Emphysema not only creates narrowing in the airways, but also causes the alveoli, the tiny air sacs in the lungs, to lose their natural elasticity, become overstretched, and rupture. The person with this disease is then only able to partially exhale. Development of an excessively enlarged chest is a characteristic side effect.

People with COPD are prone to serious respiratory diseases such as pneumonia, acute bronchitis, and influenza. Diminished air exchange also results in fatigue, a weakened immune system, and tissue fragility and cyanosis in the extremities. Tissues injure more easily and heal more slowly, with a lesser quality of repair.[11] Constant breathing difficulty and fatigue makes the patient irritable, apprehensive, anxious, depressed, and powerless. During an episode of respiratory insufficiency, people may be sleepy, restless, aggressive, panic-stricken, or confused.

Massage can benefit these patients in many ways. Narrowed airways force the respiratory muscles to overwork, most especially the muscles of the diaphragm and upper girdle, trapezius, scalenes, and sternocleidomastoid. Therefore, attention to the neck and thoracic area will be welcome. Polastri et al., also suggest in their scoping review that percussion and vibrations to the chest can enhance the clearance of mucus.[12] During times of anxiety and hopelessness, touch can soothe tension and give the person a sense of control. In addition, massage can play a part in developing relaxation skills, an important component in learning to live with a chronic respiratory problem.

Organ failure

Organ failure, which typically involves the heart, lungs, liver, or kidneys, is a common cause of dyspnea and runs along a spectrum from mild to severe. Often when the term "failure" is used, it means a diminishment in the organ's functioning, such as with congestive heart failure

or renal failure. The cause of labored breathing might be fluid around the heart or in the lungs, which would call for a distinctly different massage approach than with a patient affected by COPD. The medical staff will support the dyspneic patient in organ failure with supplemental oxygen, medications, and in some cases removal of fluid around the lungs. Touch practitioners can support the patient during bouts of anxiety that arise from dyspnea. A slow, soothing approach that instills a sense of safety can positively impact the person's sense of breathing difficulty.

Other causes of dyspnea

Shortness of breath can arise in many other circumstances, such as asthma, situational anxiety, a mood disorder, or pulmonary fibrosis. A slow, sedating approach to massage therapy is often the best in these cases. If obesity is the cause, improving the patient's positioning might improve their breathing. A collapsed lung will surely affect the breathing and brings on a panicky feeling. One patient was admitted to the hospital with a collapsed lung due to broken ribs that had caused bleeding in the pleural cavity. The patient was frightened as she tried and failed to breathe adequately. Slow, gentle foot massage soothed the patient enough to quell the struggle to breathe.

Pulmonary embolism is the most consequential of all the causes of dyspnea. However, even a person being treated for a pulmonary embolism could have calming holds with the approval of the nursing or medical staff.

Clinical considerations: Dyspnea

Pressure:

- Fatigue.
- Tissue fragility.

Site:

- Oxygen-delivery device.

Positioning:

- Fowler's position will be best in most circumstances.

Edema

Edema is the accumulation of fluid in the interstitial space between cells and can be the result of many different factors. It can be part of a disease process, such as heart or renal failure, or an obstruction, such as a blood clot or tumor. Certain medications, inflammation, or an electrolyte imbalance can be the cause. Pregnancy, too, nearly always is accompanied by swelling in the extremities, as is extended bedrest.

Edematous tissues are not only puffy but fragile. The skin integrity may be poor due to being overstretched, thereby increasing the chance of a pressure sore or skin breakdown. People with edema also often have reduced blood flow, which further increases the risk of skin breakdown.

Gentle Swedish massage in particular can be helpful to people with edema. It doesn't solve the issue, but instead gives people relief from the heavy fullness that can develop. Patients with swelling due to pregnancy, lack of ambulation, and fluid retention due to medications, such as steroids or antitumor drugs, can also safely receive gentle effleurage to the legs. So, too, can most people with renal or heart insufficiency. The key is to not place an extra demand on these systems, which can be accomplished with nonforceful pressure and shortening the length of the session.

It is still appropriate to caution against any type of massage stroke, gentle or otherwise, to areas that are edematous due to local infection or a blood clot. Swelling due to obstructions, such as a tumor, would also preclude the use of any type of touch that moves fluid. However, many hospital massage therapists have safely substituted techniques, such as Reiki or gentle holds, that do not use pressure or stroking.

The following guidelines are intended for use with patients with edema. Later in this chapter lymphedema is discussed, and in many ways the guidelines are similar. However, the two types of edema have very different causes and call for a separate discussion.

Clinical considerations: Edema

Pressure:

- Edematous tissues are fragile. Use only the amount of pressure required for lotioning, level 1–2.
- The skin in the swollen area may also have poor integrity if the edema is chronic.
- Reduced pressure may be necessary to prevent overloading major organ systems.

Site:

- Massage strokes should be avoided to limbs with an obstruction, blood clot, or infection-related edema. Resting the hands on the limb may be used instead with staff approval.
- Be watchful for areas of skin that may have thinned due to edema.
- No touch to a weeping area of the body.

Positioning:

- Elevate edematous limbs.
- Be mindful of placing the person in a side-lying position on the edematous limb, as it may be uncomfortable. Additionally, the weight of the body may create an occlusion.

Other:

- It is important when massaging limbs affected by edema that therapists adhere to the following instructions and work in the sequence given (see Figure 8.2 A–C).
  1. Stroke only towards the heart.
  2. Massage the proximal part of the limb first (upper leg or arm).
  3. Do not bring the stroke back toward the feet or hands. Always stroke toward the heart. Hand-over-hand stroking gives the feeling of continuous contact. Massaging in this sequence allows the area "upstream" to empty, thereby creating space for the fluid that will drain from the lower regions.

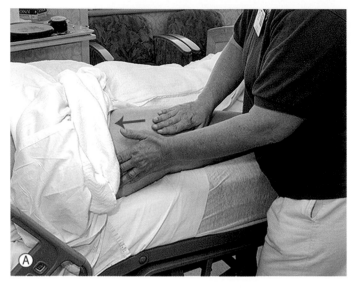

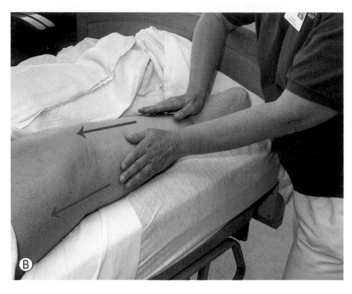

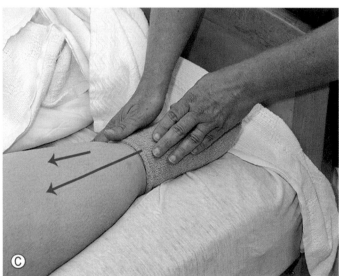

FIGURE 8.2

A Begin by massaging the most proximal section of the limb (thigh or upper arm). **B** Next move to the middle section of the limb (knee or elbow areas). Give attention to the joints, as fluid pools there. **C** End with the lower part of the extremity (ankle/foot or wrist/hand), still performing strokes toward the heart. (*Author's note:* Ideally this patient would have removed her socks, but her feet were cold, so she declined.) End with at least three long integrative strokes from the distal to proximal end of the limb to give the feeling of wholeness.

(Photos by Don Hamilton.)

Fatigue

As with many other conditions, fatigue is a multifaceted state. It may be due to a low red blood cell count, as occurs with anemia. Or poor oxygenation, a result of COPD or CHF, can also leave people feeling tired. A person's disease may be the culprit, such as MS, lupus, or Parkinson's disease. Many medications, such as cancer therapies, anticonvulsants, antacids, and certain heart medications, can contribute to a sense of being fatigued. Fatigue accompanies an infection. There is also a psychological component brought on by fear, loss of control, or hopelessness that can be a part of tiredness. Even if all of the above factors were absent, being confined to bed decreases circulation, thereby creating a sense of lethargy.

When creating the massage session plan, it is important for the therapist to hone in on the reason for the patient's sense of feeling fatigued. Are the sensations truly fatigue, or is the person experiencing lethargy, weakness, or drowsiness? Certain medications, such as those for blood pressure and heart disease, can cause a feeling of drowsiness or lethargy due to depression of the central nervous system and slowing down of the heart. This is different from fatigue related to cancer treatment or an infection. Blood pressure and heart medications, on their own, might not require a major pressure adjustment to massage strokes. However, fatigue related to chemotherapy or an infection has a different root cause and would demand a significant decrease of pressure.

For instance, Jerry, 75 years old, was affected by Parkinson's disease, which caused his muscles to be very rigid; the tension created tiredness. The rigidity also caused him to shuffle when walking and he moved very slowly. Additionally, Jerry had anemia, for which he took epoetin alfa (Procrit) to support red blood cell production. On the other hand, Jasmina, 60 years old, had high blood pressure and cholesterol for which the doctor prescribed lisinopril (Zestril) for blood pressure and atorvastin (Lipitor) for cholesterol. She reported these medicines made her feel lethargic and her thinking fuzzy. Both of these patients indicated to the therapist that they were fatigued, because fatigue is a catch-all word. However, the massage plan for Jerry would have called for greater adjustments than Jasmina, despite both people using the word fatigue to describe how they felt.

Rather than being titled fatigue, this section could have been titled "rest and healing," giving it a more positive outlook. In the past, rest was one of the primary treatments for regaining health – people undertook rest cures. One of the most significant contributions that touch therapy has to offer any patient is the chance to rest, and rest promotes healing. Patients consistently report feeling more energetic following a massage session if the level of demand on their body is properly adjusted. Some of the ways to make a session more restful is to decrease the pressure level, substitute demanding modalities for gentler ones, shorten the length of session, and minimize any agenda. This is true for all patients whether they are experiencing lethargy, exhaustion, weariness, or fatigue. And it is true no matter whether the root cause is fever, fear, COPD, or recovering from surgery. (See Table 6.1 (Pressure Scale) for more details on pressure adjustments.)

Clinical considerations: Fatigue

Pressure:
- Administer light pressure, allowing the body to rest.

Positioning:
- Severely fatigued patients may tolerate only minimal repositioning.

Other:
- During episodes of fatigue, sessions may need to be shortened.

Fever

Fever is typically associated with infection due to bacteria or virus. The patient may be admitted with it; it could have been introduced via an indwelling catheter or during surgery; a low white blood cell count from cancer chemotherapy could be the reason; or the fever could be a reaction to a blood transfusion or medication. However, there are also noninfectious fevers associated with heart attack, trauma, pulmonary embolism, alcohol withdrawal, and advanced cancers, especially leukemia and lymphoma.

Fever is taught as a strong contraindication to massage, which then is incorrectly translated to mean "do not touch." However, it must now be apparent to the reader that some form of touch therapy can nearly always be performed no matter how severe a person's medical condition. The only time a practitioner should avoid contact with a febrile patient is when the fever is caused by a communicable disease.

The patient's body systems are hard at work during a febrile episode. The heart rate increases significantly, speeding up the distribution of white blood cells, and cell wall permeability is increased, which allows for faster chemical reactions and therefore faster recovery for damaged tissues. Immune activity is stimulated, particularly T cells, B cells, and antibodies. The toxic by-products of the bacteria or virus also create side effects in the body, such as fatigue, confusion, and joint pain.[13,14]

Systematic touch that does not place a demand on the body is beneficial for febrile patients. Slow, light lotioning strokes or resting the hands on the body are well received in this circumstance. Gentle, compassionate touch will sometimes temporarily lower an elevated body temperature, giving the patient a momentary respite from the discomfort of a fever.

There will be differing opinions regarding touch therapy during fever – some institutions allow therapists to apply gentle touch, others do not. Clinically there is no reason not to support a policy of gentle touch during febrile episodes. However, some staff will be wary of it and that must be taken into consideration.

Clinical considerations: Fever

Pressure:

- Only gentle holds or light lotioning.

Immunosuppression

People in health care settings, especially hospitals, long-term care facilities, or rehabilitation centers, are especially prone to immunosuppression. Sometimes it is an outcome of advanced age, other times it can be due to medications, such as steroidal drugs or those taken for HIV and cancer. Surgery and trauma, too, can suppress the immune system,[15] as can diseases such as leukemia, aplastic anemia, AIDS, and lymphomas. This is because the level of either white blood cells or lymphocytes is lowered or not functioning normally. The principal side effect of a deficient immune system is the risk of infection. Other complications are increased risk of cancer, fungal infections, malaise, fatigue, and fever.

Two medical terms associated with lowered immunity are leukopenia and neutropenia. Leukopenia is a decreased level of all white blood cells. The normal level of white blood cells is around 4,500 and 11,000 leukocytes per cubic microliter (most often denoted as $4.5–11 \times 10^3$/microL to make the numbers more manageable.) Neutropenia is a low level of neutrophils, the white blood cells which are essential for fighting infection.[16] The

importance of infection cannot be overstated, as it is a common cause of death. The neutrophil level is measured using a lab test called the absolute neutrophil count (ANC). The normal range is between 1,500 and 8,000 cells per cubic microliter ($1.5–8.0 \times 10^3$/microL). A lab value of 1,500 or lower is considered neutropenic. A count of 500 (0.5) represents severe neutropenia, which commonly occurs in chemotherapy patients.[17]

Cancer and AIDS patients are particularly prone to immunosuppression: cancer patients because of treatment, and AIDS patients because of the disease. People who receive high-dose chemotherapy, such as precedes bone marrow or stem cell transplantation, experience the most severe immunosuppression. High-dose chemotherapy causes the white blood cell count to drop to as low as 100 (0.1). During this time, patients are at an extremely high risk of infection from micro-organisms that are benign to a healthy person – to the person with neutropenia, they can be lethal. Even fresh food and flowers are not allowed because of the bacteria and fungi on them.

The immune systems of people who go through organ transplantation are purposely suppressed with drugs, such as cyclosporine and prednisone, to prevent rejection of the new organ. The trade-off, however, for managing the rejection is that it puts the person at risk for infection. Often organ transplant patients must take immunosuppressants for the rest of their lives.[18]

Immunosuppression does not stop a person from receiving bodywork. There may be co-influencing factors that the therapist must adjust for related to age, surgery, or disease. However, the specific adjustment related to a compromised immune system is the observance of Standard Precautions.

Clinical considerations: Immunosuppression

Pressure:

- If the person is severely immunosuppressed, they generally feel unwell and have other co-influences. Undemanding pressure is called for.

continued

Inflammation

Health care patients are affected by a wide variety of inflammatory conditions, some of which are systemic and others are local. Meningitis and measles are examples of systemic conditions that have an inflammatory component, one being triggered by bacteria, the other by a virus. Systemic inflammatory conditions are characterized by fever and fatigue.

Dermatitis, surgical sites, and wounds are examples of local inflammation. Intravenous (IV) catheters and the medications given through them can also create inflammation. Phlebitis, the inflammation of a vein, and cellulitis, an acute infection of the skin and subcutaneous tissue, are common inflammatory conditions encountered in health care settings. Cellulitis develops most often in the presence of damaged skin or poor circulation.

The classic symptoms of local inflammation are **heat**, **tenderness**, **redness**, and **swelling**. Other signs are loss of function, itching, the formation of blood clots, and pus. Local inflammation, such as in phlebitis and lymphangitis, also may present with a red streak that runs proximal from the site of inflammation.[19]

The symptoms of inflammation are signals to touch practitioners that there is a condition developing, or one that is already fully matured. Because of their involvement with the skin, massage therapists may be the ones who discover cellulitis, a blood clot, or an edematous area caused by inflammation. Comprehensive skin assessment is crucial for patients in these settings. If heat, tenderness, redness, or swelling is encountered, the therapist should stop, query the patient if possible, and consult with the nursing staff when in doubt.

Clinical considerations: Inflammation

Pressure:

- Even if inflammation is local in nature, it is safest in this environment to give gentle massage to the entire body.

Site:

- Avoid contact with areas of local inflammation.

Positioning:

- An inflamed wound, such as a decubitus ulcer or unhealed wound, may preclude certain positions.
- Inflammation that triggers swelling may benefit from elevation.

Lymphedema

This section is intended to bring greater awareness of lymphedema to practitioners. It is well beyond the scope of the book to train therapists how to provide lymphatic drainage or even how to massage areas affected by serious lymphedema. Therapists are encouraged to study this topic further and become adequately trained so that they can perform relaxation massage safely.

Lymphatic basics

Lymphedema can be caused by a variety of triggers, such as congenital influences, surgery, or trauma. Most often, however, therapists will encounter lymphedema, or a risk for it, in cancer patients whose treatment involved removal of and/or radiation therapy to the lymph nodes in the **neck**, **axilla**, or **groin**. It is these three clusters that drain superficial lymph. In people whose lymphatic system is intact, lymph converges toward these three main groups of nodes. (Notice how the arrows are pointing toward these three clusters of nodes in Figure 8.3.) Three main watersheds divide the body into territories.

If some of the cervical, axillary, or inguinal nodes have been removed and/or damaged by radiation therapy, the capacity of the lymphatic system is lessened in that area. The combination of surgical removal and radiotherapy further increases the possibility of lymphedema occurring.

The lymphatic system has been likened to a sewage treatment plant with the lymph nodes acting as the filtering system for plasma protein molecules, fats, cellular debris, bacteria, and viruses. If the lymph nodes have been removed or damaged by radiation, the "sewage" contained in that part of the lymphatic system goes

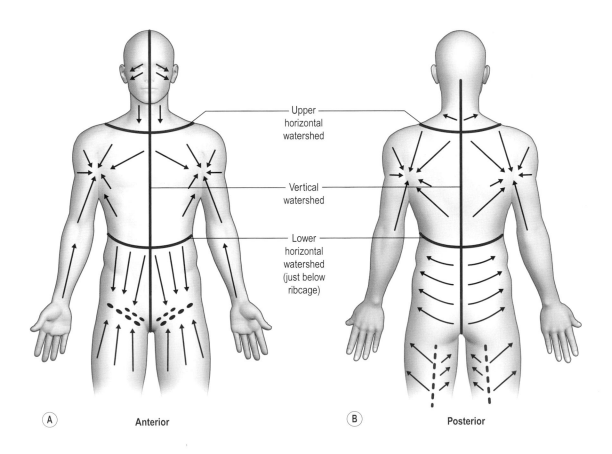

Upper horizontal watershed

Vertical watershed

Lower horizontal watershed (just below ribcage)

A   Anterior

B   Posterior

FIGURE 8.3
Superficial lymph drainage patterns. In a healthy patient, the superficial lymph converges in the body toward three main groups of nodes: the cervical, axillary, and inguinal. Two watersheds, a vertical one and the lower horizontal, divide the body into quadrants. A third watershed just above the clavicles, called the upper horizontal watershed, is the destination point for the lymph from the head and neck.

unfiltered or is poorly filtered. Movement through the system also occurs more slowly, creating a backup into the affected territory. This backup of excess fluid and protein is lymphedema. Joachim Zuther, an expert in manual lymphatic drainage, refers to lymphedema as "protein-rich edema."[20]

Unfiltered protein is one of the problematic aspects of lymphedema that sets it apart from edema. Left unfiltered, excess protein causes tissues to thicken and become fibrotic. Lymph then stagnates, providing a medium for bacterial growth and in turn increases the risk of infection. In addition, a secondary disease process is universally found in lymphedema patients which effects the skin. Research shows a thickening of the skin over time, up to 12 cells deep. This malformation of skin on the limb or quadrant greatly impacts the functions of the skin including absorption and elimination.[21]

Lymphedema is a serious condition. There is no cure for it, only constant monitoring and management. Not only are people at increased risk for infection in the affected limb, their body image, as well as activities of daily living, can be affected. The excess fluid creates heaviness in the limb, which can cause discomfort, joint pain, loss of mobility, and postural problems. Once a person has had an occurrence of lymphedema, future episodes may happen more easily and take longer to resolve. Even if people at risk for lymphedema have never had an incidence, they remain vulnerable for the remainder of their lives, which is difficult for them to comprehend.

The management of lymphedema is a complex situation and requires a great deal of training. Only practitioners with lengthy, supervised training, such as occurs with manual lymphatic drainage or lymph drainage therapy, should attempt to reroute excess, accumulated lymph. Touch practitioners without training in lymphedema management should refer clients to a specialist: most often that will be a physical or occupational therapist.

Massage adjustments

Lymphedema can occur years after cancer treatment, triggered by mosquito bites, a flu shot, or sunburn. Massage involving deep pressure has initiated an episode for some, especially those treated on an outpatient basis. For example, Mary had completed her breast cancer treatment five years prior and had never had an incidence of swelling on the treated side. One day while in the breast cancer center following a mammogram, she discouragingly showed her now swollen arm to a nurse massage therapist. The nurse quizzed Mary in an effort to trace the cause of the swelling. It transpired during the questioning that the patient had received a deep-tissue massage the day before. Although she had been given a number of massages since finishing treatment, this was the first deep-tissue session. And, while Mary reported that the bodywork felt comfortable and pleasant at the time, the nurse suspected that it was the cause of the swelling.

Vigorous massage creates the possibility of causing lymphedema or exacerbating an existing case if patients have had one or more nodes surgically removed from the neck, axilla, or groin. Deep massage triggers the inflammatory response, which releases chemicals that initiate vasodilation, causing permeability of blood capillaries and migration of plasma proteins out of the vascular system and into surrounding tissue. The affected area of a person whose lymphatic capacity has been diminished cannot always handle the greater fluid volume created by an inflammatory event, such as vigorous massage. Zuther, therefore, recommends that people with, or at risk for lymphedema, should not receive bodywork to the affected quadrant that would cause the skin to redden.[22]

Massage therapists can safely provide massage to people at risk for lymphedema or with very mild cases providing that they follow a very specific set of guidelines. These guidelines are listed in detail in the clinical considerations below. However, they can be briefly summarized as follows: 1) reduce the pressure in the affected quadrant to avoid reddening the skin; 2) stroke only toward the heart on limbs; 3) start at the upper part of the limb; 4) don't stroke into a cluster of affected nodes; and 5) stroke toward the working nodes.

Bodywork given to inpatients is usually so gentle that the risk of triggering lymphedema is profoundly less than with those being treated on an outpatient basis, such as in the radiation oncology department. People at risk for lymphedema present the most complicated scenarios for massage practitioners. They tend to be more energetic and want more vigorous massage, however, there is no way of knowing which of the at-risk patients will develop lymphedema. Many can go without an incidence in their lifetime, others have a constant level of residual fluid in the affected limb, others wax and wane, and some teeter unknowingly on the brink of lymphedema until a certain confluence of events overloads the lymphatic system. For example, a person might come down with a cold, which can be enough to cause the already overloaded lymphatic system to lose its delicate balance and develop lymphedema.

The adjustments listed below are intended to give therapists basic guidance in the administration of comfort-oriented bodywork to people at risk for lymphedema.

Clinical Considerations: Lymphedema

Pressure:

- If the patient is at risk for lymphedema, use a level of pressure on the affected area that does not cause redness. Controlled fascial release techniques that do not redden the skin are OK.
- Do not perform exaggerated stretches or twists.
- If the person has significant lymphedema, only rest the hands on the affected quadrant until guidance has been received by the patient's lymphedema specialist. The remainder of the body can be massaged with adjustments relative to the patient's general health.

Site:

- Massage the untreated side first. If it is the patient's first massage, be mindful even with the untreated side. Establishing trust is important.
- Stroke only toward the heart on the treated limb as show in the edema protocol (see Figures 8.2A–C). This is the direction that lymph is trying to flow, toward the heart.
- Massage segments of the limb sequentially using a proximal-to-distal order. For example, begin

with the shoulder and upper arm, forearm, and the hand. End with long strokes that connect the entire limb. (Again, see Figures 8.2A–C).

- Limit the amount of time to no more than a few minutes in the affected territory. This will ensure that the area is not overworked. Even gentle massage can overburden the lymphatic system by moving too much lymph. Remember, the quadrant is more than just the limb!
- Do not aim strokes at the area of nodal involvement, e.g., neck, axilla, or groin.
- Keep strokes lateral on the affected upper arm or leg (Figure 8.4A).
- If the affected quadrant is in the upper body, massage the back with strokes that move down past the rib cage (Figure 8.4B). The rib cage is the demarcation line between the upper and lower quadrants.
- The opposite is true if the lower quadrants are affected. Extending the strokes up past the rib cage, with the patient's permission, would be helpful because the lymph nodes in the upper body are undamaged.
- When the risk is in the upper quadrants, strokes that travel lateral to medial on the back are best (Figure 8.4C).

Positioning:

- Do not allow an affected arm to hang off the massage table or be occluded by the position in a massage chair.

Other:

- When massage clients are under medical care for lymphedema, confer with their lymphatic practitioner about adjustments that need to be made to the massage session. Lymphedema specialists often prefer that their patients wait until the swelling is under control before they receive massage, or they may request that the patient receive no massage in the affected quadrant.

continued

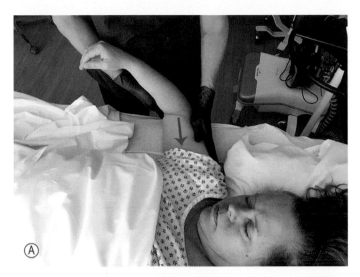

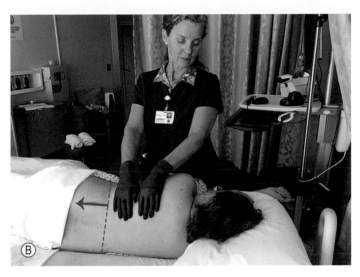

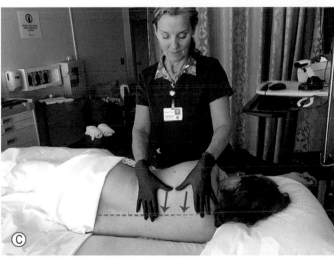

FIGURE 8.4
Massaging the person at risk for or with mild lymphedema. This patient is at risk for lymphedema due to breast cancer treatment. **A** The therapist is demonstrating a stroke on the lateral part of the arm. The strokes should not be aimed into the axilla, which has been affected by lymph node biopsy. **B** The therapist is taking her stroke down past the horizontal watershed at the bottom of the rib cage toward the working inguinal nodes. **C** The therapist is doing strokes that move lateral to medial, toward the working nodes on the opposite side.

- Monitor the amount of time spent in affected quadrants.
- Educate patients beforehand so that they understand why a lesser pressure is being used. Most people will not fuss about the lighter pressure if they understand the reasoning. These patients may be able to have firmer pressure in the non-treated areas if their general health is sufficient. When told this, most people accept the limitations on the affected side. For instance, someone treated for breast cancer can have somewhat firmer massage below the rib cage (e.g., to gluteals, hamstrings, or quadratus lumborum.) Someone treated in the lower quadrants can have firm pressure to the shoulders, scapula, and around the thoracic spine if their general health is adequate.

Nausea and vomiting

Nausea and vomiting accompany a plethora of conditions, such as anesthesia, pregnancy, cancer treatment, inner ear problems, dehydration, heart attack, fever, migraines, anxiety disorders, and liver disease. Like many other symptoms, the root causes are complex and not completely known. They can be related to mental, emotional and physical states.

The nervous system plays a role in nausea and vomiting, particularly the vagus nerve. It is the longest of the cranial nerves, extending from the brain to the intestines. The vagus nerve is the main component of the parasympathetic nervous system and supplies visceral sensation from most of the digestive tract. It communicates with the brain via signals that are triggered from mechanical and chemical stimuli.[23,24] The parasympathetic system is known as the "rest and digest" part of the nervous system, while the sympathetic section is known as the "fight or flight" part. Several studies have shown that increased sensations of nausea are associated with a decreased parasympathetic and increased sympathetic nervous system response.[23] Logically then, it would seem to be a valid notion that by increasing the parasympathetic response, nausea might be diminished. Affecting the parasympathetic system is done by giving a slow, quiet bodywork session using level 1 or 2 pressure. Additionally, Til Luchau points out that the vagus nerve surfaces at the ears and thus, attention to them might reap the benefits of stimulating this nerve.[25] Since the ears are not always a normal area to include in a session, be sure to ask the patient if they are happy to include this area and explain the possible help it might bring.

Controlling nausea and vomiting is important. Not only are they uncomfortable symptoms, but they also can lead to electrolyte imbalances, dehydration, and malnutrition. These conditions can lead to accelerated breathing and heart rate, confusion, irritability, fatigue or lethargy, dizziness, constipation, headache, and worst-case scenario, seizures.[26] Malnutrition also puts a person at greater risk of frequent illness and a longer healing time.[27]

Patients who have received massage while in a health care setting know that the style of touch is noninvasive and are more likely to want this gentle therapy, even during a bout of nausea. One way to present the idea is by saying: "Your nurse said you were feeling sick to your stomach. She thought that some very slow, gentle touch might help with that." Those whose only massage experience has been in a setting such as spa, chiropractic office, or in a therapist's private practice may decline touch therapy if they are nauseous, not realizing the difference between hospital-based massage and massage for a healthy, robust person. For some patients who don't feel well, being touched is too much to bear. They don't have the energy to receive extra people or the stimulation that massage can create. As always, the decision must be left to the patient.

Tip 8.2 Some acupressure points that may benefit nausea

Stomach 36, spleen 6, and pericardium 6, bladder 18 and 19.[8]

Clinical considerations: Nausea

Pressure:

- Pressure or force that creates movement should be avoided.
- Slow, level 1 pressure that is sedating.

Positioning:

- Self-limiting. Patients generally prefer not to reposition.

Pain

This one term, pain, is inadequate to express the overarching, intertwining nature of the many sensations called pain. This word is used to describe somatic feelings associated with many disparate conditions, such as surgical incisions, constipation, edematous limbs, nerve damage, depression, and myalgia.

Pain is often approached as a purely physiological issue, from tissue damage due to an accident or dysfunction of some aspect of the body, or bone on bone pain of a shoulder, hip, or knee, for example. Drugs and procedures are usually the first line treatments the doctor and patient try under this model. However, scientific evidence is showing that pain is determined not just by the physical, but also the social and emotional realms, known in medical parlance as biopsychosocial factors. In this approach to health care, social factors, such as cultural or religious beliefs, social support, and financial circumstances influence pain, as do aspects of the emotional domain, thoughts, depression, coping behaviors, and previous adverse experiences. There is an abundance of literature on the relationship between trauma in both childhood and adulthood and chronic pain, anxiety, depression, fibromyalgia, and other health issues.[28–31]

Students leave massage education with a focus on the musculoskeletal system, which is often addressed in an overly vigorous way. And yet, the key to success when concentrating on pain is how the therapist engages with the central nervous system: it doesn't respond favorably to force or coercion. The primitive part of the brain and the limbic system are constantly assessing the environment for danger: "Am I safe, or not safe?" Experiences from the past imprint in the neural pathways and can be re-triggered by present-time events, such as an MRI scan, surgery, childbirth, or an invasive massage. Helping patients attain the relaxation/parasympathetic response creates a secure environment. Being spacious, coaxing the body, allowing, and soothing are qualities that will build a sense of safety.

Healing occurs more readily when pain is well managed, which is why it is such a high priority to health care staff. Patients won't always admit to being in pain, however, physical clues can be found in moans, sighs, breath holding, grimacing, rigid posture, restlessness, and insomnia. Withdrawing, acting out, exhibiting depression, anxiety, irritability, confusion, or talking about death may be other indications of severe discomfort.

Various cultures approach pain differently. Some societies believe that pain should be fixed quickly and embrace the use of medication. Other cultures believe that pain should be endured, rejecting the use of drugs – sometimes to the despair of physicians. Perceptions around gender and age can also influence how patients experience pain. As always, it is not the job of a practitioner to encourage one belief over another. It is their obligation to honor a person's health decisions.

At the start of a session, massage therapists commonly query patients about their pain level, often using a 0–10

Info Box 8.1 Explaining pain

Pain is a product of brain and body working together. Multiple CNS sites contribute to the experience of pain, including: 1) cerebral cortex (thoughts); 2) limbic system (emotions); and 3) prefrontal cortex (executive and attentional processes). This means that *pain is both physical and emotional*, 100% of the time.

Pain can be acute, lasting 3 months or fewer, or chronic, persisting for 3 or more months or beyond expected healing time. Pain may become chronic for various reasons, including a process known as **central sensitization**. We get better at the things we practice over time, be it piano, tennis or puzzles. When we "practice" pain for weeks, months and years, the brain learns to be "good" at pain. When this happens, we say the brain has become "sensitive" to pain. Like a fire alarm ringing in the absence of fire, a sensitive brain sends out warning signals even in the absence of danger, when no protection is required. Therefore, *pain is not an accurate indicator of tissue damage* – rather, it's the brain's best guesstimate as to whether protection is required, and how much.

Integrative and multidisciplinary approaches are now the gold standard of pain treatment, combining biomedical and psychosocial interventions. Pain education plus nonpharmacological treatments like Cognitive Behavioral Therapy (CBT), Mindfulness-Based Stress Reduction (MBSR), biofeedback and massage can help patients turn the volume down on pain.

(Adapted from: Zoffness R. The Pain Management Workbook: Powerful CBT and Mindfulness Skills to Take Control of Pain and Reclaim Your Life. Oakland: New Harbinger Publications; 2020).

scale. However, practitioners frequently don't ask the next question: "What is causing your pain?" It is important for the massage therapist to zero in on the source of pain if possible. (Sometimes it isn't possible, as with old, trauma-related pain.) This enables the practitioner to know which tools to use from their massage kit. If structural or tissue damage caused by an injury, a myofascial technique might be best. If anxiety is contributing to physical unease, the therapist would be best to approach in a gentle, slow way, focused on the skin. This will create a sedating effect on the parasympathetic nervous system. If constipation, nausea, or edema are causing discomfort, the reader will find suggestions in those sections of this chapter. Even if a therapist has no training in a specific technique, the experience of many therapists shows that a mindful, systematic touch protocol can still help with a multitude of pains.

Clinical considerations: Pain

Pressure:

- Pain medication: the patient can't give accurate feedback.
- Take a gentle approach with guarded areas. They are best coaxed open.
- Remain focused on imparting comfort and nurturance. This will decrease anxiety and a reduction of muscular tension will follow and thus a decrease in pain.

Site:

- Painful areas often cannot be massaged directly but may be improved through attention to reflexology or acupressure points, or by using energy techniques.

Positioning:

- Self-limiting. Patients in pain can surprise the therapist with their willingness to reposition, especially to receive a back massage.
- Observing the patient's positioning in the bed and correcting postures that are contributing to pain can be as important as the bodywork

session. The most common cause of positional pain is slipping down into the bed, which causes stress on the back. Help the patient shift up so that the hips are in the fold of the semi-reclining bed.

Therapist's journal 8.2
Everyone's full attention

In the experience of pain, everyone wants to fix or end it. The pain has everyone's full attention. The stress is high. The room is tense. I want to create a resting place; a gentle place like a soft wave. A place where there is no resistance. This is achieved through grounding, centering myself, presenting relaxed body movement, gentle voice tone, and audible breathing. As I focus on my own comfort, I model a place that can then be mirrored back to me. This resting place eases tension in the room. The cycle of anxiety has been broken. The patient and health care team now have an alternative strategy for coping with pain.

Irene Smith, Everflowing
San Francisco, California

Peripheral neuropathy

Peripheral neuropathy can accompany a number of conditions, most notably diabetes as a result of decreased circulation; chemotherapy treatment for cancer, which damages nerves; or spinal stenosis compressing nerves in the narrowed area. The common sensations are numbness, tingling, pins and needles, and stabbing in the hands and feet.

Some people with diabetic neuropathy find that massage improves the condition to a certain degree, but most likely, at best, it will maintain sensation at its present level. Chemotherapy-induced peripheral neuropathy (CIPN) tends to improve the most with massage over time, as the nerves are able to wholly or partially repair. Numbness due to spinal stenosis may or may not have improvement, but at the very least, massage provides a pleasant interlude for the moment.

Clinical considerations: Peripheral neuropathy

Pressure:

- Massage is well tolerated by most patients, but they are unable to give accurate feedback.
- If the sensations are extremely painful, the pressure should be no more than the amount needed to apply lotion.
- Those affected by diabetic neuropathy may also have fragile tissue in the extremities.

Site:

- Some patients will prefer not to have affected areas touched.

Skin conditions

Private massage practitioners focus predominately on a client's musculature, observing its tone, flexibility, and tissue quality. Massage therapists who work with medically complex people must learn to move their primary attention to the skin. Not only will focusing on the skin help them to provide a comfort-oriented session, but it will give bodyworkers hints about the person's health status.

The skin of a hospital patient is breached continuously. It is affected by medications, a lack of oxygenation, and dehydration. Touch therapists need to read the skin, noticing areas that are not intact or that are inflamed, swollen, bruised, thinned, discolored, scarred, pale, or dehydrated. These areas may be an indication for pressure reduction, a site to avoid, or positioning needs. Pressure sores are an example of a need for pressure, site, and positioning adjustments.

There is a long-standing idea in both massage and nursing education that massage might prevent decubitus ulcers (pressure sores), or that it might speed up the healing time of a pressure sore. However, the evidence does not exist. Older analyses of pressure sore-related research from nursing literature questioned the benefit of massage for pressure sores.[32–34] Halfens et al.[32] and Buss et al.[33] recommend that extended, robust massage should not be used for patients at risk for developing ulcers around bony prominences and pressure areas. They also question the use of "soft, moderate, or standard massage." Anthony writes in the *Journal of Advanced Nursing*: "The belief held by clinicians in topical applications, physical treatments and massage in treating and preventing decubitus ulcers is in most cases misguided."[34] In its most recent review of this topic, completed in 2015, the Cochrane Library supported the ideas expressed in these older texts and journals. They found no studies that met eligibility and therefore concluded that it is unclear whether massage therapy prevents pressure ulcers.[35]

The use of moisturizers to treat dry skin, and barrier creams or ointments during incontinence are recommended to prevent pressure sores, along with frequent repositioning. Massage is not recommended as part of a treatment protocol by the NHS, the Mayo Clinic, the American Academy of Family Physicians, or other major institutional bodies. However, massage may be important in keeping the skin moisturized, the body correctly bolstered and boney prominences protected. Also, touch therapists play an important role in monitoring patients: they spend the majority of their time connected with the skin.

Vast quantities of information are available by assessing the skin. It will give bodyworkers hints about how the massage session needs to be adjusted or will point them toward questions that should be asked of the nurse. Qualities of unhealthy skin and their relationship to massage are described below.

Clinical considerations: Skin conditions

Pressure:

- With dehydrated or parchment-like conditions, avoid friction.
- Evidence of bruising or swelling.

continued

Site:

- Inspect tissue before making contact with it.
- If a pressure sore is suspected, even in an area that is just red, avoid until consulting with the nurse.
- Skin that is not intact should not be touched, either with or without gloves.
- Areas with vesicles should not be touched. Herpes and shingles are examples. Because of the highly contagious nature of herpes, practitioners should glove. Even if practitioners are massaging well away from the affected area, gloves should be worn because exudate from the vesicles can spread virus into the bedding.
- Shingles, which also produces vesicles, is not contagious. However, the shingles virus, varicella zoster, can spread to others and cause chickenpox in those who are not immune. The contagious period is when the rash has vesicles. After the blisters crust, the virus is no longer communicable.[36]
- Glove to massage an area affected by a fungal infection. Most often this will be the feet.
- Glove if blood or other bodily fluids are present on the skin, whether dried or moist.
- Inflamed areas affected by infection, such as cellulitis or abscess, should not be massaged.
- If an area is swollen, inquire about it from the nurse. Swelling can be a sign of a blood clot, organ dysfunction, or many other causes. The source will influence the massage session.
- Inquire about areas with rashes or raised, but intact bumps on the skin. Often the area can be massaged or receive static holds. Areas with petechiae can be mindfully massaged, for example.

Thrombosis

Thrombus comes from the Greek word for lump or clot, and thrombosis denotes the formation or presence of a thrombus. Three factors are thought to precipitate thrombosis: 1) venous stasis, which for example can result from extended bedrest, varicose veins, smoking, and obesity; 2) injury to the vessel wall, particularly in the pelvis or lower extremities: injuries can occur as a result of a hip fracture, trauma to the body, insertion of IV catheters, infusion of medications, or infection in the tissues surrounding the vessel; and 3) hypercoagulability, which causes the blood to clot more readily, either from inherited conditions or acquired ones – examples of which are certain cancers, some medications, and pregnancy (see Chapter 7).[37] The cause of a clot is not just singular, many of the factors overlap.

Thrombophlebitis and deep vein thrombosis (DVT) are two common thrombosis-related conditions. Phlebitis is inflammation of a vein. Thrombophlebitis is the occurrence of an inflamed vein, the inflammation of which leads to a blood clot. Thrombophlebitis is often a superficial condition that generally forms in veins of the legs, although a clot can manifest in the arm. It can be recognized by localized heat, redness, swelling, pain, or tenderness. The affected vein may be rope-like and hard to the touch. Often this type of clot can be diagnosed visually and through palpation.[38,39] Even though a superficial thrombophlebitis it is not as consequential or serious as a deep vein thrombophlebitis, it should be attended to by the health care staff as soon as possible.

If a thrombus occurs in the deeper veins, the potential side effect is very dangerous. A blood clot could break free and lodge in a smaller vessel, blocking the flow of blood and oxygen to the tissue fed by that vessel. Deep vein thrombosis is sometimes asymptomatic and at other times presents with edema distal to the site, often a dusky discoloration, and pain that feels like cramping or soreness that is exacerbated by activity or standing still for too long. One of the telltale signs of a thrombus is that the symptoms will be unilateral (only on one side). Ultrasound is the standard diagnostic test for DVT.

If one of these thromboemboli (blood clots that have broken free), gets stuck in the lungs, it is termed a pulmonary embolism (PE), the consequence of which is potentially fatal.[40] The signs of a PE can sometimes be a very dramatic and include sudden shortness of breath, which is a call for urgent action. Or, it can present in a more moderate way, such as chest discomfort when breathing deeply, lightheadedness, or a rapid pulse. Specialized CT or MRI scans are needed to diagnose a PE.[41,42]

There is no standard of practice regarding massage and blood clots within institutions such as the NHS in the UK or the American Hospital Association. Nor does the nursing or hospital massage therapy profession have a standard of practice on this subject. Many hospitals will choose to avoid massaging the lower limbs of someone at risk of developing a thrombus because this is the most frequent site of blood clot development. Other hospitals may elect just to massage hands and feet as a precautionary measure or to administer modalities that involve no pressure or stroking. Each institution must examine this issue and create protocols in conjunction with nursing and medical administrators and the massage therapy team. Even when hospital-wide guidelines have been established, individual nurses may have their own inclinations regarding this matter. Because massage therapists are usually accountable to the patient's nurse, the nurse's preferences must be honored.

Clinical considerations: Thrombosis

Pressure:

- When the patient is at risk for but has no known DVT, the pressure should still be gentle to avoid dislodging a possible clot.
- The patient may be taking anticoagulant or thrombolytic drugs, which cause easy bruising or bleeding.

Site:

- A person being treated for DVT should not receive touch therapy that includes stroking or pressure. Resting the hands on the limb may be permissible depending on institutional policy.

- Central IV and femoral catheters increase the risk of clot formation. Apply only holds to limbs or the chest with these catheters in place. If the catheter is in the inguinal space, a mindful, gentle foot massage has proven to be safe.
- As a preventive measure to developing a thrombus, at-risk patients will have elastic socks or a pneumatic compression device on the extremity. Do not remove these without nurse approval.

Positioning:

- Elevation of a limb affected by swelling due to the clot is usually permissible.

Summary

Symptoms are the signposts, the yellow flags that say to a therapist: "Something is happening here, slow down, go with care." There are no symptoms that prevent the administration of touch therapy. Their message is merely an indication to the practitioner to make adjustments.

Each new chapter of *Hands in Health Care* presents more factors that must be taken into account when planning a massage session. To the new practitioner, it might seem as if all of the necessary calculations would feel confining and unnatural, thereby overriding the pleasure of giving and receiving simple touch. While the major emphasis in this chapter, as well as in the book, is on "doing no harm," there should be no doubt that despite all of the precautions that must be observed when working with people who are medically complex, massage is a joyful event to both therapist and patient.

Chapter EIGHT

Case history 8.1 | Exercise

Instructions: On a piece of paper, make three columns: pressure, site, and position. List the conditions that would require pressure reduction, those that could be a site restriction, and the ones needing positioning adjustment. This is a complex case. Categorizing this patient's conditions using the pressure, site, positioning framework will help create a treatment plan for him that includes his whole body.

Mr Dominic has a history of breast cancer on the right side. Three years previous he underwent a modified radical mastectomy and axillary node dissection of 7 nodes (2 were positive). This was followed by chemotherapy for 12 weeks and then radiation. Part way through the radiation treatment, Mr D developed swelling in his right arm. His primary care physician referred him for lymphedema treatment. He will be on tamoxifen for another 7 years.

Mr Dominic is also affected by anemia, back pain, diabetes, high cholesterol, high blood pressure, obesity, shortness of breath, and both hips have been replaced. He is on a weekly dose of epoetin alfa (Procrit).

Recently Mr Dominic was diagnosed with myelodysplatic syndrome (MDS), a bone marrow disorder. His doctor feels that this is due to Agent Orange exposure when he served in Vietnam. Mr Dominic is taking part in a clinical trial of the drug azacitidine (Vidaza), which is causing nausea, thrombocytopenia, neutropenia, bruising, mild diarrhea, dizziness, a feeling of weakness and fatigue.

Test yourself

Multiple choice: Circle all correct answers. There may be more than one.

1. Which of the following conditions require close attention to the amount of pressure?

   A   Edema.
   B   Fever.
   C   Thrombocytopenia.
   D   Herpes.

2. Which of the following platelet counts demand ultralight pressure?

   A   112.
   B   78.
   C   19.
   D   6

3. Which of the following conditions require the practitioner to perform strokes only toward the heart?

   A   Constipation.
   B   Edema.
   C   Varicose veins.
   D   Lymphedema.

4. Immunosuppression is an indication for:

   A   Pressure restriction.
   B   Site restriction.
   C   Positioning restriction.
   D   Attention to Standard Precautions.

5. Which of the following patients are most at risk for developing lymphedema?

   A   Those with constipation.
   B   Those who had lymph node removal from the axilla.
   C   Those who are neutropenic.
   D   Those who had radiation therapy to the inguinal lymph nodes.

6. Which is the single most important massage adjustment for the patient with lymphedema or at risk for it?

   A   Elevating the affected limb.
   B   Decreasing the pressure.
   C   Avoiding the shoulders.
   D   No prone positioning.

7. Which of the following situations often results in peripheral neuropathy?

   A   Varicose veins.

   B   Nausea.

   C   Diabetes.

   D   Certain cancer drugs.

8. Which of the following conditions require gloving?

   A   DVT.

   B   Herpes.

   C   Constipation.

   D   Phlebitis.

9. Which of the following sites should not receive massage?

   A   Skin that is not intact.

   B   An edematous area due to a blood clot.

   C   Peripheral neuropathy.

   D   Varicose veins.

10. Which of the following puts a patient at risk for DVT?

    A   Extended bedrest.

    B   Insertion of an inguinal catheter.

    C   Thrombocytopenia.

    D   Pregnancy.

11. Which of the following are classic symptoms of inflammation?

    A   Heat.

    B   Tenderness.

    C   Redness.

    D   Congestion.

12. The vagus nerve:

    A   Is part of the sympathetic nervous system.

    B   Communicates with the brain.

    C   Is hypersensitive to heat.

    D   Has an influence on nausea.

13. Pain is influenced by:

    A   The nervous system.

    B   Cultural beliefs.

    C   Isolation.

    D   Financial matters.

References

1. Herrine SK. Ascites. 2018. Available from: https://www.merck-manuals.com/home/liver-and-gallbladder-disorders/manifestations-of-liver-disease/ascites.

2. Medicine Net. Ascites. 2019. Available from: https://www.medicinenet.com/ascites/article.htm

3. Mayo Clinic. Thrombocytopenia. 2018. Available from: https://www.mayoclinic.org/diseases-conditions/thrombocytopenia/symptoms-causes/syc-20378293

4. Baby Centre. Should I worry if I have low platelets? 2017. Available from: https://www.babycentre.co.uk/x542273/should-i-worry-if-i-have-low-platelets-gestational-thrombocytopenia

5. McClurg D, Walker K, Aitchison P, Jamieson K, Kickinson L, Paul L, Hagen S, Cunnington AL. Abdominal massage for the relief of constipation in people with Parkinson's: A qualitative study. Parkinson's Disease. 2016. Available from: https://www.hindawi.com/journals/pd/2016/4842090/

6. Yildirim D, Can G, Koknel Talu G. The efficacy of abdominal massage in managing opiod-induced constipation. European J of Oncology Nursing. 2019;41. Available from: https://www.ncbi.nlm.nih.gov/pubmed/31358243

7. MS Trust. Abdominal massage for constipation. 2018. Available from: https://www.mstrust.org.uk/research/research-updates/181204-abdominal-massage-constipation

8. Sohn T, Sohn R. Amma Therapy. Rochester, VT: Healing Arts Press; 1996.

9. WebMD. Dyspnea (Shortness of Breath). 2019. Available from: https://www.webmd.com/lung/shortness-breath-dyspnea#1

10. Mayo Clinic. Pulmonary hypertension. 2017. Available from: https://www.mayoclinic.org/diseases-conditions/pulmonary-hypertension/symptoms-causes/syc-20350697

11. Mayo Clinic. COPD. 2017. Available from: https://www.mayoclinic.org/diseases-conditions/copd/symptoms-causes/syc-20353679

12. Polastri M, Clini EM, Nava S, Ambrosino N. Manual massage therapy for patients with COPD: A scoping review. Medicina. 2019;55. Available from: https://www.ncbi.nlm.nih.gov/pmc/articles/PMC6572655/

13. Understanding the pathophysiology of fever. 2008. Available from: https://journals.lww.com/nursing/Fulltext/2008/08000/Understanding_the_pathophysiology_of_fever.45.aspx

14. Scientific American. What causes a fever? 2005. Available from: https://www.scientificamerican.com/article/what-causes-a-fever

15. Stoecklein VM, Osaka A, Lederer JA. Trauma equals danger—damage control by the immune system. Jrnl of Leukocyte Biology. 2012;92. Available from: https://www.ncbi.nlm.nih.gov/pmc/articles/PMC3427603/

16. Stoppler MC. Neutropenia causes, symptoms, ranges, levels, and treatment. MedicineNet. 2017. Available from: https://www.medicinenet.com/neutropenia/article.htm#what_is_neutropenia

17. Shiel WC. Definition of absolute neutrophil count. Medicine Net. 2018. Available from: https://www.medicinenet.com/script/main/art.asp?articlekey=20030

18. WebMD. Living with immunosuppression after an organ transplant. 2019. Available from: https://www.webmd.com/a-to-z-guides/organ-transplants-antirejection-medicines-topic-overview#1

19. Inflammation. Encyclopedia Britannica. Available from: https://www.britannica.com/science/inflammation

20. Zuther J, Norton S. Lymphedema Management, 3rd Ed. New York and Stuttgart: Thieme Medical Publishers; 2013, p. 113

21. Rockson S. Lymphatic Education & Research Network Symposium. 2018. Available from: https://www.youtube.com/watch?v=AlXS0RM-rCg&feature=youtu.be.

22. Zuther J. Traditional massage therapy in the treatment and management of lymphedema. Massage Today June 2002:1.

23. Singh, P, Yoon SS, Kuo B. Nausea: a review of pathophysiology and therapeutics. Therapeutic Advances in Gastroenterology. 2016. Available from: https://www.ncbi.nlm.nih.gov/pmc/articles/PMC4699282/

24. Breit S, Kupferberg A, Rogler G, et al. Vagus nerve as modulators of the brain-gut axis in psychiatric and inflammatory disorders. Frontiers in Psychiatry. 2018. Available from: https://www.ncbi.nlm.nih.gov/pmc/articles/PMC5859128/

25. Luchau T. Working with the vagus nerve. Massage and Bodywork Magazine. 2017. Available from: https://www.abmp.com/textonlymags/article.php?article=1777

26. Holland K. Healthline. All about electrolyte disorders. 2019. Available from: https://www.healthline.com/health/electrolyte-disorders#symptoms

27. Brazier Y. Malnutrition: Symptoms, causes, diagnosis, and treatment. Medical News Today. 2017. Available from: https://www.medicalnewstoday.com/articles/179316.php#symptoms

28. Mayo Clinic. Pain and depression. Is there a link? 2019. Available from: https://www.mayoclinic.org/diseases-conditions/depression/expert-answers/pain-and-depression/faq-20057823

29. Harvard Health Publishing. Chronic pain and childhood trauma. 2018. Available from: https://www.health.harvard.edu/blog/chronic-pain-and-childhood-trauma-2018033012768

30. Annals of Behavioral Medicine. The impact of social isolation on pain. 2019. Available from: https://www.ncbi.nlm.nih.gov/pubmed/29668841

31. Harvard Health Publishing. The pain-anxiety-depression connection. Available from: https://www.health.harvard.edu/healthbeat/the-pain-anxiety-depression-connection ;

32. Halfens R, Eggink M. Knowledge, beliefs, and use of nursing methods in preventing pressure sores in Dutch hospitals. Int J Nurs Stud. 1995;32(1):16-26.

33. Buss IC, Halfens R, Abu-Saad HH. The effectiveness of massage in preventing pressure sores: A literature review. Rehabil Nurs. 1997;22(5):229-242.

34. Anthony D. The treatment of decubitus ulcers: A century of misinformation in the textbooks. J Adv Nurs. 1996;24(2):309-316.

35. Zhang Q, Sun Z, Yue J. Massage therapy for preventing ulcers. Cochrane Library. 2015. Available from: https://www.cochrane.org/CD010518/WOUNDS_massage-therapy-for-preventing-pressure-ulcers.

36. Shingles transmission. 2019. Available from: https://www.cdc.gov/shingles/about/transmission.html

37. Cleveland clinic. Blood clotting disorders. 2019. Available from: https://my.clevelandclinic.org/health/diseases/16788-blood-clotting-disorders-hypercoagulable-states

38. Web MD. What is phlebitis? 2018. Available from: https://www.webmd.com/dvt/phlebitis#1

39. Mayo Clinic. Thrombophlebitis. 2017. Available from: https://www.mayoclinic.org/diseases-conditions/thrombophlebitis/symptoms-causes/syc-20354607

40. Medicine Net. Medical definition of thrombosis. 2018. Available from: https://www.medicinenet.com/script/main/art.asp?articlekey=25023

41. Mayo Clinic. Deep vein thrombosis—symptoms and causes. 2018. Available from: https://www.mayoclinic.org/diseases-conditions/deep-vein-thrombosis/symptoms-causes/syc-20352557

42. CDC. Diagnosis and treatment of venous thromboembolism. 2019. Available from: https://www.cdc.gov/ncbddd/dvt/diagnosis-treatment.html

Additional resources

Pain: Considering complementary approaches. Available from: https://files.nccih.nih.gov/s3fs-public/Pain-eBook-2019_06_508.pdf

Rattray F, Ludwig L. Clinical Massage Therapy: Understanding, Assessing and Treating Over 70 Conditions. Toronto, Canada: Talas Inc., 2000.

Werner R. Massage Therapist's Guide to Pathology, 7th Ed. Boulder, CO: Books of Discovery; 2019.

What's that beeping? Medical devices and procedures

It sounded like gentle waves on the beach when your arm passed on the sheets below my shoulders. The bed became the ocean and I was floating on the waves. I forgot all about being here.

Lupus patient after massage session.

The sounds of pumps, alarms, oxygen bubblers etc., all become routine and hardly noticeable after some time working in health care settings. However, it is important to understand a bit of what is behind the beeping. Entering a patient's hospital or treatment room always presents a practitioner with many unknowns. In addition to assessing the patient's primary diagnosis and what types of medications are being administered, touch therapists will want to have a basic understanding of what tests or treatment the patient is receiving. These may also cause side effects that need to be taken into consideration when planning the hands-on session. For example, how might the tubes, wires, and monitors affect the session? Have recent procedures left incisions that will need positioning adjustments?

Two important topics are discussed in this chapter: common medical devices and frequently administered medical tests or treatments, collectively known as medical procedures. When massage therapists have a general understanding of these topics, they can feel more confident about the appropriate adjustment decisions they make and feel enabled to provide a safe and effective touch session. Therapists showing an understanding of these topics tend to build trust in the patient and medical staff alike. Over-confidence, however, is not an appropriate strategy. If one is not familiar with a device or procedure, don't fake it. If available, use a smart phone or device to search for basic information. It is an easy way to collect foundational information, but follow up with the patient's nurse or doctor for remaining questions.

Medical devices

The massage adjustments required to accommodate medical devices will become second nature. Assessments and treatment plans will literally build around these devices. Safety is the primary consideration: safe handling, safe distance, and safe pressure will ensure a safe and effective session. When considering safety precautions with medical devices, keep the following goals in mind:

- Infection control.
- Avoid dislodging or inappropriately moving equipment.
- Avoid interruption in device function.

Some devices necessitate specific guidelines to protect against harming the patient. For instance, many intravenous (IV) catheters and the accompanying procedures call for keeping a safe distance from the device, which is an entry site into the body. A safe distance will help protect against the introduction of lotion or other foreign substances into a physical opening. Gentle touch is a safety practice because of the possibility of bleeding or blood clots around the internal IV line.

The names and functions of commonly encountered devices along with their safety guidelines are provided here. Familiarity with this equipment fosters the ability to speak the same language as other care providers and to continue to build trust with patients. Table 9.1 lists types and examples of medical equipment.

TABLE 9.1 Types and examples of medical equipment	
Type	**Examples**
Diagnostic	Medical imaging machines: ultrasound, MRI, fMRI, PET, CT, x-ray.
Treatment	Infusion pumps and IV poles, medical lasers, PICC and central catheters.
Life support	Ventilators, incubators, anesthetic machines, heart–lung machines, dialysis machines.
Monitors	Vital signs, ECG, EEG, blood pressure, oxygen saturation.
Laboratory equipment	Analyze blood, urine, genes, dissolved gases in blood.
Therapeutic	Continuous passive range of motion, sequential compression devices.
Bedside care	Emesis basins and bags, urinals, patient alarms, transfer equipment, positioning and protectors (foam boots, slings, splints, body wedges), foley catheters, NG tubes (feeding), nasal cannulas.
Infection control	Sharps containers, personal protection equipment, biohazard disposal containers.

Collection devices

These items are the most basic hospital equipment. Bed-pans and urinals are used for patients who are unable to get out of bed to use the toilet or commode (a portable toilet placed near the bed). An emesis basin is an open, plastic container that patients use when they need to vomit or expel oral secretions. A newer option commonly provided is an expandable plastic bag with a smooth, firm rim at the mouth opening. The patient can simply hold the bag with the rim to the mouth, which results in much less splatter or mess (Figure 9.1).

Clinical considerations: Bedpan, urinal, emesis bag

Other:

- Collection devices such as urinals are commonly used and easily avoided during a massage therapy session. Urinals, toilet collection cups, or commodes should never be emptied by the massage practitioner for several reasons: most importantly, input and output measurements are routinely monitored by medical staff. If a basin needs to be moved, use a gloved hand to move the item; remove glove and wash hands before proceeding.

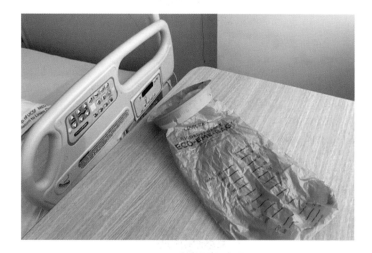

FIGURE 9.1
Emesis bag that can be brought up to the mouth if the patient needs to vomit. The smooth plastic rim provides ease of use and the elongated bag helps prevent splattering fluid.

(Photo by Carolyn Tague.)

Catheters

A catheter is a hollow, flexible tube that can be inserted into the body for a variety of purposes. The process of inserting a catheter is referred to as catheterization. The most common uses are for administering medications and fluids, collecting body fluids, monitoring physiological functions, and performing medical procedures.

Catheters have a variety of designs depending on their purpose. Some, such as the Foley and the Swan-Ganz, are referred to as balloon-tipped catheters because they have an inflatable sac at the end that holds the device in place. Catheters used during a procedure to remove plaque from coronary vessels have a blade tip that cuts and shaves. Intravenous catheters have openings to the exterior that allow blood to be drawn or medications to be given without the skin being punctured each time. Other catheters are equipped with an electrical cautery wire, which can be used for such procedures as opening the bile duct to allow extraction of kidney stones.[1]

Foley catheter

The Foley catheter, commonly referred to as a urinary or in-dwelling catheter, is a balloon-tipped catheter. It is inserted into the patient's bladder to allow the drainage and collection of urine into a bag that hangs off the side of the bed, usually near the floor (Figure 9.2). The balloon, which is filled with sterile water, holds the tube in place. Most commonly, a Foley is used to drain urine before and after surgery when a patient is not expected to ambulate.

Clinical considerations: Foley catheter

Pressure:

- Extra gentle touch if working on the abdomen so as not to cause irritation to the bladder or push on the location of the tube.

Site:

- The collection bag will generally be hooked on a lower bed rail, allowing gravity to help with elimination. Extra care is needed to avoid touching the bag. It should not be elevated above the body because of potential backflow.

Positioning:

- Educate patients to use extra care when repositioning so as not to pull on or dislodge the inserted balloon-tipped tube.

External urinary catheters

Because incidence of urinary tract infections (UTIs) are high among patients with Foley catheters, efforts to remove the catheters as soon as possible have been employed in recent years. One newer option for men is

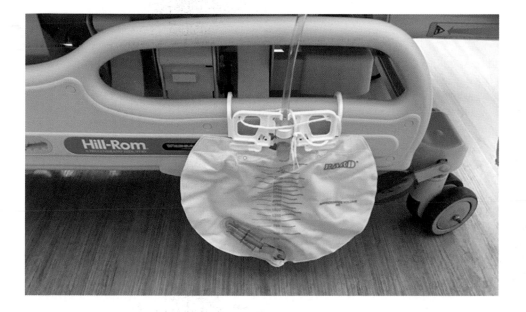

FIGURE 9.2
Foley catheter collection bag. It clips onto the side rail and has measuring lines for easy reading of output.

(Photo by Carolyn Tague.)

called an external urinary catheter (condom catheter) which is a type of modified catheter worn over the penis.

Intravenous catheters (IV)

Intravenous catheters allow the administration of fluid directly into a patient's veins such as medications, nutrients, water, or electrolytes. These devices also may serve in blood withdrawal.

A variety of intravenous catheters are used depending on the need. A peripheral line is inserted by needle into a vein on an extremity. The most common insertion sites are anywhere on the arm or hand, and rarely on the foot. Peripheral lines are used in situations in which a temporary IV catheter is needed, such as postoperatively. Practitioners may hear the term "hep lock" in relation to peripheral lines: they are sometimes referred to in this way because a heparin solution is placed in the catheter to prevent it from closing up when not in use.

There are several types of central venous catheters, also known as central lines or central venous access devices. Tunneled devices, such as a Hickman, Broviac, and Groshong, are inserted into a central vein, usually the subclavian, by tunneling under the skin. The insertion site may be in the chest, usually on the right side (in the upper arm, or the antecubital space). Central catheters inserted into the arm are referred to as peripherally inserted central catheters (PICCs). PICCs are placed into one of the central veins, such as the subclavian or superior vena cava, via the larger upper arm veins, the basilic, brachial, or cephalic. It is usually left in place for an extended period of time for patients receiving chemotherapy, organ transplant, and intensive care unit (ICU) patients.

Implanted IV devices, such as a Portacath, also known as a "port", are reservoirs that are placed under the skin and hooked to a catheter that travels subcutaneously to the vein. They aren't visible from the outside, although the therapist will see a bulge at the placement site. The nurse accesses these devices with a special needle that has a 90° angle.

Intravenous fluids can be infused into the patient through external or internal means. The traditional external method is to hang bags of solution on an IV pole, allowing them to be drip-fed by gravity. Computerized pumps attached to the IV pole are another method of delivery. These pumps allow fluids to be infused at a certain volume per hour. Pumps also can be implanted under the skin, usually in the lower left quadrant of the abdomen, to continuously deliver medications or chemotherapy.[1]

A patient's story 9.1　　Nuances of touch

Lying on the massage table, too tired to speak, I silently asked my therapist to stop talking. As she did, I relaxed enough to feel her presence next to me. A Healing Touch practitioner, her hands began above me and joined me at times during our session with holds, gentle strokes or rest positions on my body. This was manageable. Even the thought of a comfort-oriented massage flooded my body with too much information and felt overwhelming. I recognized I was far, far beyond my normal threshold for receiving touch.

As we settled into each other's presence I momentarily wished for a "good rub" on my shoulders. This thought however instantly brought a startled response in awareness of my port. A deep breath offered relief, allowing me to let go of my concern that her touch might disrupt my access device. When her hands did rest gently there above my clothes, I had to ask her to lighten pressure, as the simple weight of her hands was too much to bear. I am mother to my cub, my port; my portal that brings treatment to sustain and regain my life.

It is an odd juxtaposition: to feel starved for touch yet hypersensitive to it. I remind myself that my body is in hyperdrive at a molecular and biochemical level. The chemo has destroyed my veins while helping clear my cancer.

continued

What's that beeping? Medical devices and procedures

The immunotherapy offers support to my immune system while at the same time suppressing my ability to fight infections. My skin is so sensitive I find comfort only in my softest fleece robe or a tepid bath. This is not the "me" I have known. Now, I measure everything in life with a question: what can my body, mind and spirit handle today? Right now?

Healing Touch offered in reverence and compassion opens my soul's awareness of the many layers of life that reside within and beyond my body. Here, new horizons carry me in streams of energy that join physical and nonphysical aspects simultaneously. When resting in a space of trust with a therapist who adjusts to my needs, I heal. I heal within and beyond. My soul finds hope that I will walk into a new way of being.

Meg
Rochester, New York

Clinical considerations: IV catheter

Pressure:

- Only use gentle pressure on the extremity containing an IV due to the increased risk of clot formation. This is true more often of central lines, including ports, where the development of a blood clot in the arm is not an unusual occurrence. Swelling and warmth are common signs.
- Bodyworkers must make it part of their intake routine to ask the nurse if patients have an IV, what type, and whether they are exhibiting any signs of a thrombus.

Site:

- Do not touch IVs or the area several inches around them. This will help to prevent the introduction of bacteria into the area and to avoid accidentally dislodging the catheter or causing bruising or discomfort to the patient.
- Massage distal to central lines or ports; avoid massage to areas with catheter tubing.
- Limbs containing peripheral lines can be massaged lightly over the extremity, but avoid the area around the insertion point and medial soft tissue where catheter lines are in place.
- Phlebitis, which presents as a red streak on the skin, can develop in the limb containing an IV.

Not only can the catheter itself be irritating to the vein but so too can the medications being infused. The hands can rest on a phlebitic limb, but modalities that require stroking movements, such as effleurage, should not be performed in the affected area.

Positioning:

- Usually, patient comfort will be the guiding influence on positioning. Some people are comfortable lying on their IV catheters, others are not.
- A small towel or washcloth placed just above the proximal border of a port can allow the patient to comfortably lie prone. Do not place the padding directly under the port, as this compresses the catheter into the chest wall.
- For catheters such as Groshong and Hickman that have tubing external to the body, small towels positioned both medial and distal around the catheter to allow space without putting any pressure on it may create enough comfort to allow the patient to lie prone.
- Care must be taken of IV tubing, which often is quite long. When moving bedrails or repositioning the patient, be certain the lines don't become wedged in the bedrails, occluded, or create a tugging sensation in the patient at the insertion site.

Chapter NINE

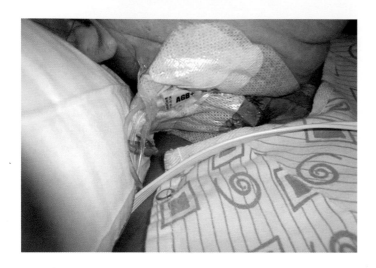

FIGURE 9.3
Central line catheter. Note the protective bandaging and clear tape to hold it securely in place without openings being exposed.

(Photo courtesy of Baptist Health, Lexington, Kentucky.)

Therapist's journal 9.1
The IV change

Mr PB needed to have his IV changed. He had been in the hospital for a couple of weeks, and this was not the first time that he needed an old IV removed and a new one placed. He was nervous, and his nurse asked me if I could come in as an extra support. I was able to gently massage his feet and had music playing in the background as the IV was changed. Mr PB was so grateful, noting how much easier it was compared to the previous experience. The nurse was also very appreciative, as she wanted her patient to have an easier experience with less pain and anxiety. Definitely a win-win all round!

Mary Aguilera-Titus LMT
Silver Spring, Maryland

Cardiac catheters and devices

The heart may be catheterized for a number of reasons, such as to perform diagnostic procedures, or to treat conditions. Diagnostically, heart catheters can collect important information such as pulmonary blood flow, pressures in the heart chambers, oxygen saturation, and valve function. As treatment interventions, hearth catheterization may be used to perform angioplasty or an atherectomy, both of which are done to improve blood flow in the coronary vessels. An angiogram is usually performed in conjunction with heart catheterization. During this part of the process, an x-ray contrast fluid is injected into the coronary blood vessels, which allows the cardiologist to view the heart's anatomy on a fluoroscopic screen. If narrowing is apparent (stenosis), the doctor may perform a balloon angioplasty to compress the plaque against the vessel wall or an atherectomy to grind the plaque into small bits. Laser angioplasty is also an option commonly used. During this procedure, amplified light waves are transmitted via a fiberoptic catheter. The laser beam heats the catheter tip and vaporizes the plaque. Further treatments, such a stent placement may be done during the procedure.

Stents

Stents are common treatment devices used in the heart catheterization lab for patients who have a blockage or narrowing of the blood vessels of the heart or other parts of the vasculature. Typically, the narrowing or blockage is caused by atherosclerosis. The device is made of wire or plastic mesh, and is placed via balloon catheterization through the groin or arm to keep a blood vessel open. It can also be used in other areas, such as the ureter or carotid artery.[2,3]

Clinical considerations: Cardiac devices

Pressure:

- Patients are at risk of bleeding, especially if a femoral catheter was used and because of anticoagulant or thrombolytic medications. Therefore, no deep pressure should be applied anywhere on the body.
- If a femoral catheter was used, avoid massage to the leg that may cause a circulatory effect. Apply only noncirculatory techniques to the legs,

continued

lower back, and gluteals. Catheters inserted at the groin can potentially cause bleeding into the back, known as retroperitoneal bleeding. The patient affected by a retroperitoneal bleed may complain of back, thigh, or groin pain. However, it is a problem that cannot be addressed by massage.

Site:

- Patients lie on an examining table for a prolonged period during this procedure, which takes a toll on the back. Special attention to this area is often appreciated.

Positioning:

- To prevent bleeding or dislodgment of the catheter, the affected extremity is immobilized for up to 24 hours following the procedure. If the arm was involved, it will be placed in a sling. Side-lying on the opposite arm will be possible in some instances.
- Catheterization into the groin requires immobilization in a supine position for at least 4 to 6 hours.[1] After this time, side-lying may be possible. However, the puncture site will be tender for days, possibly eliminating the use of prone position.

Pacemakers and defibrillators

Despite amazing technological advances, such as the micro-sized pacemaker, many cardiac treatments still require a surgical intervention. Standard pacemakers and defibrillators are typically placed surgically under the skin on the left side of the chest, just below the clavicle. Insulated wires are threaded through the blood vessels into the heart chambers. The pacemaker provides an electrical stimulus to the heart to regulate its beat. A defibrillator can act as a pacemaker, but it can also be programmed to deliver a high-energy shock to correct more serious arrhythmias, such as tachycardia or fibrillation.

The main positioning protocol for these patients is that the arm on the affected side cannot be lifted any higher than the shoulder to prevent dislodgement of the device. For the first 24 hours after the procedure, they will wear a sling on the side of the placement.[4]

Micra pacemakers

Recent technologies have produced "leadless" pacemakers that may be an appropriate treatment for bradycardia (slow or irregular heart rhythm), which is a common but serious heart condition that puts one at higher risk for fainting, heart failure or sudden cardiac arrest.[5] "The Micra Transcatheter Pacing System is a miniaturized single chamber pacemaker that is implanted directly into the right ventricle, eliminating the subcutaneous pocket and creating a leadless pacemaker system."[6] Additional leadless devices for other heart conditions are also being developed. Pericardial effusion and device dislodgement are still risk factors, but compare well to complications of traditional pacemakers.[7]

Clinical considerations: Pacemakers and defibrillators

Pressure:

- Gentle massage is generally permissible to the unaffected area of the upper body. For example, if a device is placed in the left side of the chest, gentle massage to the right side is permissible. Moderate or deep force is not advisable to ensure that the leads will not be dislodged. Two months are needed for them to become embedded in the body.
- Within reason, the patient can have self-limiting pressure from below the rib cage to the lower extremities.
- Pain medication will affect the ability of the patient to give accurate feedback.

Site:

- The entire affected area (shoulder, upper back, upper chest and arm) should be avoided for the first day or two.

continued

- If a leaded device is placed on the right side, do not massage either side of the upper body. When devices are implanted in the right side of the body, the lead wires are still brought across to the left side, so the entire upper body needs to remain stable.

Positioning:

- Following the placement of mechanisms with wires, patients are on bedrest for 24 to 48 hours, and the extremity nearest to the device must be immobilized. This allows the leads in the heart to stabilize, thereby preventing dislodgment.

Jacket defibrillator

A vest or jacket defibrillator may be worn close to the skin around the chest. Monitors will sound an alarm if the heart rate indicates a serious problem, and a defibrillator in the jacket will send a shock to restore a normal heart rhythm.[8,9]

Clinical considerations: Jacket defibrillator

Pressure:

- Generally, avoid strokes toward the heart for patients with cardiac conditions. Increased fluid or circulation intent is too much and unnecessary in medical settings.
- Level 0–2 pressure is appropriate for distal areas. If swelling or edema is present use level 0–1. (See Chapter 6.)

Site:

- Avoid lotion anywhere on or near the jacket or vest.

Positioning:

- Head above heart positioning is recommended for acute cardiac conditions.
- Avoid prone positions.

Swan-Ganz catheter

A Swan-Ganz catheter, commonly referred to as a "swan," is a balloon-tipped catheter that monitors heart function. Most commonly, it is used in patients with congestive heart failure or those who have had a severe myocardial infarction (MI) or heart surgery. The device is threaded into the heart and ultimately wedged into a pulmonary artery where it can measure heart rate, pressures in the heart chambers, cardiac output, and blood volume. The entrance site most often is at the side of the neck, but can also be at the antecubital space. These devices are left in place for about a week or less. The risk of infection is higher with catheter types such as the Swan-Ganz or a central line, which have an external opening. In this situation, an infection would be serious because the catheter leads directly into the heart.[1]

Clinical considerations: Swan-Ganz catheter

Pressure:

- Gentle massage only to side of neck without the device.

Site:

- Massage to the unaffected parts of the neck may be very welcome since the patient must lie for an extended period with the head turned to the side in a static posture while the catheter is placed.
- The site of the catheter should be avoided. If it is placed on the side of the neck, the back of the neck, as well as the entire opposite side of the neck, can be gently massaged. The remainder of the body also can be massaged with relevant adjustments for other conditions.

Positioning:

- Positioning will be restricted to supine and side-lying on the side opposite the catheter.

continued

- Even after the initial 24 hours, movement of the affected side is limited, especially over-the-head motions, which are not allowed for the first week.[1]

Compression devices

While walking and getting out of bed is generally encouraged as soon as possible, compression devices may be used to prevent edema and to promote circulation in the extremities. Sometimes they are simple elastic garments that fit tightly on the arms or legs; in other cases, an air-filled tube is used to create the compression. The latter are generically referred to as pneumatic compression devices (Figure 9.4). The air can be maintained at either a constant low pressure or be rhythmically inflated and deflated. Rhythmic inflation/deflation promotes circulation and prevents deep vein thrombi from forming in the legs.[1]

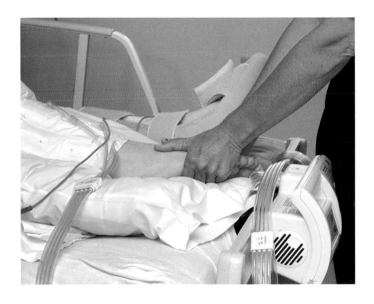

FIGURE 9.4

A commonly used compression device. Foot massage and reflexology can easily be applied.

(Photo by Don Hamilton.)

Clinical considerations: Compression devices

Pressure:

- Compression devices can be taken off in order to massage the legs if the nurse is in agreement. As stated in the thrombosis section of Chapter 8, there is no standard of practice within the massage or nursing professions with regard to rubbing the legs of patients at risk for developing a blood clot. The decision to massage patients with compression devices must be made on a case-by-case basis. If approval is given, the pressure should be light.

Site:

- While it is possible to remove elasticized compression hose, a great deal of effort is required, which is fatiguing to the patient. Although skin-to-skin contact is beneficial, it is often better to leave the stockings on and stroke over them without lotion, assuming, of course, that the nurse has given approval.

- Pneumatic devices, on the other hand, are removed easily. However, since these devices must be replaced in a certain way, have the nurse put them back onto the patient's leg or foot.

- If the nurse does not want the pneumatic compression device removed from the legs, it is sometimes acceptable to massage the feet, which extend beyond the apparatus as in Figure 9.4.

Positioning:

- Generally self-limiting.

Drains, tubes, and shunts

Drains

Besides being used as catheters, tubes are also used as drains, feeding tubes, and shunts. A drain is used to remove fluid that collects in a cavity or wound. It can be as simple as a wick of gauze, or it can be made of tubing attached to a suctioning machine. The drained fluids are then collected in a bag or other container. The Jackson-Pratt (or J-P tube) and Pleurevac are commonly encountered drainage systems.

Drains may be used following surgery to allow drainage from an internal organ to the outside. The T-tube, which drains bile, is an example, along with the gastrostomy, jejunostomy, and nephrostomy tubes. These last three drain the stomach, middle portion of the small intestine, and kidneys, respectively.

Tubes

Some tubes are employed as both a drain and a feeding tube. The nasogastric (NG) tube is an example of this. The patient who is unable to eat may have an NG tube, which is inserted into the nose, guided down the esophagus, and into the stomach. Food and medications can then be delivered through this route. The NG tube also can be used to suction out irritating stomach secretions that cause nausea or ulcers. An orogastric tube is similar, but the tubing is inserted into the mouth instead of the nose. Several drains mentioned earlier, such as the gastrostomy and jejunotomy tubes, are also used to administer nutrition. They often are referred to simply as "feeding tubes." The feeding tube is connected to a pump on the IV pole that paces the delivery of the nutritional formula contained in a hanging bag. Some people will be discharged with a feeding pump system in place for long-term use.

Other tubes assist the breathing process. An endotracheal tube creates a passage from the mouth or nose into the trachea and is used to provide an open airway, to prevent aspiration of intestinal contents, and to suction out secretions. A tracheostomy tube is surgically inserted directly into the trachea from the outside and is used when there is an obstruction in or damage to the airway.

Shunts

A shunt is a tube placed internally to divert fluid from one compartment of the body to another, and is therefore not visible from the outside. For example, an arteriovenous shunt is placed in the arm of a person needing hemodialysis. The device connects an artery to a vein, usually in the forearm.

Brain shunts

In patients with hydrocephalus, a shunt is used to divert cerebrospinal fluid (CSF) away from a blocked area in the brain. Newer devices have an externally controlled or programmed valve for keeping CSF drainage at the correct pressure.[10,11] Extracranial shunts such as a ventriculoperitoneal (VP) shunt, divert CSF to another part of the body, such as the peritoneum.[1]

There are several types of shunts that can be surgically implanted in the brain to drain and maintain proper CSF pressure and flow. Significant to the hospital-based massage therapist is the incision site, generally above or behind an ear and the thin tube that will be in the neck subcutaneously and therefore palpable.

Clinical considerations: Drains, tubes, and shunts

Pressure:

- Force or movement that places pressure on the tubes should be avoided.

- For brain shunts, use gentle overall pressure as any brain surgery may affect physical and mental function.

Site:

- The site of the tube and surrounding area should be avoided. One reason is that tubes opening to the outside are susceptible to bacterial infections. Avoiding contact with the site will decrease the chance of introducing further bacteria into the area.

- When working around drains, bodyworkers must be mindful of the possibility of leakage onto the bedding or gown and apply the appropriate Standard Precautions.

- Patients often complain about significant throat irritation from NG or tracheal tubes. Of course, the throat cannot be directly touched when these devices are in, but holding the hands several inches above the throat, as is done with Therapeutic Touch or Reiki, may reduce the discomfort. This in turn increases the patient's overall comfort level.

continued

Positioning:

- Most drains and tubes preclude using the prone position.
- Side-lying may be acceptable if there are no other influencing factors with regard to the patient's general health.

Other:

- Hospital length of stay will depend on the patient, but several precautions are advised, including not showering for several days, and keeping the incision site well-tended to avoid infection. Long-term precautions include avoiding close head contact with magnets as the programmable valve could be unintentionally changed.[11]

Resections and collection bags

Much could be discussed regarding surgeries to correct blockages or diseased organs in the gastrointestinal tract and the waste management system. Issues pertinent to the devices a touch therapist may encounter are the focus here.

Colostomy bags

Following intestinal surgery, perhaps to remove a tumor or because of an ischemic or inflamed bowel, a variety of surgeries may be performed to "resection" the bowel. Some resections require the bowel to be diverted to the surface of the abdomen with a stoma. For colon resections, a replaceable colostomy bag is affixed around the stoma for fecal matter collection (Figure 9.5). The stoma and its colostomy bag are generally located in the lower quadrants of the abdomen. The stoma is a part of the intestine and will appear red or pink, moist, soft and can change in size up to several inches. Typically, stomas have no feeling when touched. Because the organ is made of involuntary muscle, its functions are uncontrollable by the patient. If slight bleeding is seen in or around the stoma, the client and caregiver should be informed.

Ileostomy and urostomy bags

A similar surgical process can be performed to other areas of the bowel and urinary tract. If the affected area is the

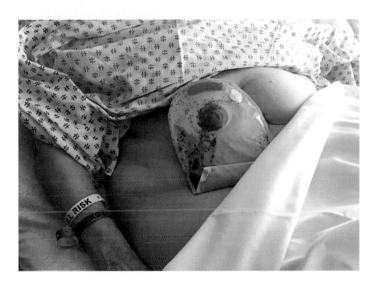

FIGURE 9.5
Colostomy bag and stoma. Output is involuntary and bags need to be emptied on a regular basis. The bag is affixed to the skin around the stoma with double sided adhesive rings. Bags need to be changed every few days.

(Photo by Carolyn Tague.)

ileum, an ileostomy bag collects waste from that part of the bowel; a J-pouch is used to collect the contents of the jejunum. When surgery is performed to divert the flow of urine from the bladder to a path outside the body, a urostomy bag is placed over the stoma to collect urine. Often, these procedures are temporary and serve to allow the affected area to heal. When this has been accomplished, the bowel or ureters are restored with a "take down" surgery.[1]

Clinical considerations: Collection bags

Pressure:

- Generally self-limiting unless affected by other health conditions.

Site:

- If the patient is comfortable with it, there is no medical reason not to give gentle touch in the general area containing the collection bag. Avoid lotion for several inches around the bag adhesive.

continued

- Leakage may occur around the stoma, causing irritation and possibly breakdown of the surrounding skin. Colostomies on the far right side of the colon and ileostomies tend to have more leakage because the fecal matter is looser and more watery in these areas. If leakage has occurred, practitioners should glove when massaging the site.

Positioning:

- Patients differ in their comfort level with regard to lying on or near their collection bag. Many people who have had a colostomy for a number of years are at ease lying in all positions. Others will want to minimize repositioning. The neck, feet, and hands are good starting places because no repositioning is required.

- Patients with a collection bag on the far side of the abdomen may need to confine their positioning to the opposite side and supine.

- As patients become more trusting of the bag and familiar with the accompanying sensations, they will be more comfortable trying a variety of positions.

Other:

- Invariably, people with a collection bag suffer initially from body-image issues. The acceptance of touch therapy may be difficult but can go a long way toward healing the emotional impact of their medical condition.

- Odors, noises, and output is uncontrollable and may lead clients to feel embarrassed or self-conscious. Normalizing these natural bodily functions is helpful, especially to people with new ostomies.

Monitors

When continuous measurement of some aspect of a patient's health is necessary, an electronic monitor might be used. Some monitors use telemetry, which transmits information by wire or radio signals to another location, such as the nurses' station. An example of this is cardiac telemetry, in which the heart's pressures and electrical activity data are sent to a monitor somewhere distant from the patient. The information about pressures is gathered by a Swan-Ganz catheter (see above). An electrocardiograph (ECG) monitors the electrical activity of the heart via electrodes attached to the patient's chest.

Massage practitioners may encounter many other types of monitors. The electroencephalograph, or EEG, measures the electrical activity in the brain. A variety of cranial monitors are used to measure pressure inside the skull if the person has suffered head trauma.[1]

Pulse ox

The amount of oxygen in the blood is monitored by a pulse oximeter, known as a "pulse ox" (Figure 9.6). A pulse oximeter works by passing a specific wavelength of light through a vascular bed, usually a finger, and measuring the absorption of light by oxygenated (red) and deoxygenated (blue) blood. The relationship between these two can be used to determine if the blood is carrying enough oxygen. Practitioners can see the digital readout of the monitor, which is near the patient's bed. Oxygen saturation above 90% is the desired level.

Fetal monitor

In childbirth, a fetal monitor is used to measure the fetus's heartbeat and the mother's abdominal tension during uterine contractions. Fetal monitors can be external or internal. Internal types, which are inserted into the uterus, are more accurate than external ones, which are placed on the outside around the woman's abdomen.

Continuous glucose monitors

These monitors are inserted under the skin in the upper arm by a primary care physician and can be used to read blood glucose for up to three months. The sensor under the skin transmits the blood glucose level to a hand-held receiver; in this way patients can avoid the traditional finger-prick method. Other monitors are

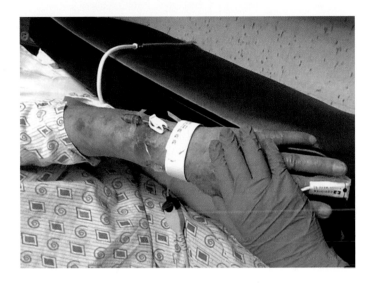

FIGURE 9.6
A pulse ox is a small device clipped or taped onto a fingertip – the middle finger in this instance. The blood oxygen saturation is measured; oxygen levels need to stay above 90%.

(Photo courtesy of Baptist Health, Lexington, Kentucky.)

becoming more user-friendly such as self-applied sensors that can last for a few weeks. Smart device applications or hand-held readers can be used to check blood glucose readings in seconds, at any time.[12]

Clinical considerations: Monitors

Pressure:

- Force or movement that could displace the monitor should be avoided.

Site:

- Therapists must be mindful when massaging around sites containing a measurement device, such as the belly of a woman connected to a fetal monitor, the neck of someone with a Swan-Ganz catheter, the chest of a person with ECG electrodes, the upper arm site of a blood glucose monitor, or the finger containing a pulse ox monitor.

Positioning:

- Positioning will be affected by most of these medical devices. However, repositioning is nearly always possible. The necessary adjustments are usually apparent by using common sense.

Orthopedic devices and equipment

When a patient has disease or trauma to the musculoskeletal system, it may be necessary to immobilize the affected body part(s) to allow bones and other connective tissues to heal. This is accomplished through the use of splints, braces, casts, slings, fixators, and traction devices. There are a variety of relatively simple devices that stabilize an area. Splints act to immobilize a joint or joints through the use of a rigid framework bound to the body. A brace is similar to a splint, but it usually allows some movement of the joint, often with the use of hinges. A cast can be made of plaster, plastic, or fiberglass and is molded to fit the body part that needs to be immobilized. A sling is a supporting bandage used to immobilize a limb, most commonly a loop suspended from the neck to support the forearm. New products are in development that show promise in reducing skin degradation during the healing process and for being generally more user-friendly, but availability and adoption of new materials by doctors may vary. Patients can expect to wear a cast for several weeks and have to be careful not to get them wet. Transitioning to a splint or brace for several additional weeks is also common.

Another group of apparatus is more complex and often involves surgery. A fixator uses a combination of pins, nails, screws, and plates to hold bones together and can be either internal or external. Lumbar fusion and bone grafting surgeries have been used for over 100 years. Combining these techniques with the addition of fixator equipment is common today.[10]

Traction devices, which are a system of ropes, pulleys, and weights, bring injured body parts into alignment by pulling on them and holding them in place. A continuous passive motion device is often used to passively move a joint after surgery, to maintain its range of motion.[1]

Clinical considerations: Orthopedic devices and equipment

Pressure:

- Avoid force or movement that could displace the body's alignment.

Site:

- Casts must be protected from becoming soiled or wet. Moisture causes plaster to soften, which can then cause skin breakdown.
- The skin at the edge of a cast or other orthopedic device can become irritated.

Positioning:

- An orthopedic apparatus severely limits the positioning possibilities for a massage session.
- Maintaining proper alignment of the affected areas is vital. Practitioners should work closely with the nursing staff to ensure that this happens. Any touch technique that affects alignment must be avoided.

Other:

- Study the orthopedic section in Chapter 7 for further massage adjustments related to the patient's general condition.

Oxygen delivery devices

If the patient's blood oxygen level is low, oxygen will be given from an external source. This can be through a simple face mask that fits over the nose and mouth or through a pronged tube in the nose known as a nasal cannula. The latter device delivers a low oxygen flow. If this amount of extra oxygen does not keep the saturation levels high enough, masks that deliver a higher concentration of oxygen are used.

When patients don't have the energy to breathe, but the doctor does not want them on a mechanical ventilator, they may be put on a continuous positive airway pressure (CPAP) mask or BiPAP mask. This provides positive airway pressure during both inhalation and exhalation. The CPAP or BiPAP mask is sometimes not well tolerated by patients because it must be sealed tightly against the face in order to maintain pressure.

Oxygen is sometimes administered directly to the trachea through an endotracheal tube, a tracheostomy tube, or a catheter that is placed directly into the trachea. The placement of an endotracheal tube is referred to as intubation: removal of the tube is extubation. If a patient is unable to breathe on their own, a mechanical ventilator, or vent, is attached to the endotracheal tubing. Patients on ventilators are nearly always in the ICU due to the high amount of expertise required to monitor these devices.[1]

Hospitalized patients with oxygen support may feel more restricted to the bed and unnecessarily avoid moving to the chair or walking. A nasal cannula may easily slip out of the nostrils without the patient's awareness. Most devices will have a vaporizing "water bubbler" attached on the wall to keep the oxygen moist and avoid damaging the sensitive tissue inside the nose. Without moisture, prolonged use of oxygen could degrade the tissue to the point of open wounds.

Clinical considerations: Oxygen delivery devices

Positioning:

- Positioning will be the main adjustment needed. However, this is not caused so much by the oxygen delivery devices in and of themselves. It is the general condition of the patient that will dictate positioning restrictions.
- Those with a nasal cannula, face mask, or tracheal device may be able to lie on their side for a back massage.
- The mechanical ventilator does not prevent the patient from side-lying, but the overall condition of this group of patients usually is very acute. Often, they are in a comatose or sedated state.
- Repositioning, whenever possible, will help maintain skin integrity.

continued

Other:

- Massage is beneficial, for both the health of the skin and breathing difficulties. Relaxation can create greater openness in the chest and, therefore, increase the delivery of oxygen.
- Some patients with tracheal devices or on a ventilator will be unable to speak. Several of the communication suggestions in Chapter 7 will help touch therapists in their interactions with these patients. A "communications board" works well, allowing the patient to write requests or responses.

Pain management devices

Pain management is a serious topic in medical centers and is discussed more fully in other chapters. Here the focus is on medical devices. Currently, pain is most often managed pharmacologically and if not given as an oral medication, is delivered via IV and/or epidural devices. Some systems allow the patient to control the amount of pain medication given, a method called patient-controlled analgesia (PCA). The person with a PCA pump can press a button when pain relief is needed. The PCA system is computerized, which controls the maximum amount of medication that the patient can receive in a given time period. Pain medication can also be injected into the epidural space in the lumbar spine for pain in the lower extremities and abdomen. Epidural anesthesia is frequently used during childbirth and spinal surgery.

Electrical stimulation is sometimes used to relieve pain. Transcutaneous electrical nerve stimulation (TENS) is a system that delivers electric currents to the surface of the skin, relieving pain in underlying areas. A TENS unit can be worn continuously to relieve chronic pain. For deeper stimulation, a percutaneous electrical nerve stimulator can be surgically placed around a nerve. An internal receiver is implanted under the skin, and the patient activates an external transmitter when pain relief is needed. In similar systems, electrodes can also be placed in the spinal cord or brain.[1]

Clinical considerations: Pain management devices

Pressure:

- Massage strokes administered to people receiving systemic pain relief should not be forceful because the medication will affect the ability of the patient to give accurate feedback about the pressure.
- When the pain-control system treats only a localized area, gentle pressure should be applied to that area.

Site:

- IV and epidural catheter sites and the area surrounding them should be avoided. This is especially true of an epidural catheter, which is placed near spinal nerves and the spinal canal.
- Any stroke that creates excessive movement also should be avoided to prevent any displacement of the epidural. This is also true for electrical stimulation devices.

Positioning:

- Generally self-limiting.

Procedures

This section will familiarize the touch therapist with common medical procedures and the equipment used during them. It is useful for practitioners to know the basics of procedures as they pertain to the massage treatment plan, but also understand what the patient has experienced. Some procedures are part of the treatment process, others are diagnostic in nature. Massage therapy can be helpful as the patient undergoes certain procedures, such as hemodialysis or a PICC placement, or following procedures, such as a heart biopsy or endoscopic procedure. Massage therapists have also been employed to provide patient distraction and comfort during brain surgery when patients are kept awake. Hand massage and attentive communication with the patient helps to induce a relaxation response in the patient and allows the surgical team to assess the effects of the surgery in real time.

Biopsy

A biopsy is most commonly used as a diagnostic assessment. Tissue from the area in question is removed and then sent for analysis by a pathologist. The pathologist treats the sample chemically, slices it in thin sections, and then examines it under a microscope.

Most often, the procedure is performed with a needle that aspirates a small portion of the desired tissue. Needle biopsies are frequently employed for assessing lumps in the breast and lesions in the thyroid, liver, kidney, and lungs. The needle often can be inserted directly into the questionable area. In other instances, such as a tumor deep in the body, an x-ray is used to locate the lesion and then guide placement of the needle into the biopsy area. Tissue also can be excised surgically but this is not preferred unless necessary, due to the greater invasiveness of surgical procedures. Fiberoptic instruments, such as bronchoscopes or colonoscopes, also can be used to collect tissue samples.

Bone marrow is also biopsied in the diagnosis of blood disorders, such as leukemia or aplastic anemia, or to monitor the course of an illness, such as multiple myeloma, and its response to treatment. Usually, bone marrow is aspirated with a needle from the iliac crest or sternum. This particular biopsy is painful because the doctor must pass a somewhat large outer metal sleeve through bone before entering the cavity that produces the marrow. The needle that removes the bone marrow sample is inserted into the outer sleeve.[1,13]

Patients may report pain or soreness in the area of the biopsy for up to several days after the procedure. Redness or bruising is rare but there may be a small incision site that will need time to heal.

Clinical considerations: Biopsy

Pressure:

- Risk of clot formation due to insertion of needles, especially the large-bore type.

Site:

- Biopsy site due to tenderness or bruising.
- Be mindful of bleeding at the biopsy site, and observe appropriate Standard Precautions.

Positioning:

- Most often, positioning will be self-limiting.
- Biopsies of certain organs, such as the kidney and liver, may require positioning adjustments away from the biopsied area.

Cardiac procedures

Arrhythmia treatments

The touch therapist will encounter arrhythmia patients in the hospital when medications no longer can control the problem. Some admissions, such as to the heart catheterization lab, will be a day procedure, but others will require an overnight stay. Common treatments are the placement of a pacemaker or implantable cardioverter-defibrillator (ICD). The ICD monitors the rhythm of the patient's heart, using an electrical impulse if an abnormality is detected. Another procedure is cardiac ablation, which uses high-frequency electrical energy via a catheter to disconnect the pathway causing the abnormal rhythm. There are several other types of arrhythmias and treatments, which the reader is encouraged to research.[14,15]

Catheterization

The "heart cath" lab in any hospital is one of the busiest outpatient areas. A catheterization procedure is used to diagnose and treat certain heart diseases, such as narrowed arteries, heart valve problems, arrhythmias, blockages, to perform a biopsy, or measure the pressure and oxygen levels in the heart. The catheterization process involves the physician inserting a long, thin catheter into a vessel in the groin, neck, or arm and threading it into the blood vessels of the heart.

Many heart treatments from the past were highly invasive but can now be accomplished in the cath lab. For instance, some patients qualify to have their aortic valve replaced via catheterization rather than by standard open-heart surgery. The physician does this by threading a catheter into the groin, up into the heart, and placing a bovine heart valve on top of the patient's damaged valve.

Open heart surgery

Open heart surgery is commonly performed to replace a valve, repair the aorta, or graft new blood vessels onto the heart. Open-heart surgery is invasive and carries with it many risks. In a traditional coronary artery bypass graft (CABG), or other open-heart operation, the sternum is cut and the patient is often placed on a heart–lung machine to circulate the blood while the heart is stopped. However, some people may qualify for a less invasive CABG procedure, of which there are two types: 1) the physician accesses the coronary arteries via small incisions in the thorax without cutting the sternum; or 2) the use of a sternotomy but without placing the patient on the bypass machine: this is referred to as a beating heart surgery.[16]

Open-heart surgery has a number of risks: infection, renal and cardiac insufficiency, decreased oxygenation, breathing difficulties, coagulation problems, blood clots, hypotension, fever, edema, and anxiety. There will be a multitude of medical devices for the therapist to be mindful of, such as chest drains, IV lines in the arm, an oxygen source, sequential compression devices on the legs to maintain circulation, and a urinary catheter. Patients will be on a number of medications including blood thinners to prevent blood clots, pain medication, drugs to regulate the heart's rhythm, and antihypertensive drugs, such as beta-blockers, calcium channel blockers, and vasodilators. Despite the rigors of this operation, the survival rate is very high.

Typically, the first night post-op will be spent in the ICU and the remaining days on a cardiac care unit. People can have touch therapy in either unit. The patient will have significant sternal pain as well as leg pain if blood vessels were removed to provide new coronary vessel grafts. They may have throat pain from the endotracheal tube inserted during surgery and sore rhomboids as a result of their arms being retracted to a 90° angle during the operation. The rhomboids can be very gently given acupressure when the patient is able to be in semi-reclining position. Patients can sit semi-reclining for a couple of hours at a time, but not completely upright until the physician approves. They may lie flat, but legs must be uncrossed at all times.[17]

Tip 9.1 Special note about patients with a recent catheterization procedure

Often, heart catheterization procedures are done as day treatments. Those who have had catheterizations for such interventions as an angiogram, stent placement, or an ablation, lie supine on a hard surface for long periods during the treatment. If the catheter is inserted via the groin, the patient will have to lie flat on their back for a number of hours following the procedure. The reason for this is to give the artery time to heal and avoid serious bleeding.[18] This is a tedious position to maintain. Touch therapy is a welcome distraction, however, the therapist will need to give the session without repositioning the patient. Most commonly, massage is given to the feet, but the head, neck, hands, and arms are acceptable too. If the access site is via the radial artery, that area should be avoided. If the access point was the groin, avoid bodywork to the catheterized leg, including the foot until the patient has been cleared by the healthcare team.[2]

Clinical considerations: Cardiac procedures

Pressure:

- Post-op sedation or significant pain medications indicate gentle pressure.
- Edema: CHF patients may be affected by fluid in the lungs, body cavities, and lower extremities.
- Fatigue.
- Fever.
- Pain medication.
- Light massage to the legs is often OK with staff approval.
- The need to minimize cardiac output. Maintain awareness of heart rate and distension of jugular vein.
- Risk of bruising or bleeding due to thrombolytic and anticoagulant medications.
- Blood clot risk.
- Possible cardiac and kidney complications.
- Psychological fragility.

Site:

- Avoid touch to recent incision sites, which may include the arm, groin or neck.
- Electrodes on chest common in MI and heart surgery.
- IV catheters.
- Chest tubes.
- Oxygen delivery device.
- Pacemaker or defibrillator site.
- Mindfulness when doing leg massage due to increased risk of blood clot or swelling.
- Sternal incision common in open-heart surgery.
- Leg incision (CABG surgery).

Positioning:

- Head above heart for several days after surgery may be recommended.
- Semi-reclining position if the patient is short of breath or had open-heart surgery.
- Elevate extremities if edematous. The feet should not be elevated above the heart to avoid stressing it through too much venous return.
- Right side-lying, if the patient can tolerate it, puts less strain on the heart.
- Patient should rise slowly from supine position.
- When rising from bed to a seated position, patient should sit with feet on the floor for a moment to minimize orthostatic hypertension.
- Need to lie flat for a number of hours after an inguinal catheterization.

Other:

- Some patients may be on water restriction. They may also be on diuretics and need to use the bathroom frequently. This may also lead to muscle cramps due to an imbalance in electrolytes.

Endoscopy

Endoscopy is a method of examining internal organs that are hollow or have a cavity, such as the lungs or stomach. The instruments, generically referred to as endoscopes, are made of a hollow tube that may be flexible or rigid. A lighted optical system allows the tissues to be seen on a video screen or through a telescopic eyepiece.

Each scope is specifically designed for the part of the body to be viewed. Pulmonary specialists employ a bronchoscope to examine the trachea and bronchial tree for such conditions as tumors, constrictions, bleeding, or pulmonary diseases such as tuberculosis. A gastroenterologist uses a gastroscope to view the stomach, intestines, and other digestive organs. A sigmoidoscopy allows the sigmoid portion of the colon to be inspected, while a colonoscope allows visual examination of the entire colon. The doctor can inspect for such conditions as tumors, polyps, ulcerative colitis, or bleeding.

These scopes also have the capacity to provide treatment. For example, a laser beam can be directed through a channel of the scope to stop bleeding from a lesion. Another channel in the scope allows the passage of instruments that can take a biopsy, remove a foreign object, or excise polyps. Narrowed areas, such as in the esophagus, can be stretched to ease swallowing.

A number of other endoscopes are available for use in other areas of the body. A cystoscope is used to inspect the bladder and prostate gland, an arthroscope allows a view into joints, a laparoscope provides a way to inspect the abdomen, and the colposcope examines the vagina and cervix.[1] Generally, patients do not experience significant discomfort from these procedures. A sedative or anesthesia will provide pain avoidance during the procedure and once complete, is generally not a cause of pain. Bloating, gas, or cramping may occur[18] but the procedure is generally well tolerated.

As we take massage therapy into the welcoming and heady atmosphere of "integrative medicine," let's not be hesitant to promote the most important aspect of our work: touch for the sake of touching. Touch comforts patients and caregivers. Touch makes invasive procedures more tolerable for patients who may be afraid, restless, out-of-control, in pain, and/or doubting their very touchableness. The undivided attention and compassionate human touch we bring to them is the most important "stroke" in the massage therapist's repertoire.

Teddi Dunn and Marian Williams[19]

Clinical considerations: Endoscopy

Pressure:

- Pain medication or sedatives will interfere with the ability to give accurate feedback.

Site:

- Usually, the scope is inserted through an orifice, so there are no site restrictions. One exception is a laparoscopic procedure in which a small incision is made near the umbilicus.
- Depending on the type of procedure, the positioning may have created discomfort, especially in the neck or back.

Positioning:

- Generally self-limiting.

- As part of some scoping procedures, such as a laparoscopy and esophagogastroduodenoscopy, air is inserted to permit better visualization or to separate the intestines from the pelvic organs. This manipulation of the intestines can cause bloating, abdominal discomfort, and difficulty passing gas or having a bowel movement.

Gastric stimulator

A gastric stimulator device may be placed in the stomach to help move food out and through the digestive tract. Devices are likely to stay implanted for several days, depending on how acute the patient's illness is. People who have this device commonly have type 1 diabetes.

Hemodialysis

Hemodialysis, a process that cleanses the blood of accumulated waste products, is used for people with chronic, end-stage renal failure or temporarily for patients whose acute illness has shut down the kidneys. If the patient's general health is good enough, the procedure can take place in the hemodialysis unit. Other patients, often those in the ICU, are dialyzed with a portable machine at the bedside. Those with stable kidney problems will receive dialysis in an outpatient center. Blood is accessed in several different ways. An oversized central line called a permacath may be placed in either the subclavian, internal jugular, or femoral vein. Another method of creating an access point is via an arteriovenous fistula (also termed anastomosis) (Figure 9.7). A fistula is created by suturing an artery and a vein, usually the radial artery and cephalic vein in the non-dominant arm. Two large-bore needles are then inserted into the vessel, one to obtain blood, the other to reinfuse it. A synthetic tube can also be grafted between an artery and vein to serve as an access point.

Blood is pulled from one of these access points and directed through a semipermeable dialyzer, which performs the filtering function of the kidneys. When the process is finished, usually in about 4 hours, the blood is returned to the body through the patient's access site.

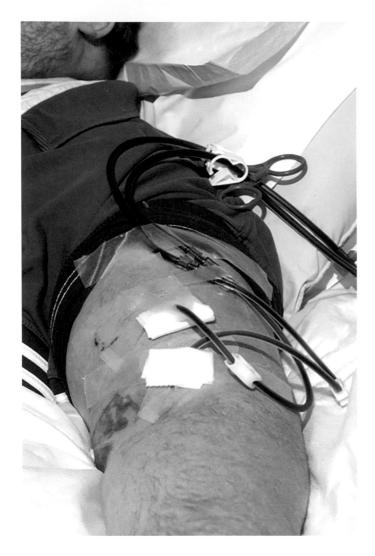

FIGURE 9.7
Arteriovenous fistula.

(Photo by Richard York, Oregon Health and Science University.)

The hemodialysis patient may experience the following complications:

- Cramping may occur if too much fluid is taken too quickly for the body to adjust to. The caregiver staff will often give fluids to counteract the cramping. Massage holds to temporarily affected areas is indicated and may be greatly appreciated. Pain and anxiety related to cramping is common and gentle massage therapy may be helpful.

- Blood sugar levels can drop rapidly on dialysis. Notify the nurse immediately if any the following signs appear:
  - Breaking out in a sweat.
  - Trembling or shaking.
  - Difficulty concentrating.
  - Dizziness or weakness.

- Vomiting or severe nausea is a risk factor during the treatment. Clients are advised not to eat before their appointment.

- Low blood pressure may occur. Watch for reports of dizziness or seeing spots in the eyes.

- Loneliness and anxiety are common side effects of the treatment. Sessions typically last around four hours and are needed 3 times per week for most.[12]

It must be remembered that the person undergoing hemodialysis usually has a complex medical history. Many of these patients are diabetic or have heart conditions. Touch therapists should also study the sections in the book related to those subjects.

Clinical considerations: Hemodialysis

Pressure:

- Potential for homeostatic disequilibrium. Massage should not be demanding to the body.

- Fatigue.

- Easy bruising.

- Fragile skin.

- Heparin (blood thinners).

- Hypertension.

- Neuropathy.

- Central line catheters, such as a permacath, or shunts increase the risk of clot formation. Massage the extremity nearest to the central line or shunt very gently. For instance, if the permacath is in the subclavian vein, massage the arm on the side very lightly.

Site:

- Do not perform circulatory touch techniques to the arm containing a permacath or fistula
  continued

because of the possibility of clot formation. Also, it is important not to risk dislodging or damaging the device.

- Lotioning the patient's hand is usually permissible.
- Avoid permacath site.

Positioning:

- Because of the potential for hemodialysis patients to "crash", do not have them sit at the edge of the bed.
- No prone positioning.
- Side-lying only on the opposite side from the access device.

Incision and drainage of wounds

Many people present to the Emergency Department (ED) with abscesses, wounds that are not healing and infections in soft tissues. Poor circulation, injection sites and neurological disorders that lead to poor health and hygiene may contribute to the causes. If infections are not treated, the condition can develop into septic shock, threatening vital organs and the person's life. Sepsis is defined: "as life-threatening organ dysfunction caused by a dysregulated host response to infection."[20] Patients will often be treated with intravenous antibiotics, but also, wounds will be incised, drained and dressed.

Clinical considerations: Incision and drainage of wounds

Pressure:

- Level 0–1 and avoid direction of strokes that might affect circulation.

Site:

- Completely avoid wound area, including bandaging or dressings. No lotion within 3 inches of bandages.

Positioning:

- Avoid body weight or pressure on any wound whenever possible.
- Extra pillows that elevate affected limbs in order to reduce swelling may be recommended.

Lumbar puncture

A lumbar puncture, also known as a spinal tap, is performed between two lumbar vertebrae, usually the third and fourth, with a thin, hollow needle that is inserted into the spinal canal. It usually takes about 30 minutes. Two common purposes for a lumbar puncture are to measure pressure in the cerebrospinal fluid (CSF) or to take a sample of spinal fluid for analysis. A number of

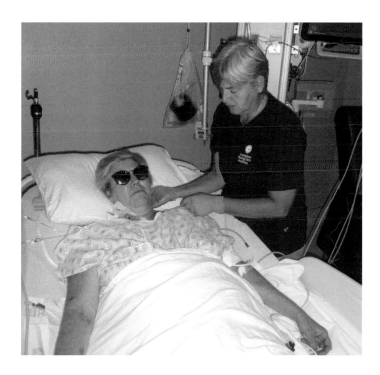

FIGURE 9.8
Massage therapist with complex patient. Note central catheter in the neck, PICC, and monitors.

(Photo courtesy of Baptist Health, Lexington, Kentucky.)

diseases or conditions may be diagnosed from the sample: multiple sclerosis, Guillain-Barré syndrome, meningitis, brain abscess, Reye's syndrome, and AIDS-related conditions. The presence of blood in the spinal fluid also can be determined.

A lumbar puncture may also be performed to inject a contrast dye or radioactive substance as part of creating a diagnostic image of the CSF. Antibiotics and anti-cancer drugs, as well as spinal anesthesia, may be placed in the spine by this process. A new use of the procedure is to determine levels of the tau protein and beta-amyloid, two substances associated with Alzheimer's disease.[1] Patients may report significant pain around the procedure site and have difficulty finding a comfortable position to lie down or sleep in.

Clinical considerations: Lumbar puncture

Pressure:

- Patients usually feel unwell afterward and have increased muscular tension. Headaches are not uncommon. Therefore, soothing pressure is called for.
- Pain medication will interfere with the ability to give accurate feedback.

Site:

- The puncture site will be very tender.
- Bleeding or CSF leakage may occur at the puncture site following the procedure.
- The patient may have sore muscles as a result of the position that must be maintained to open the lumbar vertebrae: side-lying, curled into a tight ball with the knees pulled to the chest.

Positioning:

- The patient must lie flat for 2 hours following the procedure.

Scans

Body scans allow the examination of internal organs and structures. The x-ray has been used for over a century, while computed tomography (CT) scans, ultrasound,

magnetic resonance imaging (MRI) scans, and functional MRI (fMRI) are more recent methods of assessment.

X-rays

X-rays are high-energy electromagnetic waves that have the ability to penetrate most solid matter and to act on photographic film. These rays often are used to assess the health of the skeletal structure but can be used to visualize certain soft-tissue areas, as with a mammogram.

Special procedures combine the use of a contrast dye and x-rays to obtain a clearer picture of the affected area. For example, to better see the functioning of a joint, dye that is opaque to x-rays is placed in the joint and then x-rayed, a process called arthrography. This same process can be used to examine arteries in the brain, which is known as a cerebral arteriograph or angiography. Kidneys, bile and pancreatic ducts, and the space around the spinal cord also can be assessed using this procedure.[1]

Clinical considerations: X-rays

Pressure:

- Adjustments to pressure will not be necessary because of a simple x-ray but may be required when dye is injected into the body.
- Some patients have a reaction to the dye, such as nausea, headache, dyspnea, hives, increased heart rate, and numbness in the extremities.
- Sedatives will interfere with the ability to give accurate feedback.
- The process of threading a catheter through the veins can dislodge a clot or plaque deposit. In light of that risk, only superficial massage should be administered.

Site:

- Bleeding at the catheter site.
- Certain parts of the body may feel strained from lying in awkward positions. Massage to them might be helpful.
- Certain procedures require the insertion of a catheter in the inguinal area. Massage should be

continued

avoided to that extremity due to the increased risk for a thrombus. The patient may have groin pain from the use of this type of catheter.

- IV catheter sites.
- Pain at the site where dye was injected.

Positioning:

- Generally self-limiting.

CT, MRI and fMRI scans

Many of the x-ray techniques have become supplemental with the advent of less invasive CT and MRI scans. CT scans employ ultrathin x-rays to analyze soft-tissue structures. The x-rays are beamed through segments of the body and picked up by the CT equipment to create a three-dimensional composite representation of the body. The information is fed into a computer that converts the data into a video or photographs. Contrast dyes are sometimes used to enhance the contrast of the image. CT scans are particularly useful for imaging brain disorders such as strokes, hemorrhages, injuries, tumors, swelling, and fluid accumulation.

An MRI is also a computerized scanning technique. Unlike a CT scan, which uses x-rays, the MRI machine employs a strong magnetic field that measures the response of the body's hydrogen atoms, which are abundantly present in water. MRIs, because of their ability to give high-resolution pictures, are useful for assessing the spinal cord and nerve fiber disorders such as multiple sclerosis. Functional magnetic resonance imagining (fMRI) is a tool for mapping brain activity. The process is considered noninvasive and safe.[1,21]

A touch practitioner cannot be in the room during a CT scan because of the use of x-rays. An MRI tube is extremely confining and, despite the use of sedatives, very anxiety producing. Previously, the presence of a family member or massage therapist who is holding their feet was allowed in some hospitals. Today however, safety guidelines strictly limit entry into the MRI room.[22]

Clinical considerations: CT, MRI and fMRI scans

Pressure:

- Pain medication or sedatives will interfere with the ability to give accurate feedback.

Site:

- If contrasting dye was administered, there will be an IV site.
- Patients are required to lie flat on their back during the scan, sometimes for hours. Attention to the back will soothe tensed musculature.

Positioning:

- Self-limiting.

Other:

- The contrast dyes are absorbed into the bloodstream and eliminated through urine. They pose no risk to practitioners. Patients must, however, be well-hydrated before and after procedures using contrast agents to protect the kidneys. More frequent trips to the bathroom are common.

Nuclear and PET scans

Nuclear imaging employs small amounts of radioactive isotopes that are attached to a drug or chemical. The two together are referred to as radiopharmaceuticals. These substances, which can be swallowed, inhaled, or injected into the body, are designed to concentrate in a certain organ. The radioisotope gives off radioactive energy that in turn produces an image of the organ showing its size, shape, and functioning. Some damaged tissue will have an increased uptake of the radioactive material, suggesting an abnormality, while other tissue will show an irregular distribution. Bones, lungs, liver, brain, thyroid, heart, and blood can be scanned in this way.

Positron emission tomography (PET) scans are one particular type of nuclear scan, and combine the use of radioisotopes, called positrons, with computer imaging techniques. A glucose-like solution is mixed with mildly radioactive tracers, which are injected or inhaled into the body. The PET scanner measures how quickly tissues absorb the radioactive isotopes, an indication of cellular metabolism based on patterns of glucose utilization. In the brain, areas of decreased metabolism indicate dysfunction. However, when testing for a cancer, just the opposite is true: quick absorption of the solution indicates an area containing cancer because tumors need increased nutrition to remain viable, greedily absorbing the sugary solution.[1]

The multiple gated acquisition (MUGA) scan is another diagnostic procedure that employs nuclear technology. It assesses the function of the heart by withdrawing a small amount of blood from the patient, inserting a radioactive substance into the sample that attaches to the red blood cells, and then reinjecting the cells back into the bloodstream. A gamma camera placed above the patient detects the low-level radiation being given off by the radiolabeled cells and is able to produce an outline of the heart's chambers and accurately measure the output of the left ventricle.[23]

Clinical considerations: Nuclear scans

Pressure:
- Generally self-limiting.
- Some people have a sense of malaise or slight fatigue afterward.
- Some scans, such as PET, require the patient to lie very still for more than an hour while the nuclear material circulates through the body. Generalized muscular tension will be evident. Gently coaxing the muscles into relaxation is the best approach.

Site:
- Usually, when the nuclear material is injected, it is done through a peripheral IV catheter. Tenderness will be present at the site.

- Depending on the part of the body that requires scanning, the patient may have to lie in an awkward position, such as with the arms over the head, for a prolonged period. Attention to the affected areas will be welcomed.

Positioning:
- Generally self-limiting

Ultrasound

This technology uses sound waves to create an image of the body. A wand-like device sends high-frequency sound waves into the tissue, which reflect back and form an image that can be displayed on a screen. Most people are familiar with the use of ultrasound to monitor the progress of a fetus in utero. It also can be used to detect tumors, examine abdominal organs, the thyroid, and prostate gland. IV nurses who specialize in the placement of PICC lines use ultrasound to locate a vein suitable for inserting the catheter. Additionally, it can measure the flow of blood in veins and arteries.[1]

Generally, scans are well tolerated by patients physically. Stress due to diagnostic testing and anxiety around health issues is often acute after these procedures. Wait times for test results while hospitalized can feel extralong for patients and their families and friends.

Summary

Medical devices and procedures add yet another dimension when planning a massage session with a person who is in a health care setting. While this chapter does not give exhaustive information for all the various devices and procedures a therapist may encounter, it does provide a good foundation for the critically thinking practitioner.

Case history 9.1 | Exercise

Instructions: On a piece of paper, make three columns: pressure, site, and position. List the conditions that apply to each category.

CY is a 43-year-old man who suffered a severe stroke while teaching English as a second language in Thailand. Upon return to his home in California, he was admitted to a long-term care facility because he does not have family who can meet his care needs. CY has an indwelling catheter for urine collection, he has wrist braces to help control his hand spasticity and ambulates by wheelchair. While he is not at all cognitively impaired, his speech is very slurred and so he uses a communications board to point to letters and spell out his words and sentences. Today, CY has a procedure scheduled to replace his catheter. Infection is a risk as are pressure sores from being in the wheelchair most of the day.

Acknowledgments

The authors thank the following reviewers and contributors: Carol Baillie RN, CMT; Jill Cole BAS, LMT, BCTMB; Amie Mascarinas-Galleri RN; Sanjay Reddy MD; Cathrine Weaver MSN, RN.

Test yourself

Multiple choice: Circle all the correct answers. There may be more than one.

1. Which of the following reasons are indications for gentle pressure when massaging a person undergoing hemodialysis?

   A The potential for a complex medical history that often includes heart disease or diabetes.

   B The potential for blood clot formation around the access device.

   C The potential for increased fatigue.

   D Risk of increased pain in lower extremities.

2. Patients with PICC lines require the following session adjustments:

   A Head above heart positioning.

   B Avoid any touch to the insertion area and several inches around it.

   C Deeper pressure because of increased risks of stasis.

   D Offer water after the session due to dehydration risk.

3. Match each of these procedures to the correct definition below.

   1. Bone marrow biopsy.
   2. fMRI.
   3. Hemodialysis.
   4. Angioplasty.
   5. Tracheotomy.

   A Tube inserted directly into trachea to bypass airway blockage or dysfunction.

   B Cleans the blood of waste and toxins when the kidneys are unable.

   C Compresses or dislodges plaque in a heart vessel.

   D Take a sample of tissue from inside a bone for diagnostic purposes.

   E Scan of living tissue, such as the brain, for diagnostics.

Chapter NINE

References

1. Nettina S. The Lippincott Manual of Nursing Practice. Philadelphia: Lippincott Williams & Wilkins; 2001; 2018.

2. American Heart Association. What is coronary angioplasty. Available from: https://www.heart.org/-/media/data-import/downloadables/f/7/a/pe-abh-what-is-coronary-angioplasty-ucm_300437.pdf

3. MedLine Plus. Angioplasty and stent placement—carotid artery. Available from: https://medlineplus.gov/ency/article/002953.htm

4. Weaver C. Personal communication, 20 August 20 2019.

5. Mayo Clinic. Bradycardia. Available from: https://www.mayo-clinic.org/diseases-conditions/bradycardia/symptoms-causes/syc-20355474

6. Wiles B, Roberts P. Design and evaluation of the Micra transcatheter pacing system for bradyarrhythmia management. Future Cardiol. 2019; 15(1):9–15. doi: 10.2217/fca-2018-0077.

7. Bhatia N, El-Chami M. Leadless pacemakers: a contemporary review. J Geriatr Cardiol. 2018; 15(4):249–53. doi: 10.11909/j.issn.1671-5411.2018.04.002.

8. WebMD. Vest defibrillator may help heart attack survivors. Available from: https://www.webmd.com/heart-disease/news/20180313/vest-defibrillator-may-help-heart-attack-survivors

9. Maier S. Wearable defibrillator lowers sudden cardiac death, but only when you wear it. Available from: https://www.ucsf.edu/news/2018/09/411876/wearable-defibrillator-lowers-sudden-cardiac-death-only-when-you-wear-it

10. Hunter TB, Yoshino MT, Dzioba RB, et al. Medical devices of the head, neck, and spine. Radiographics 2004; 24(1):257–85.

11. Beaumont Health. Brain shunt. Available from: https://www.beaumont.org/treatments/brain-shunt?related=treatment

12. Baillie C. Personal communication, 27 Oct 2019.

13. Larson DE. Mayo Clinic Family Health Book. New York: William Morrow and Company; 1990.

14. American Heart Association. About arrhythmia. 2016. Available from: https://www.heart.org/en/health-topics/arrhythmia/about-arrhythmia

15. Cleveland Clinic. Arrhythmia treatments. 2019 Available from: https://my.clevelandclinic.org/health/treatments/16751-arrhythmia-treatments

16. Michigan Medicine. Coronary artery bypass surgery: minimally invasive methods. 2018. Available from: https://www.uofm-health.org/health-library/ue4718abc

17. Weaver C. Personal communication, 12 August 12 2019.

18. Mayo Clinic. Upper endoscopy. Available from: https://www.mayoclinic.org/tests-procedures/endoscopy/about/pac-20395197

19. Dunn T, Williams M. Massage Therapy Guidelines for Hospital and Home Care (4th edition). Olympia: Information for People; 2000.

20. Singer M, Deutschman CS, Seymour CW, et al. The Third International Consensus Definitions for Sepsis and Septic Shock (Sepsis-3). JAMA 2016; 315(8):801–10. doi:10.1001/jama.2016.0287.

21. UC San Diego School of Medicine. Center for Functional MRI. What is fMRI? Available from: http://fmri.ucsd.edu/Research/whatisfmri.html

22. UC San Francisco Department of Radiology and Biomedical Imaging. Access restriction. Available from: https://radiology.ucsf.edu/patient-care/patient-safety/mri/access-restriction

23. Verywell Health. The MUGA scan. Available from: https://www.verywellhealth.com/the-muga-scan-1745247

Additional resources

- Most hospitals and rehabilitation centers will have some teaching materials and often "teaching labs". Ask a nurse in your facility for information on access and opportunities that might be available to you.

- On-line teaching videos are available for free on virtually any device or procedure. Be a critical thinker and consider the sources when reviewing new material.

Chabner DE. The Language of Medicine. Philadelphia: W.B. Saunders; 1996.

Kalani L, Aghababaeian H, Majidipour N, et al. The effects of acupressure on severity of depression in hemodialysis patients: a randomized controlled trial. Available from: https://japer.in/storage/models/article/J60vJnfllkcVmyrzlJ3o-Q3qK8Lj9nJA5xHRdWtphyRLA2qKrvWuIerSerE00/the-effects-of-acupressure-on-severity-of-depression-in-hemodialysis-patients-a-randomized-control.pdf

Krames Patient Education. Understanding Coronary Artery Procedures. Krames Health and Safety Education, The Stay Well Company; 2000.

Memorial Sloan Kettering Cancer Center. About your ventriculoperitoneal (VP) shunt surgery. Available from: https://www.mskcc.org/cancer-care/patient-education/about-your-ventriculoperitoneal-vp-shunt-surgery

Pulse Heart Institute. Micra pacemaker. Available from: https://www.pulseheartinstitute.org/how-we-help/electrophysiology/micra-pacemaker/

Roth E, Falck S. What is a ventriculoperitoneal shunt? 2017. Available from: https://www.healthline.com/health/ventriculoperitoneal-shunt

Pharmaceutical factors: Adjustments for medications

Learn voraciously and surrender constantly. It doesn't matter how much you know or what your fancy hands can do. You will always be in very good company at the threshold of ignorance. The greatest service in which you can engage will be inspired by true curiosity, genuine humility and generous collaboration.

Lauren "Cal" Cates CMT

Co-founder Healwell, Arlington, Virginia

For many manual therapists, discussions about medications and pharmacological considerations cause a glazed-over, blank stare. The language, which is literally Greek and Latin or at best "market-speak," requires a mental focus that can feel very distant from hands-on work. This is understandable, however, becoming familiar and competent in the basics of pharmacology is, in fact, one of the skillsets that sets apart the hospital-based massage practitioner. It is not expected that touch therapists in health care settings will be able to define the class of drug or understand specific mechanisms of action. It is inherent in medical settings, though, that providers of any direct patient care are familiar with how drugs may affect a patient's physical stability, cognition, and activities of daily living (ADLs). The good news is, because the touch work is adjusted for pressure, site and position, the intervention can be safely provided while medications are being taken.

By becoming acquainted with the material in this chapter and knowing resources that are available from any smart device, massage therapists will gain the basic knowledge required. For example, practitioners will recognize easy bruising can be caused by prednisone, heparin, or anticancer therapies; rashes may happen because of many medications; or that "fall precautions" are the possible result of narcotics or benzodiazepines.[1]

It should be noted that while in the acute care setting, therapists can turn to nurses for advice. However, outpatient or private practice settings also require the massage therapist to have a functional knowledge of

---

Info Box 10.1 Top 25 most prescribed drugs[1]

Lisinopril (Antihypertensive)
Levothyroxine (Hypothyroidism)
Atorvastatin (Antihyperlipidemic)
Metformin (Antidiabetic)
Simvastatin (Antihyperlipidemic)
Omeprazole (Anti-GERD)
Amlodipine (Antihypertensive)
Metoprolol (Antihypertensive)
Acetaminophen, hydrocodone (Opioid analgesic)
Albuterol (Bronchodilator)
Hydrochlorothiazide (Diuretic)
Losartan (Antihypertensive)
Gabapentin (Anticonvulsant)
Sertraline (Antidepressant)
Furosemide (Antihypertensive)
Acetaminophen (Analgesic)
Atenolol (Antihypertensive)
Pravastatin (Antihyperlipidemic)
Amoxicillin (Antibiotic)
Fluoxetine (Antidepressant)
Citalopram (Antidepressant)
Trazadone (Antidepressant)
Alprazolam (Antianxiety)
Fluticasone (Nasal corticosteroid)
Bupropion (Antidepressant)

---

medications and access to quick reference sources for immediate consultation. It is these clients who more often push therapists for vigorous bodywork, not realizing that their health condition and their medications place a demand on the body that may preclude forceful massage. Many of the drugs taken by outpatients, such as analgesics, corticosteroids, and heart medications, are examples of pharmaceuticals that require the implementation of massage precautions.

The purpose of this chapter is to present frequently prescribed categories of drugs, their common uses, and their side effects. The side effects are then categorized into the clinical framework that revolves around pressure, site and positioning considerations. Information on drugs could fill volumes. This chapter presents a broad overview rather than a lengthy listing of minute details. A medications reference manual or smart-phone app[2] can supply the remaining information (see additional resources at the end of this chapter.)

TABLE 10.1 Common medications reference table for manual therapists[1]

Drug groups	Side effects	Common drug names	Massage indications
Antianxiety drugs	Sedation, dizziness, GI reactions, confusion	Diazepam (Valium), lorazepam (Ativan), alprazolam (Xanax)	Pressure restriction Positioning assistance
Antibiotics	GI reactions	Amoxicillin, trimethoprim/sulfamethoxazole (Bactrim), ciprofloxacin (Cipro), levofloxacin (Levaquin), erythromycin, cefaclor (Ceclor), vancomycin	Self-limiting
Anticoagulants	Bruising, GI reactions	Heparin, warfarin (Coumadin), aspirin	Pressure restriction
Anticonvulsants	GI symptoms, drowsiness, CNS effects	Carbamazepine, gabapentin (Neurontin), phenytoin (Dilantin)	Pressure restriction Positioning assistance
Antidiabetics	Hypoglycemia	Glipizide (Glucotrol), metformin (Glucophage), rosiglitazone (Avandia), pioglitazone (Actos), chlorpropamide (Diabinese)	Pressure restriction
Antiemetics	Sedation, headache, constipation, depression	Prochlorperazine (Compazine), metoclopramide (Reglan), droperidol, promethazine (Phenergan), haloperidol, ondansetron (Zofran)	Pressure restriction Site restriction
Antifungals	GI reactions, fatigue, headache, dizziness, rash, itching	Fluconazole (Diflucan), nystatin	Pressure restriction Positioning assistance
Antilipemics	Headache	Atorvastatin (Lipitor), simvastatin (Zocor), pravastatin (Pravachol), lovastatin (Mevacor)	None
Antiplatelet medications	GI reactions, headache, dizziness, bleeding	Clopidogrel bisulfate (Plavix), tirofiban (Aggrastat), eptifibatide (Integrilin), abciximab (ReoPro), aspirin	Pressure restriction
Antispasmodics	Sedation, dizziness, fatigue, hypotonicity, GI reactions	Cyclobenzaprine (Flexeril), diazepam (Valium), dantrolene (Dantrium), succinylcholine	Pressure restriction Care when stretching Positioning assistance
Antitumor drugs	Fatigue, thrombocytopenia, neutropenia, GI reactions, neuropathy, edema, organ toxicity, hair loss	Cyclophosphamide (Cytoxan), 5FU, cisplatin, carmustine, methotrexate, etoposide, vincristine, vinblastine	Pressure restriction Site restrictions Positioning considerations

continued

TABLE 10.1 Common medications reference table for manual therapists[1] *continued*

Drug groups	Side effects	Common drug names	Massage indications
Antivirals	GI reactions, fatigue, headache, rash	Acyclovir, zidovudine (Retrovir), AZT, foscarnet, ganciclovir	Pressure restriction
Beta-blockers	Hypotension, bradycardia	Propranolol (Inderal), metoprolol (Lopressor)	Positioning assistance Heat precautions
Cardiac glycosides	Fatigue, weakness, hypotension	Digitalis, digoxin (Lanoxin)	Pressure restriction Positioning assistance
Corticosteroids	Mood changes, euphoria, insomnia, skin problems, bruising, osteoporosis	Prednisone, dexamethasone (Decadron), methylprednisolone (Solu-medrol)	Pressure restrictions Site restrictions
Diuretics	Frequent urination, dehydration, electrolyte imbalance, dizziness, fatigue, hypotension	Furosemide (Lasix), mannitol, chlorothiazide (Diuril)	Pressure restriction Positioning assistance
Fluid replacement	Itching, anaphylactic shock	Saline, Ringer's, blood components	Normally, minimal restrictions
Hematopoietic drugs	Bone pain, fatigue, headache, rash, edema	Epoetin alfa (Procrit, Epogen) filgrastim (Neupogen), sargramostim (Leukine), oprelvekin (Neumega)	Self-limiting Pressure restrictions
Immunosuppressants	Tremor, risk of infection, fever, thrombocytopenia, neutropenia, increase in blood pressure, hirsutism	Tacrolimus (Prograf), azathioprine (Imuran), cyclosporine (Gengraf), mycophenolate mofetil (CellCept), prednisone	Strict Standard Precautions Pressure restrictions Site restrictions Positioning restrictions
Laxatives	GI reactions	Docusate (Colace), Fleet enema, senna (Senokot), psyllium (Metamucil)	Self-limiting
Narcotics	Sedation, hypotension, nausea, constipation	Morphine, codeine, hydromorphone, oxycodone	Pressure restriction Fall precaution
Nonnarcotic analgesics	GI reactions, easy bruising	Aspirin, acetaminophen (Tylenol)	Pressure restriction
NSAIDs	GI reactions	Celecoxib (Celebrex), ibuprofen (Advil), naproxen (Aleve), indomethacin (Indocin)	Pressure restriction
Sedatives and hypnotics	Sedation, weakness, confusion, CNS depression	Lorazepam (Ativan), flurazepam (Dalmane), temazepam (Restoril), zolpidem (Ambien), zaleplon (Sonata), barbiturates	Pressure restriction Positioning assistance
Thrombolytics	Bleeding, urticaria, headache, GI reactions	Streptokinase, urokinase, alteplase, anistreplase	Severe pressure restriction

Abbreviations: CNS, central nervous system; GI, gastrointestinal; NSAIDs, nonsteroidal anti-inflammatory drugs.

Each hospital or health care organization has a formulary from which physicians must prescribe drugs. Differences will exist from institution to institution. Presented in the "Selected drug names" sections are the more frequently used medications.

In the US, brand names are used because they are easier to pronounce and remember than the generic names. In other countries, generic names are more common. For example, docusate is a generic stool softener, but doctors and nurses most often refer to it as Colace, the brand name. Another example is ondansetron, a therapy prescribed for nausea. However, the medication a therapist might hear more often is Zofran. When the name of a drug is capitalized, it reflects a brand-name medication; those beginning with a lowercase letter are generic names. Coumadin, for example, is a brand-name anticoagulant; warfarin, on the other hand, is the generic medication. In this text, the generic drug is listed first with the brand name in parentheses, for example: docusate (Colace) and warfarin (Coumadin).

People are often on medications from more than one category; someone who has cardiac problems may not only be on medications to support the heart but also on medications to control anxiety, blood pressure and cholesterol, and anticoagulants.

The massage precautions presented in this chapter relate only to drugs. The patient's health condition, medical devices, age, and other variables will also impact the touch therapy session. Additionally, the focus is on massage adjustments that may occur with some regularity rather than on an infrequent basis. The study of drug reactions in pharmacological documentation might lead a touch practitioner to believe that the person on medications is so complex and fragile that massage would always be contraindicated. However, the majority of drug side effects listed in reference manuals occur on a limited basis. Dizziness is a good example: it is commonly listed as a drug reaction to scores of medications. In reality, dizziness is not a widespread phenomenon, which is also true of many other symptoms.

Info Box 10.2 The main side effects[3,4]

Common medication side effects to look out for include:

Bruising
Confusion
Decreased pain sensation
Edema
Fall risk
Fatigue
GI problems such as nausea, diarrhea, vomiting or
    constipation
Headache
Orthostatic hypotension
Skin changes

Warning labels on most medications list extreme risks, including death. Rare side effects must be listed and usually are labeled "rare". Common side effects are also listed as such and should be taken into consideration when planning any type of touch session. Use mobile apps for quick reference such as WebMD or RxList.

One additional note: many touch practitioners gravitate toward natural healing concepts, and a few may have a bias against drugs. However, it is imperative to honor a patient's treatment choices. It is the massage therapist's job to provide only massage therapy. Advising the patient to alter the dosage or stop a medication is well outside the bodyworker's scope of practice, as is making suggestions about herbs, vitamins, or other supplements.

How to use this section

The most common medication types are listed below. There will be a brief description of the purpose for the medication and a general explanation of its mechanism of action, which simply means what changes or effects the chemicals have on the structure of cells and tissues. According to Wikipedia, the definition is:

Info Box 10.3 Special interest: Opioid crisis in America

Every day, more than 130 people in the United States die after overdosing on opioids.[5] The misuse of and addiction to opioids, including prescription pain relievers,[6] heroin,[7] and synthetic opioids such as fentanyl,[8] is a serious national crisis that affects public health as well as social and economic welfare.

The Centers for Disease Control and Prevention estimates that the total economic burden of prescription opioid misuse alone in the United States is $78.5 billion a year, including the costs of health care, lost productivity, addiction treatment, and criminal justice involvement.[5]

Info Box 10.4 Joint Commission guidelines and reference material[9]

"The hospital provides nonpharmacologic pain treatment modalities.

While evidence for some nonpharmacologic modalities is mixed and/or limited, they may serve as a complementary approach for pain management and potentially reduce the need for opioid medications in some circumstances. The hospital should promote nonpharmacologic modalities by ensuring that patient preferences are discussed and, at a minimum, providing some nonpharmacologic treatment options relevant to their patient population. When a patient's preference for a safe nonpharmacologic therapy cannot be provided, hospitals should educate the patient on where the treatment may be accessed after they are discharged. Nonpharmacologic strategies include, but are not limited to: physical modalities (for example, acupuncture therapy, chiropractic therapy, osteopathic manipulative treatment, massage therapy, and physical therapy), relaxation therapy, and cognitive behavioral therapy."

"In pharmacology, the term mechanism of action (MOA) refers to the specific biochemical interaction through which a drug substance produces its pharmacological effect. A mechanism of action usually includes mention of the specific molecular targets to which the drug binds, such as an enzyme or receptor."[10] Beyond this brief information, several specific drug names will be listed and their common side effects. A "Clinical considerations" section will offer quick reference for the touch practitioner working with clients and patients reporting use of these medications. Further resources can and should be consulted.

Analgesics

Analgesics are prescribed for pain reduction. The type of pain reliever administered is dependent mostly on the severity of pain. Narcotics, which are derived from opium or opiate-like substances, provide the strongest pain relief, but are also addictive. The other two categories, nonnarcotic analgesics and nonsteroidal anti-inflammatory drugs, control pain by inhibiting prostaglandins or decreasing inflammation.

Narcotics: Opioid analgesics

Purpose: Management of moderate to severe pain and anesthesia.

Uses: Induces sleep and tranquilizes the central nervous system (CNS) before invasive procedures such as surgery, provision of local anesthesia, relief of moderate to severe pain, cough suppression, narcotic withdrawal (methadone), and labor pain.

Basic mechanism: Binds with opiate receptors in the CNS, altering perception and emotional response to pain. Local anesthesia is caused by the inhibition of nerve impulses from sensory nerves. The cough reflex is suppressed by action on the cough center in the brain.

Selected drug names: Morphine, codeine, hydromorphone (Dilaudid), methadone, oxycodone (OxyContin), fentanyl (anesthesia), pethidine (Demerol), buprenorphine (Buprenex), tramadol.

Common side effects: Sedation, dizziness, light-headedness, gastrointestinal (GI) reactions, respiratory depression, constipation, euphoria, hallucinations, anxiety, decreased mental alertness, confusion, weakness, hypotonic muscles, and depressed neural responses. Anesthesia can also cause tremors, restlessness, hypotension, and flatulence.[11–13]

Clinical considerations: Opioid analgesics

Pressure:

- Analgesic effect makes feedback about pressure inaccurate.
- Apply stretching techniques carefully due to hypotonic muscles and decreased neural responses. It is easy to overstretch joints and muscles during this time.

Site:

- GI reactions are common from narcotics and may require avoiding the abdomen. If tolerated, attention to abdominal reflexes may help diminish nausea and constipation.
- Narcotics are sometimes delivered via a transdermal patch so avoid massaging the area containing a patch. Also, heat caused by fever or environmental influences, such as heating pads or hot tubs, can increase the delivery of the analgesic in a transdermal patch and cause toxicity.

Positioning:

- Narcotics cause a number of side effects that make the patient a fall risk. Information concerning fall precautions is presented in Chapter 12.
- Weakness, confusion, or constipation may make repositioning difficult.

Other:

- Unless contraindicated, encourage deep breathing following surgery, which promotes elimination of anesthesia.

- Because many medications can suppress cognition and responsiveness, persistent inquiry may be needed. Be sure to obtain the information and consent that is needed prior to the touch session.

Non-narcotic (non-opioid) analgesics and antipyretics

Purpose: These drugs have mild pain-relieving, anti-inflammatory, and fever-reducing effects. Antipyretic is the medical term for the ability to reduce a fever.

Uses: Mild to moderate pain from arthritis, prevention of thrombosis, reduction of myocardial infarction (MI) risk in patients with previous MI or angina, inflammatory conditions, fever.

Basic mechanism: These drugs are thought to block pain impulses by inhibiting prostaglandin synthesis in the CNS. Prostaglandins contribute to the inflammatory response by causing vasodilation and by intensifying the effect of histamines and kinins, other chemicals that are part of the inflammatory response. By inhibiting prostaglandins, inflammation is decreased. Fevers are believed to be reduced by acting on the heat-regulating center of the hypothalamus to produce vasodilation, which allows heat to dissipate.

Selected drug names: Aspirin, acetaminophen (Tylenol).

Common side effects: Easy bruising, mild GI reactions, rash.[11–13]

Clinical considerations: Non-opioid analgesics

Pressure:

- Patient may not give accurate feedback due to analgesic effect.
- Easy bruising.

Positioning:

- Patient should remain in upright position for 15–30 minutes after administration.

A patient's story 10.1	Acetaminophen and massage

I am a 56-year-old man recovering from radical neck surgery. The 12-hour operation for cancer took place in two spots along the left carotid artery. The doctors replaced about 5 inches of the carotid with a Gortex stent. They took a muscle from my stomach and used it to replace a muscle in my neck. They also grafted some skin from the right thigh to cover the new neck muscle. I have a feeding tube implanted in my stomach. Because of the neck surgeries, I am learning how to swallow again because half of the esophagus is non-responsive. On top of that, my left shoulder, neck and part of the larynx and tongue are numb because the nerves were cut during surgery. I am also experiencing headaches and back pain as a result of the surgery, which I've never had.

Originally, I was on IV morphine for pain, which caused severe nausea. The risk of nausea and potentially vomiting was dangerous for me because it could lead to aspiration. The staff tried hydrocodone, oxycodone, and a fentanyl patch, all of which caused nausea. The only pain medication that I could take that did not cause nausea was acetaminophen and celecoxib (Celebrex). Even with them, I was still experiencing pain between 3–4 on the pain scale. The doctor and nurse providing my home care prescribed a muscle relaxant, which was totally ineffective. With that, they said there was nothing else they could do for the shoulder pain, back spasms, neck pain and headaches.

Life changed when a friend paid for a massage therapist to come give me a massage. I was skeptical about the approach at first. I had had only two massages in my life, but none in the last 15 years. After the first massage I noticed a difference. My pain level was way down; my back started relaxing and the headaches were less severe. The effect lasted about 36 hours. After the second massage, the effect lasted several days. After three weeks, my pain level was at 1 or 2 or none at all. Part of the benefit was that I did not know how tense I was until I learned how it felt to be relaxed during the massages. Now when I feel myself getting pain I know how to relax, allowing the pain to subside.

George Douglas
Portland, Oregon

Nonsteroidal anti-inflammatory drugs (NSAIDs)

Purpose: Reduction of inflammation, pain, and fever.

Uses: Mild to moderate relief from osteoarthritis, rheumatoid arthritis, pain, ankylosing spondylitis, gout, bursitis, tendonitis, dysmenorrhea.

Basic mechanism: NSAIDs inhibit an enzyme that decreases prostaglandin synthesis.

Selected drug names: Celecoxib (Celebrex), ibuprofen (Advil/Motrin), naproxen (Aleve), indomethacin (Indocin).

Common side effects: GI reactions, including bleeding and ulcers. [11–13]

Clinical considerations: NSAIDs

Pressure:

- Patient may not give accurate feedback due to analgesic effect.
- If the patient is under treatment for GI side effects, they will most likely prefer gentler pressure.

Site:

- If the patient is under treatment for GI side effects, refrain from abdominal massage.

Antianxiety medications

Purpose: To control anxiety, including general anxiety disorder (GAD).

Uses: Anxiety, GAD, panic disorders, acute alcohol withdrawal, preoperative apprehension, conscious sedation before short diagnostic or endoscopic procedures, sedation of intubated patients in critical care settings.

Basic mechanism: They are thought to most likely potentiate the effects of gamma-aminobutyric acid (GABA), an inhibitory transmitter that depresses the CNS.

Selected drug names: Long-lasting: diazepam (Valium), lorazepam (Ativan), midazolam (Versed), clonazepam (Klonopin); short-lasting: chlordiazepoxide (Librium), alprazolam (Xanax). Antianxiety medications are also referred to as anxiolytics or benzodiazepines.

Common side effects: Sedation, lethargy, dizziness, GI reactions, ataxia, confusion, slurred speech, memory impairment.[11–13]

Clinical considerations: Antianxiety medications

Pressure:

- Patient may not give accurate feedback if drowsy or lethargic.

Positioning:

- If the patient is dizzy, take care during repositioning or when the patient is rising from the table or bed.

Anti-Alzheimer's drugs

Purpose: Agents may temporarily improve cognitive function and therefore improve quality of life.

Basic mechanisms: All agents act by increasing the amount of acetylcholine in the central nervous system.

Selected drug names: 1) Cholinesterase inhibitors: donepezil (Aricept), galantamine (Razadyne), rivastigmine (Exelon); 2) memantine (Namenda).

Common side effects: Nausea, vomiting, diarrhea, loss of appetite, weight loss, confusion, agitation, headache, dizziness.[11–13]

Clinical considerations: Anti-Alzheimer's drugs

Pressure:

- Confusion, inability to give feedback.

Positioning:

- Nausea, vomiting.

Antibiotics: Anti-infectives

Purpose: To prevent and treat bacterial infections.

Uses: Sinus infections, pneumonia, otitis media, urinary tract infections (UTIs), respiratory infections, acne, cellulitis, bacterial infections such as meningococcus, staphylococcus, *Escherichia coli*, gonorrhea, and syphilis.

Basic mechanisms: Each group of antibiotics acts differently to inhibit the growth of bacteria. They can act to disrupt bacterial cell walls or cell membranes, inhibit bacterial protein synthesis, or block specific steps in bacterial metabolism.

Selected drug names: There are several groups of antibiotics, including:

1. Penicillins: penicillin, amoxicillin, ampicillin, dicloxacillin, nafcillin, oxacillin.
2. Aminoglycosides: streptomycin, gentamicin, neomycin.
3. Cephalosporins (Ceclor): cefotaxime (Claforan), cefotetan (Cefotan), cefoxitin, ceftazidime (Fortaz), ceftriaxone.
4. Sulfonamides: trimethoprim/sulfamethoxazole (Bactrim, Septra).

5. Tetracyclines: doxycycline.

6. Fuoroquinolones: ciprofloxacin (Cipro), levofloxacin (Levaquin).

Other miscellaneous antibiotics are erythromycin, vancomycin, and bacitracin. Most antibiotics are derived from a living organism (e.g., penicillin is derived from mold). Others, such as the sulfonamides, are derived from organic chemicals.

Common side effects: GI reactions.[11–13]

Clinical considerations: Antibiotics

- Standard Precautions are indicated due to infection risk. Check with nurse or signage outside of patient rooms for any further precautions.
- The side effects of antibiotics are seldom severe enough on their own to force any adjustments in a touch therapy session.

Anticoagulants

Purpose: To prevent the formation of blood clots.

Uses: Deep vein thrombosis (DVT), pulmonary embolism, various cardiac conditions such as atrial fibrillation, surgery, dialysis, apheresis, prevention of clot formation related to central IV catheters.

Basic mechanism: Inhibits conversion of prothrombin to thrombin or lowers levels of prothrombin. This ultimately interferes with the production of fibrin, which forms a delicate net that entangles red blood cells, white blood cells, and platelets. These trapped cells can then become a clot. Anticoagulants are often referred to as "blood thinners," which is a misnomer. More accurately, they defend against platelet aggregation or dissolve thrombus. Warfarin reduces clotting in the blood by preventing vitamin K from working properly.

Selected drug names: Heparin, warfarin (Coumadin), aspirin, apixaban (Eliquis), enoxaparin (Lovenox), rivaroxaban (Xarelto), alteplase (Activase).

Common side effects: Bruising, nosebleed, bleeding gums, GI reactions, headache and dizziness (Plavix).[11–13]

Clinical considerations: Anticoagulants

Pressure:

- People on a therapeutic dose of anticoagulants are at increased risk for bruising. Those on a prophylactic dose are at no more risk of bruising than people not on the drugs. The elderly are an exception to this. They are at risk even on a preventive dose.

Anticonvulsants

Purpose: Inhibiting or decreasing the amplitude, frequency, and duration of seizures. Depresses abnormal neuronal discharges in the CNS.

Uses: Epileptic and nonepileptic seizures, Bell's palsy, migraines, diabetic neuropathy, trigeminal neuralgia, ventricular dysrhythmias.

Basic mechanism: Inhibits nerve impulses by limiting the transport of sodium ions across the cell membrane in the motor cortex. Sodium is necessary for the transmission of nerve impulses.

Selected drug names: Phenytoin (Dilantin), valproic acid (Depakene), fosphenytoin (Cerebyx), carbamazepine (Tegretol), gabapentin (Neurontin), divalproex sodium (Depakote). Barbiturates and benzodiazepines are also used as anticonvulsants. Information about barbiturates is given in the "Sedatives and hypnotics" section. Benzodiazepines are listed under the "Antianxiety drugs" heading.

Common side effects: GI symptoms, rashes, CNS effects such as nystagmus, ataxia, slurred speech, mental confusion, and drowsiness.[11–13]

Antidepressants

Purpose: Generally used to treat depression and anxiety, chronic pain syndromes, smoking cessation, bulimia, social anxiety disorder.

Uses: Obsessive-compulsive disorder, panic disorders, posttraumatic stress disorder, migraines, chronic headaches, chronic pain, peripheral neuropathy, attention deficit disorder, bedwetting in children.

Basic mechanism: Affects the level of dopamine, norepinephrine, and serotonin.

Selected drug names: The commonly prescribed antidepressants are divided into:

1. Tricyclics: amitriptyline, imipramine (Tofranil), nortriptyline (Pamelor), doxepin (Silenor).
2. Selective serotonin re-uptake inhibitors (SSRIs): fluoxetine (Prozac), paroxetine (Paxil), sertraline (Zoloft), citalopram (Celexa).
3. Serotonin-norepinephrine reuptake inhibitors (SNRIs): venlafaxine, duloxetine (Cymbalta), fluvoxamine (Luvox).

Two miscellaneous antidepressants are trazodone and bupropion (Wellbutrin).

Common side effects: Tricyclics: sedation, dry mouth, blurred vision, orthostatic hypotension; SSRIs: sexual dysfunction, GI reactions, mild sedation, overstimulation of CNS; SNRIs: dizziness, nausea, dry mouth, insomnia.[11-13]

Tip 10.1 Drug combinations

Almost 55% of adult Americans take an average of 4 medications daily. Not only do the side effects of the medications need to be taken into consideration, but also the complexity of the comorbidities when assessing your patient or client.

Antidiabetics

Purpose: Stabilization of blood glucose level.

Uses: Diabetes.

Basic mechanism: Insulins decrease blood sugar by increasing the transport of glucose into cells. Insulin can be delivered by injection (syringe or insulin pens) or via an insulin pump. Usually, the oral hypoglycemics also contribute to lowering blood sugar levels, but in a variety of ways. Sulfonylureas stimulate the beta-cells in the pancreas to release insulin; biguanides act on the liver to decrease glucose production and improves insulin sensitivity by increasing peripheral glucose intake; TZDs promote the increase of glucose uptake in the muscles and in the liver; and starch blockers inhibit the enzyme alpha-glucosidase, which delays the digestion of ingested carbohydrates, resulting in a smaller rise in blood glucose. DPP-IV inhibitors (such as sitagliptin) and GLP-1 receptor agonists (such as exenatide) decrease blood glucose by stimulating insulin from beta-cells and increasing insulin sensitivity. SGLT-2 inhibitors reduce glucose reabsorption and increase urinary glucose excretion.[11–13]

Selected drug names: There are several classifications of antidiabetic drugs: insulins, oral hypoglycemic drugs and other injectable medications. The medication, excluding insulin, is composed of seven groups of drugs:

1. Sulfonylureas: glipizide (Glucotrol).

2. Biguanides: metformin (Glucophage).

3. Alpha-glucosidase inhibitors: acarbose (Precose) (also known as a starch blocker).

4. Thiazolidinediones (TZDs): rosiglitazone (Avandia), pioglitazone (Actos).

5. DPP-IV inhibitors: sitagliptin (Januvia).

6. GLP-1 receptor agonists: exenatide (Byetta), liraglutide (Victoza).

7. SGLT-2 inhibitors: empagliflozin (Jardiance), dapagliflozin (Farxiga).[11–13]

Common side effects: Hypoglycemia is the most common side effect. Other possible side effects from various drugs are fatigue, edema, headaches, GI symptoms, nausea, vomiting, and yeast infections.[11–13]

Info Box 10.5 Common diabetes drug combinations (for severe cases)

Antianxiety medication or antidepressant
Anticoagulants
Antihypertensive
Digoxin
Diuretic
Insulin or oral lipid-lowering agent

Clinical considerations: Antidiabetics

Pressure:

- Easy bruising.
- Edema.
- General fatigue and weakness.
- Muscle cramps, weakness, numbness, and tingling.

Site:

- Rashes and other skin sensitivities (sulfonylureas).
- Be mindful of injection or testing sites that may be sensitive or painful.
- Exercise caution around insulin pump sites so they are not accidently dislodged from the body.

Other:

- Be aware of the possibility of metabolic instability due to hypoglycemia. Common signs are sweating, shaking, weakness, tingling in the fingers, blurred vision, difficulty concentrating, and increased perspiration. Discuss with the patient ahead of time the action that should be taken if hypoglycemia occurs.

Antiemetics

Purpose: To control nausea and vomiting.

Uses: Nausea and vomiting associated with cancer treatment or surgery, anesthesia, motion sickness, vestibular disorders, GI disorders, Parkinson's symptoms, reduction of secretions before surgery.

Basic mechanisms: Most antiemetics act by blocking neurotransmitter receptors for serotonin or dopamine in regions of the brain or the periphery, such as the small intestine, that are involved in the control of vomiting. For example, serotonin, which is released from certain cells in the GI mucosa, causes afferent transmission to the CNS via the vagal and spinal sympathetic nerves. Blockage of these receptor sites inhibits the stimulation of these peripheral nerves.

Selected drug names: Two main groups: 1) Drugs that block dopamine receptors (dopaminergic antagonists): prochlorperazine (Compazine), chlorpromazine, metoclopramide (Reglan), promethazine (Phenergan); 2) Drugs that block serotonin receptors (5-HT3 antagonists): ondansetron (Zofran), granisetron (Kytril), dolasetron (Anzemet). Drugs from other categories are also used to control nausea or are used in conjunction with other antiemetics: cannabinoids (marijuana, Dronabinol, Marinol); dexamethasone, a glucocorticoid (Decadron); benzodiazepines such as lorazepam (Ativan); antihistamines such as dimenhydrinate (Dramamine); and scopolamine, an anticholinergic.

Anticholinergics reduce the effect of acetylcholine, a neurotransmitter that stimulates skeletal muscle contraction.

Common side effects: Sedation is the most common, followed by restlessness, dizziness, headache, constipation, and dysphoria. Prolonged use of corticosteroids can cause many adverse side effects (see "Corticosteroids"). Cannabinoids can cause distorted perceptions, such as euphoria and dysphoria.[11–13]

Clinical considerations: Antiemetics

Pressure:

- Distorted perceptions (cannabinoids).
- Sedation.

Antifungals (systemic)

Purpose: To destroy fungal infections.

Uses: Histoplasmosis, cryptococcosis, blastomycosis, phycomycosis, aspergillosis, candida, skin infections.

Basic mechanism: Antifungals perform their job by binding to sterol in the fungal cell membrane. This alters cell permeability, which allows potassium, sodium, and cell nutrients to leak out, causing fungal cell death. Sterols, such as cholesterol, are in the lipid family.

Selected drug names: Nystatin, fluconazole (Diflucan), itraconazole (Sporanox), amphotericin, ketoconazole.

Common side effects: Fatigue, GI reactions (can be moderate to severe), itching, rash, headache, dizziness, edema.[11–13]

Clinical considerations: Antifungals

Pressure:

- During fungal cell die-off, clients do not feel well.
- Edema.
- GI reactions.

Site:

- Rashes.

Antispasmodics (skeletal muscle relaxants)

Purpose: Reduction of muscle tone in skeletal muscles.

Uses: Muscle hypertonicity and pain in musculoskeletal conditions (injury, inflammation, fibromyalgia); spasticity in multiple sclerosis, stroke, spinal cord injury, and cerebral palsy; during surgery to prevent muscle spasms; facilitation of endotracheal intubation and orthopedic manipulations.

Basic mechanism: Centrally acting muscle relaxants work on the brain and/or spinal cord to suppress nerve impulses on motor pathways. Peripherally acting muscle relaxants act either on the muscle cell itself by blocking calcium channels or on the neuromuscular junction by blocking the effects of acetylcholine, a neurotransmitter that stimulates skeletal muscle contraction.

Selected drug names: Dantrolene (Dantrium), cycloben, succinylcholine, diazepam (Valium), baclofen, carisoprodol (Soma), methocarbamol (Robaxin).

Common side effects: Sedation, dizziness, weakness, fatigue, hypotonicity of muscles, GI reactions, respiratory depression, hallucinations, and confusion.[11–13]

Clinical considerations: Antispasmodics

Pressure:

- Drowsiness.
- Weakness and fatigue.
- Hypotonic muscles can be easily overstretched. Range-of-motion techniques should be performed with slow tenderness, taking care not to over-stretch joints and muscles.

Positioning:

- Fall precaution if dizzy.

Antitumor (antineoplastic) medications

Purpose: To destroy cancer cells and/or prevent tumor growth.

Uses: Tumors, leukemias, lymphomas.

Basic mechanism: There are several different mechanisms of action: 1) alkylating drugs, antimetabolites, and antitumor antibiotics disrupt the synthesis and function of DNA and RNA; 2) mitotic spindle drugs impair cell division by preventing formation of the mitotic spindle; 3) hormonal agents affect tumor growth in cancers dependent on hormones; 4) interferons help activate the body's immune system against cancer cells.

Selected drug names: Antineoplastics are grouped by:

1. Alkylating agents: busulfan, carmustine, cisplatin.
2. Antimetabolites: doxorubicin, etoposide, fluorouracil (5FU).
3. Antibiotic agents: bleomycin, dactinomycin, methotrexate.
4. Mitotic impairment agents: vinblastine, vincristine.
5. Hormonal agents: breast cancer – tamoxifen, letrozole, anastrazole; prostate cancer – goserelin (Zoladex).
6. Miscellaneous agents: rituximab (Rituxan), arsenic trioxide, gemcitabine.

Common side effects: Most cancer drugs cause thrombocytopenia, leukopenia or neutropenia, anemia, and fatigue. Other common side effects are nausea, vomiting, diarrhea, hair loss, peripheral neuropathy, rashes, skin sensitivity, skin fragility, edema, anorexia, seizures, cardiotoxicity, kidney toxicity, liver toxicity, osteoporosis, fever, and chills.[11–13]

Clinical considerations: Antitumor/ antineoplastic medications

Pressure:

- Edema.
- Fatigue.
- Fever.
- GI symptoms.
- Leukopenia/neutropenia.
- Organ damage and toxicity.
- Osteoporosis.
- Peripheral neuropathy.
- Skin problems (sensitivity and fragility).
- Thrombocytopenia.

Site:

- Areas affected by osteoporosis.
- Peripheral neuropathy.
- Rashes and other skin disorders.
- IV site: catheter, port, or pump.

Positioning:

- Nausea.

continued

Other:

- Be sensitive to the patient's feelings regarding hair loss.
- The antitumor drug, thiotepa, is excreted through the skin. Therapists should glove within 24 hours of treatment.
- Sessions may need to be shortened if fatigue is severe.

Antiviral and antiretroviral medications

Purpose: To prevent replication of viruses.

Uses: HIV/AIDS, herpes, encephalomyelitis, influenza, shingles, cytomegalovirus, chronic hepatitis B.

Basic mechanism: Antivirals disrupt the enzymes that cause the DNA synthesis necessary for viral replication. Antiretrovirals, a specific type of antivirals, are used primarily in the treatment of HIV. Two of the main groups of antiretrovirals interfere with an enzyme known as reverse transcriptase. This enzyme is needed by HIV to infect healthy cells and reproduce itself in a person's body.

Protease inhibitors, another type of antiretroviral medication, block protease, an enzyme that breaks down protein. Protease also is one of the enzymes HIV uses to reproduce itself.

Selected drug names: Antivirals (used for influenza, herpes, shingles, cytomegalovirus retinitis): ganciclovir, foscarnet, famciclovir (Famvir), acyclovir (Zovirax), docosanol, valacyclovir (Valtrex), cidofovir (Vistide), oseltamivir (Tamiflu), zanamivir (Relenza).

Antiretrovirals:

1. Reverse transcriptase inhibitors: zidovudine (Retrovir), nevirapine (Viramune), emtricitabine/tenofovir disoproxil fumarate (Viread), lamivudine (Epivir), efavirenz (Sustiva), ritonavir (Norvir).
2. Protease inhibitors: amprenavir, atazanavir (Reyataz), lopinavir/ritonavir (Kaletra).
3. Multiclass combination drugs: Atripla, Triumeq, and Complera.
4. Integrase inhibitors: raltegravir (Isentress).

Common side effects: GI reactions, fatigue, headache, dizziness, fever, muscle aches.[11–13]

Clinical considerations : Antiviral and antiretroviral medications

Pressure:

- General fatigue and weakness.

Site:

- Rashes.
- If treatment is for herpes, be aware of the possibility of herpes lesions as well as drug reactions.

Tip 10.2 Medications lists

When working with medically complex clients, it is helpful to review their medications lists. On intake forms it is also helpful to ask "reason for taking" as many medications are used "off label."

Cardiovascular medications

Several groups of medications support heart and vascular function. Some, such as the beta-blockers and cardiac glycosides, work directly on the heart. Others cause changes in the blood vessels either by relaxing them or by interrupting substances that contribute to constriction of the vessels. Increasing vessel diameter reduces peripheral resistance, thereby easing the heart's burden. Vasodilators and ACE inhibitors are examples of these. Anticholesterol medications are also prescribed for heart patients to reduce the risk of an MI or stroke. In addition, patients will take drugs from groups mentioned in other sections of the chapter, such as anticoagulants or diuretics.

Antilipemics

Purpose: To lower lipid levels.

Uses: Reduce the risk of coronary artery disease; reduce the risk of MI, cardiovascular accident (CVA), or transient ischemic attack (TIA) following MI or with familial hypercholesterolemia.

Basic mechanism: Inhibition of an enzyme needed for cholesterol synthesis.

Selected drug names: Atorvastatin (Lipitor), lovastatin (Mevacor), simvastatin (Zocor), pravastatin (Pravachol).

Common side effects: Headache, muscle pain, weakness, joint pain, stuffy nose, and sore throat.[11–13]

Clinical considerations : Cardiovascular medications

Pressure:

- Muscle pain may be significant.

Antiplatelet medications

Purpose: Prevention of platelet aggregation.

Uses: Treat and prevent thromboembolic events such as stroke and MI.

Basic mechanism: Platelet inhibition is sometimes described as a mild form of "blood thinning." The mechanism is slightly different for each drug. In general, the chemicals prevent adenosine diphosphate (ADP) from binding to its platelet receptor, inhibit the enzyme phosphodiesterase III, or bind to certain glycoprotein receptors, each of which inhibits platelet aggregation.

Selected drug names: Clopidogrel bisulfate (Plavix), aspirin, ticlopidine (Ticlid), cilostazol (Pletal), eptifibatide (Integrilin), tirofiban (Aggrastat).

Common side effects: GI reactions, headache, dizziness, bleeding, leg pain, itching, and rash.[11–13]

Clinical considerations: Antiplatelet medications

Pressureing:

- Bleeding.

Positioning:

- If the patient is dizzy, be prepared to assist with positioning or rising from the table or bed.

Beta-blockers

Purpose: To relieve cardiac stress by slowing cardiac contractions, improving rhythm, and reducing blood vessel constriction.

Uses: Hypertension, angina pectoris, dysrhythmias, MI, migraines, anxiety and tremors.

Basic mechanism: Prevents sympathetic stimulation by competing with sympathetic neurotransmitters for beta-receptor sites.

Selected drug names: Propranolol (Inderal), metoprolol (Lopressor), atenolol, labetalol.

Common side effects: Orthostatic hypotension, bradycardia, mild GI reactions. Individual drugs may cause cough, insomnia, dizziness, and dry mouth.[11–13]

Clinical considerations: Beta-blockers

Positioning:

- Dizziness and orthostatic hypotension may require the patient to take care when repositioning and/or require the therapist to assist the patient in rising from the table or bed. Encourage the person to move more slowly to allow the blood pressure to reestablish itself. When rising from the bed or table, the patient should stay sitting for a minute or so before standing.

Other:

- Interventions that cause vasodilation, such as hot stones, hydrocollators, or body wraps, should be greatly moderated or avoided with these patients.
- Patients taking beta blockers may be unaware if their blood glucose drops too low.

Cardiac glycosides

Purpose: To reduce the workload of the heart by slowing the heart rate and increasing the efficiency of the cardiac cycle.

Uses: Congestive heart failure (CHF), atrial dysrhythmias.

Basic mechanism: Alters the sodium/potassium pump, resulting in influx of calcium into cardiac muscle cells, which causes more forceful contractions. Also reduces the conduction rate of electrical impulses at the AV node and increases vagus stimulation to slow the heart rate.

Selected drug names: Digitalis, digoxin (Lanoxin).

Common side effects: Fatigue, general muscle weakness, GI reactions, rash, headache, dizziness, confusion.[11–13]

Clinical considerations: Cardiac glycosides

Pressure:

- Fatigue and weakness.

Positioning:

- Be mindful of dizziness.

Vasodilators

Purpose: To decrease blood pressure by increasing vessel diameter of peripheral blood vessels, which decreases peripheral resistance.

Uses: Angina pectoris, hypertension, tachycardia, CHF, dysrhythmia.

Basic mechanism: 1) Nitroglycerin causes smooth muscle relaxation by forming nitrous oxide; 2) calcium channel blockers block the influx of calcium into smooth muscle cells, which then causes the muscle tone in the vessel walls to relax; 3) angiotensin-converting enzyme (ACE) inhibitors prevent the formation of angiotensin II, a substance that causes vasoconstriction; 4) alpha-receptor drugs act on alpha-sympathetic receptors to reduce the vasoconstrictive effects of sympathetic stimulation.

Selected drug names: These drugs can be grouped into four categories:

1. Vasodilators: nitroglycerin.
2. Calcium channel blockers: nifedipine (Procardia), verapamil, diltiazem (Cardizem).

3. ACE inhibitors: captopril (Capoten), enalapril (Vasotec), lisinopril (Zestril).
4. Alpha-receptor drugs: prazosin (Minipress), doxazosin (Cardura), clonidine (Catapres), methyldopa.

Common side effects: Hypotension, dysrhythmia, headache, flushing, edema, mild GI reactions, drowsiness.[11–13]

Clinical considerations: Vasodilators

Pressure:

- Drowsiness.
- Edema.

Site:

- Nitroglycerin is sometimes administered via a transdermal patch. Therapists should avoid getting the ointment on their fingers, as it will cause vasodilation.

Positioning:

- Hypotension (the patient should take care when repositioning or rising from the table or bed.)

Other:

- Interventions that cause vasodilation, such as heated stones, hydrocollators, or body wraps, should be greatly moderated or avoided with these patients.

Info Box 10.6 Common cardiac drug combinations

Analgesic
Antianxiety medication or antidepressant
Anticholesterol
Anticoagulant
Antihypertensives
Cardiac glycosides
Diuretic

> ### Info Box 10.7 Common congestive heart failure drug combinations
>
> Antianxiety medication or antidepressant
> Antihypertensives (sometimes several)
> Digoxin
> Diuretic
> Dobutamine
> Dopamine
> Sedative

Corticosteroids

Purpose: Glucocorticoids reduce inflammation and suppress the immune response; mineralocorticoids affect fluid and electrolyte balance.

Uses: Glucocorticoids: autoimmune disorders (rheumatoid arthritis, lupus), inflammatory disorders (arthritis, tendonitis, bursitis), allergic disorders and hypersensitivity reactions, GI disorders (ulcerative colitis, hepatitis, inflammatory bowel disease,) respiratory disorders (asthma, emphysema, tuberculosis), cancer, and tissue and organ transplant rejection. Mineralocorticoids are given for certain adrenal conditions.

Basic mechanism: Corticosteroids act directly on the nucleus to stimulate the production of specific proteins. These proteins, primarily enzymes and messengers, cause a variety of effects, such as decreased production of prostaglandins, histamine, kinins, and other inflammatory substances. Capillary permeability is decreased, inhibiting the migration of white blood cells into injured areas and reducing the quantities of circulating white blood cells. This group of drugs causes increased breakdown of cell proteins and fat in order to increase blood glucose through gluconeogenesis in the liver. Fibroblast and osteoblast activity also are decreased, as is calcium absorption from the intestines.

Selected drug names: Glucocorticoids: cortisone, dexamethasone (Decadron), hydrocortisone (Solu-Cortef), prednisone, prednisolone, methylprednisolone (Solu-Medrol), fludrocortisone.

Common side effects: GI irritation, changes in mood and behavior, euphoria, insomnia, poor wound healing, edema, flushing, sweating, easy bruising. Long-term use can cause osteoporosis, skin fragility, and weakened connective tissue.[11–13]

> ### Clinical considerations: Corticosteroids
>
> *Pressure:*
>
> - Easy bruising.
> - Edema.
> - Osteoporosis.
> - Skin and connective tissue fragility.
> - Decreased inflammation can make an injury appear less acute. Patients may not give accurate feedback.
>
> *Site:*
>
> - Areas of fragile skin or poor wound healing.
> - Areas that have received cortisone injections over a period of time are susceptible to poor tissue integrity. Also, the area may be tender from receiving injections.

Diuretics

Purpose: To decrease fluid volume in the body by increasing the output of urine.

Uses: Hypertension, edema due to CHF or other causes, ascites, liver disease, pulmonary edema, glaucoma.

Basic mechanism: Diuretics act in different places in the kidneys to increase urine output. Most act by increasing sodium and chloride excretion, which causes water to follow through osmosis.

Selected drug names: Chlorothiazide (Diuril), furosemide (Lasix), spironolactone, mannitol, hydrochlorothiazide.

Common side effects: Urinary frequency, dehydration, electrolyte imbalance (particularly low potassium), dizziness, fatigue, rash, mild GI reactions, orthostatic hypotension.[11–13]

Clinical considerations: Diuretics

Pressure:

- Dehydration.
- Electrolyte imbalance.
- Fatigue.

Tip 10.3 Scheduling around diuretics[14,15]

Patients who have just been given a diuretic, such as Lasix, will typically experience the need to urinate more frequently over several hours. Diuretics are recommended to take during the day so patients can sleep at night. Scheduling sessions around this medication may be difficult; expect interruptions! Normalizing the side effect and appreciating its importance for the patient's health is a great way to build therapeutic relationships and provide support beyond the touch session.

Fluid replacement

Purpose: To balance the fluid levels in the body.

Uses: To maintain or replace stores of water, electrolytes, or blood components, or to restore acid–base balance.

Basic mechanism: These fluids work via osmotic pressure in which fluid or substances move from an area of stronger concentration to weaker concentration.

Types of fluids: Saline, Lactated Ringer's (an electrolyte solution of calcium chloride, potassium chloride, sodium chloride, and sodium lactate in water), D5W, and blood components, most commonly whole blood, red blood cells, platelets, plasma, or plasma expanders (Plasmanate). Individual electrolytes can also be given.

Common side effects: Most often there are no side effects from receiving fluids. Infused blood products

can cause reactions sometimes, often within 5 minutes of infusion. Itching is the most common symptom, but infused blood products can infrequently cause hives, a swollen throat, fever or severe allergic reactions.[11–13]

Clinical considerations: Fluid replacement

Pressure:

- Avoid area of IV site. Do not place patient on the same side as the IV site.
- If a patient were having a severe reaction to blood products, a massage would not be allowed during that time.

Positioning:

- If affected by orthostatic hypotension or dizziness, the patient should take care when repositioning, especially when getting up and down from the table or bed. These side effects put the patient at risk for falling.

Hematopoietic drugs

Purpose: Stimulation of blood cell growth.

Uses: Red blood cell stimulants are prescribed for anemia caused by antitumor, HIV-related, and immunosuppressive drug regimens, as well as end-stage renal disease and bone marrow disorders. Patients undergoing antitumor or other immunosuppressive therapies that decrease white blood cell levels, such as occurs with organ transplantation, may be given drugs to boost the white blood cell count to decrease the risk of infection. These same groups of patients may also need support to induce platelet production.

Basic mechanism: Each of the different types of hematopoietic drugs stimulates tissue in the bone marrow to create the early precursors, or stem cells, of the various blood cells. For example, Neupogen encourages proliferation of a certain type of white blood cell, the neutrophils. The drugs also act as a growth factor that enhances production of red blood cells, white blood cells, or platelets. Leukine, for example, contains granulocyte macrophage colony-stimulating factor, a substance that supports white blood cell production.

Selected drug names: Red blood cell production: epoetin alfa (Procrit, Epogen); white blood cell production: filgrastim (Neupogen), sargramostim (Leukine); platelet production: oprelvekin (Neumega).

Common side effects: The most common among all three types of hematopoietic drugs is bone pain. Others are upper respiratory infections, fatigue, headaches, GI symptoms, chest pain, rash, edema, and hypertension. Within 12 hours of the injection, chills and sweating can occur.[11-13]

Immunosuppressants

Purpose: To suppress the immune system.

Uses: To prevent rejection of organ transplants and bone marrow transplants, rheumatoid arthritis, and psoriasis.

Basic mechanism: These drugs inhibit proliferation and function of T lymphocytes and release of lymphokines.

Selected drug names: Cyclosporine (Gengraf), azathioprine (Imuran), tacrolimus (Prograf), muromonab-CD3, sirolimus, mycophenolate mofetil (CellCept). Prednisone, too, is often part of the immunosuppressive drug regimen.

Common side effects: Common to many of the immunosuppressant drugs are candida infections, tremors, headache, hyperglycemia, hirsutism, risk of infection, leukopenia, thrombocytopenia, fever, GI reactions, increased blood pressure, and decrease in kidney and/or liver function. In addition to some of the above side effects, muromonab-CD3 commonly causes tachycardia and chest pain. Sirolimus can result in back and joint pain, myalgia, breathing and respiratory disorders, rash, and acne.[11-13]

Clinical considerations: Immunosuppressants

Pressure:

- Fever.
- GI reactions.

- Myalgia and joint pain.
- Potential organ toxicity.
- Tachycardia and chest pain.
- Thrombocytopenia.

Positioning:

- Bone pain.
- Chills or sweating.
- Fatigue.
- Breathing difficulties.
- Chest discomfort.

Site:

- Skin disorders.

Other:

- Perhaps most important is the need for strict observation of Standard Precautions due to the patient's immunosuppressed status.
- Patients may feel embarrassed if they have experienced increased hair growth generally throughout the body, known as hirsutism.
- Tremors are a universal byproduct of many immunosuppressants. Massage may slightly reduce them temporarily for an hour or two.

Info Box 10.8 Organ transplantation drug combinations

Before transplantation:
Anticoagulant (heart)
Antihypertensive
Immunosuppressants
Insulin (if diabetic)
Lactulose (liver)
Prednisone

After transplantation:
Analgesics
Antibiotic
Anticholesterol

continued

Chapter TEN

Anticoagulant
Antifungal
Antihypertensive
Antiulcer
Calcium supplements
Diuretic
Hematopoietic drugs
Immunosuppressants (usually several)
Laxative
Magnesium supplements

Laxatives

Purpose: To soften stools or increase peristaltic movement in the bowel.

Uses: Constipation, preparation for childbirth, surgery, colorectal exam, and stool softening.

Basic mechanism: Some laxatives increase water retention in the stool or draw water into the intestine, allowing for easier passage. Others promote peristalsis.

Selected drug names: Castor oil, docusate (Colace), psyllium, methylcellulose, senna (Senokot), glycerin, magnesium salts, lactulose, bisacodyl.

Common side effects: Nausea, abdominal cramping, and diarrhea.[11-13]

Clinical considerations: Laxatives

Pressure:

- Abdominal discomfort makes the entire body uncomfortable. Forceful pressure is not usually welcome.

Site:

- Direct touch on the abdomen often will be refused.
- Attention to the digestive reflex points may be helpful.

Positioning:

- Abdominal discomfort.

Pregnancy-related drugs

Drug reference books do not contain a category known as pregnancy-related drugs. This section presents information on a variety of drugs that are used during high-risk pregnancy or labor and delivery but that come from other drug categories.

Preterm labor: Preterm labor drugs act by interfering with smooth muscle contractions. During acute preterm labor, the patient is usually given terbutaline, a short-term, fast-acting drug. The side effects can be nervousness, restlessness, tremors, headache, insomnia, pulmonary edema, angina, hypertension, MI, nausea, vomiting, hypokalemia, increased heart rate, increased blood sugar, and hypersensitivity to the environment.[11,13] Vistaril, an antianxiety medication, is given to counteract the side effects of terbutaline. Massage would probably not be approved during this acute event, which generally lasts a few hours.

Magnesium sulfate and nifedipine (Procardia), a calcium channel blocker, are used to quell less intense early labor. The side effects of magnesium sulfate can be muscle flaccidity, hypotension, depressed reflexes, difficulty moving, sedation, and GI symptoms. Potential massage adjustments would be a decrease in pressure due to sedation and muscle flaccidity and positioning adjustments due to hypotension and difficulty moving. Procardia has side effects including muscle cramps, headache, GI symptoms, and dizziness. Methergine is administered to stop bleeding; it can trigger GI symptoms, headache, dizziness, and hypotension. These side effects call for the use of noninvasive pressure and care in repositioning.

Labor: Oxytocin (Pitocin) is used to induce labor. Medically, there are no reasons to adjust the variables of a massage session. However, the drug triggers contractions that are harder and faster than normal, lessening the mother's ability to cope with the intensified situation.

Nausea: Nausea is sometimes controlled with promethazine (Phenergan). It commonly has a sedating effect on people, which is an indication for gentle touch and care during repositioning.

Pain management: The narcotic fentanyl is used during labor. Massage cautions for narcotics can be found in the "Analgesics" section earlier in the chapter. Patients with an epidural will have greatly diminished sensation distal to the epidural site, a pressure caution with regard to massage.[11-13]

Sedatives and hypnotics

These two drug categories have been grouped together because they function in a similar manner and are used for common reasons.

Purpose: To sedate, and relieve anxiety or insomnia.

Uses: Insomnia, preoperative sedation, before endoscopic procedures or biopsies to calm the patient, muscle spasms, psychiatric disorders, seizures.

Basic mechanism: These medications work in a variety of ways. Some act on the limbic, thalamic, and hypothalamic regions to depress the CNS. Others, such as barbiturates, also depress brain cell activity in certain parts of the brain stem, thereby decreasing impulse transmission to the cerebral cortex.

Selected drug names: Triazolam (Halcion), lorazepam (Ativan), diazepam (Valium), temazepam (Restoril), zolpidem (Ambien), zaleplon (Sonata); barbiturates: pentobarbital (Nembutal), secobarbital (Seconal), phenobarbital.

Common side effects: Sedation, CNS depression, ataxia, impaired coordination, decreased mental alertness, confusion, muscular weakness.[11–13]

Clinical considerations: Sedatives and hypnotics

Pressure:

- CNS depression.
- Confusion or decreased mental alertness.
- Muscular weakness.
- Sedation.

Positioning:

- Take care when repositioning patients who are sedated, confused, or have an unsteady gait associated with ataxia.

Thrombolytics

Purpose: To break down blood clots.

Uses: DVT, pulmonary embolism, arterial thrombus and embolism, break down coronary artery thrombi after MI, acute ischemic CVA, acute, evolving transmural MI.

Basic mechanism: Thrombolytics convert plasminogen to plasmin, which then breaks down the clot.

Selected drug names: Streptokinase, urokinase, alteplase, reteplase, tenecteplase.

Common side effects: The most common side effects of these drugs are decreased hematocrit, urticaria, headache, and nausea. Therapists also need to be aware of an increased risk of surface bleeding and GI, genitourinary, intracranial, and retroperitoneal bleeding.[11–13]

Clinical considerations: Thrombolytics

Pressure:

- Risk of bleeding.

Other:

- Most often, thrombolytics are administered in the emergency department during a highly acute event. If a massage therapist were to work during such a time, they would most likely hold the patient's hand or stroke their head.

Tip 10.4 A starting place

A place to start studying medications is with the following list of drugs, which are commonly prescribed to a variety of patient populations. Investigate their purpose, side effects, and necessary massage adjustments.

- Acetaminophen
- Ativan
- Benadryl
- Colace
- Coumadin and heparin
- Ibuprofen
- Lasix
- Morphine and its derivatives
- Prednisone
- Valium
- Vicodin

Chapter TEN

A patient's story 10.2 | Benadryl cocktail

My first IV Benadryl cocktail was a hoot to experience. I was trying to use my phone to let my family know where I was in the clinic, but my slurred speech-to-text was incomprehensible and my fingers keyed bizarre words. My nurse, cousin and I were laughing heartily as return text messages were emojis of happy faces, rolled eyes and question marks. I was punch drunk. Medications speak to me and I listen. This informs me of who I am in the moment and informs my care team how best to help me heal.

Meg
Rochester, Minnesota

Case history 10.1 | Exercise

Instructions: On a piece of paper, make three columns: pressure, site, and position. List the conditions that apply to each category.

BF is a 62-year-old man with a very complex medical history which includes 4 major surgeries in the gastrointestinal system. As a young man, BF was misdiagnosed as having psychosomatic stomach pain due to stress and family trauma. After years of medication treatments and exploratory surgeries, he was diagnosed with a congenital blockage in the duodenum. BF is currently admitted for infection with fever and vomiting. BF has an IV for antibiotics and pain management. Because of a long history of opioid use for pain management, there is concern of dependence and potential over-prescription with poor pain control. He has a strict diet to control poor digestion and is advised to avoid solid foods at this time.

Summary

Pharmacology is an enormous field of science and can feel overwhelming to practitioners and patients alike. In addition, the use of medications "off label" make it unlikely for a therapist to master the field. Know your resources! Included at the end of this chapter are online resources that can be consulted whenever questions arise. As always, consulting client's physicians is recommended.

Possession of basic pharmaceutical knowledge deepens the touch practitioner's understanding of a patient's overall health. It especially brings greater awareness of the demands that medications place on the body. Many medications commonly cause GI symptoms such as constipation; skin problems; organ toxicity, in particular the liver and kidneys; sedation; and decreased cognition and alertness. When these new layers of information are factored into the massage treatment plan, it gives an additional reason to take great care when working with people who have compromised health.

Acknowledgment

The authors thank Carol Baillie RN and Hannah Baillie RN for their significant contributions to this chapter.

Test yourself

Multiple choice: Circle the correct answer. There may be more than one.

1. Anticoagulants call for the following touch session adjustments:

   A   No side-lying.
   B   Head above the heart.
   C   Pressure limits.
   D   All of the above.

2. A patient experiencing nausea from other medications or a procedure will likely be given the following drug type:

   A Anticonvulsants.
   B Antiemetics.
   C Antispasmodics.
   D Laxatives.

3. Common medication side effects include all except:

   A Skin changes.
   B Fatigue.
   C Hair growth.
   D Edema.

4. Sedatives and hypnotics are often used for patients with insomnia, muscle spasm, or anxiety. Positioning adjustments would include:

   A Extra care and time.
   B Extra bolstering.
   C Less lotion.
   D Less draping adjustments.

5. Beta-blockers are used for:

   A Low platelets.
   B Hypertension.
   C Nausea and vomiting.
   D Stabilizing blood glucose level.

6. The mechanism of action for nonsteroidal anti-inflammatory drugs (NSAIDs) is:

   A To reduce pain and fever.
   B Provide mild to moderate relief.
   C Inhibit an enzyme that decreases prostaglandin synthesis.
   D To cause gastrointestinal (GI) reaction or ulcers.

7. The purpose of anticonvulsant medications is to:

   A Decrease blood pressure.
   B Block the influx of calcium into smooth muscle tissue.
   C Inhibit seizures.
   D Reduce edema.

8. Clients taking immunosuppressant medications indicate the following massage therapy adjustment:

   A Increased pressure.
   B Strict Standard Precautions.
   C Positioning side-lying only.
   D All of the above.

9. Patients taking diuretics may be best advised to do the following prior to a manual therapy session:

   A Wash their hands.
   B Drink water.
   C Use the restroom.
   D Eat something.

10. Supplements may interact and or interfere with conventional medications.

    A True.
    B False.

References

1. Fuentes AV, Pineda MD, Venkata K. Comprehension of top 200 prescribed drugs in the US as a resource for pharmacy teaching, training and practice. Pharmacy (Basel) 2018; 6(2):pii:E43. doi:10.3390/pharmacy6020043.

2. Epocrates. Medical reference app. 2019. Available from: http://athenahealth.prod.acquia-sites.com/epocrates/products/features

3. MedlinePlus. Drug Reactions. Available from: https://medlineplus.gov/drugreactions.html

4. CDC. Medications linked to falls. 2017. Available from: https://www.cdc.gov/steadi/pdf/STEADI-FactSheet-MedsLinkedto-Falls-508.pdf

5. National Institutes of Health. National Institutes on Drug Abuse. Opioid overdose crisis. Available from: https://www.drugabuse.gov/drugs-abuse/opioids/opioid-overdose-crisis#one

6. National Institutes of Health. National Institutes on Drug Abuse. Misuse of prescription drugs. Available from: https://www.drugabuse.gov/publications/misuse-prescription-drugs/what-classes-prescription-drugs-are-commonly-misused

7. National Institutes of Health. National Institutes on Drug Abuse. Heroin. Available from: https://www.drugabuse.gov/drugs-abuse/heroin

8. National Institutes of Health. National Institutes on Drug Abuse. Fentanyl. Available from: https://www.drugabuse.gov/drugs-abuse/fentanyl

9. The Joint Commission. R3 Report Issue 11: Pain Assessment and Management Standards for Hospitals. Available from: https://www.jointcommission.org/standards/r3-report/r3-report-issue-11-pain-assessment-and-management-standards-for-hospitals/

10. Wikipedia. Mechanism of action. Available from: https://en.wikipedia.org/wiki/Mechanism_of_action

11. Vallerand A, Sanoski C, Deglin JH. Davis's Drug Guide for Nurses (15th edition). Philadelphia: FA Davis; 2017.

12. Chiampas TD. HIV treatments: list of prescription medications. Healthline; 2019. Available from: https://www.healthline.com/health/hiv-aids/medications-list

13. Kizior RJ, Hodgson KJ. Saunders Nursing Drug Handbook. Philadelphia: Elsevier Health Sciences; 2019.

14. Ogbru A. RxList: Diuretics. Available from: https://www.rxlist.com/diuretics/drug-class.htm#What are

15. WebMD. Diuretics (water pills) for high blood pressure. 2017. Available from: https://www.webmd.com/hypertension-high-blood-pressure/guide/diuretic-treatment-high-blood-pressure#1

Additional resources

Australian Medicines Handbook. Available from: https://shop.amh.net.au/support/downloads.

British National Formulary (BNF). Available from: www.bnf.org.

Davis's Drug Guide (mobile app; subscription).

MedScape (mobile app; free).

Mosby's Nursing Drug Reference (mobile app; subscription).

Preidt R. Americans taking more prescription drugs than ever. HealthDay News. 3 August 2017. Available from: https://consumer.healthday.com/general-health-information-16/prescription-drug-news-551/americans-taking-more-prescription-drugs-than-ever-survey-725208.html

11

May you embrace the beauty in what you do and how you stand like a secret angel between the bleak despair of illness and the unquenchable light of spirit that can turn the darkest destiny towards dawn.

"For a Nurse" by John O'Donohue[1]

Every facility needs to have a system for communicating which patients are to be seen for a session, and why. Whether the massage requests are collected by the nurses, or doctors place an order, or there is a sign-up sheet in a designated place, the process should be standardized and easy to follow for everyone. The Referrals and Orders sections below discuss how manual therapists receive requests and the approval to see patients. The Intake section, also known as consultation, will offer ideas and samples of how to obtain the important specific medical information for why each patient is referred, and to compile pertinent information for assessing how best to offer the touch therapy. Patient–practitioner discussions, as well as examples of how to document the most relevant information will be presented.

Moving from understanding the process to efficiently implementing the workflow takes practice, practice and just a little more practice. Therapists working in rehabilitation facilities, assisted living homes, or memory care units will benefit from the information presented here, but will likely find much less formal structure in place for their service. Independent contractors or private outcall therapists have more responsibility for maintaining good records and creating appropriate workflow to balance the confidential information restrictions for the safety of the client. Inpatient settings where manual therapy is a recognized intervention will require practitioners to follow regulations adapted by the institution in order to keep legal compliance. In the US, the Joint Commission is a third-party industry accrediting body that audits member facilities for policy and procedures compliance. Policies will vary from institution to institution and country to country.

Referrals

Depending on the specific medical center's guidelines, a massage therapy session might be requested by doctors, nurse practitioners, staff or by patients themselves, their family, or friends. Regardless of how the referral is made, the therapist must still obtain permission from the patient. Touch therapy should never be forced or undue pressure exerted on anyone to try massage if they are not interested. Many patients feel a lack of control when in the hospital. The opportunity to say "no" to massage therapy may actually be empowering, and practitioners can respectfully honor that choice as part of the service. The only exception may be the patient who is semiconscious or sedated. Consent should then be sought from the patient's legal representative, usually a family member. Interestingly, even people who are unable to communicate consciously will often signal their acceptance or rejection of touch via nonverbal means. They may pull away when

---

Tip 11.1 Gauging the "weather"

When first walking onto a hospital unit or into an acute care facility, I teach my students to take a metaphorical "weather report," to put a finger into the air, so to speak, and gauge how hard the wind is blowing and from which direction. Stated another way, how busy does the floor feel? What is the level of stress? How fast are people walking? Are they smiling or making eye contact?

These factors will influence how the massage therapist trying to collect referrals or patient information relates to the nurses. Manual therapists must adapt to their environment because it will rarely adapt to the therapist. If the "weather" is stormy and fast-moving, bodywork practitioners will need to be more assertive and obtain their information in a succinct, business-like manner. At other times, the atmosphere will be sedate, and therapists can move and speak with the staff in an unhurried manner.

Gayle MacDonald

touched, become agitated, or their rate of breathing may speed up if they do not wish to be massaged.

A variety of referral processes are used in medical care settings. At many institutions, patients self-refer. During the admission process, they may be given informational brochures about the massage therapy service or see flyers posted in common areas. Those patients desiring a session may be instructed to call a designated phone number within the hospital to place their massage request, or they may be directed to ask their nurse to place the request. Many more hospitals now use the electronic health record (EHR) through which authorized staff, such as doctors, nurse practitioners, nurses, rehabilitation therapists, and social workers, can place a referral, usually called an "order." The orders are accessed by

the massage therapist as their referral list for that day's shift. If the massage therapist does not have privileges on the EHR system, the charge nurse or other designated person will print out an orders list. Patient confidentiality regulations will likely prohibit routing information from the EHR via email if the practitioner does not have access to the medical records.

Other alternatives to a computer-generated referral are telephone, pager or voicemail where the therapist would pick up referrals over the phone. Keeping a secure paper log is recommend in these situations so that data is kept safely in one location and can be stored on site or destroyed prior to leaving the hospital campus. When the hospital experience is part of an educational program rather than a professional service, the massage school supervisor will seek the referrals from the nursing staff ideally before the student's arrival. This method of gathering referrals also works well for facilities that have a limited, part-time massage program. In long-term care facilities, massage requests may happen on the spur of the moment as the therapist passes by the nurses' station. "Do you have time for one of my residents?" a nurse will ask.

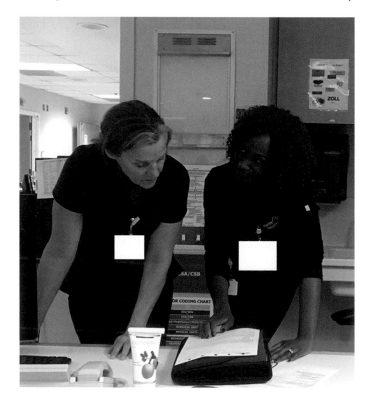

FIGURE 11.1
Hospital-based massage therapist Kate Phelan CMT, obtains intake information from her patient's nurse at Marin Health Medical Center in Marin, California.

Orders

In most medical centers, if a request is made by the patient or family, the affiliated practitioner must obtain permission from a health care team member. These authorizations, as introduced above, are known as "orders." They generally come from a physician, nurse practitioner or nurse. Good coordination of care is critical to the overall safety and wellbeing of each patient. Coordination includes managing medications, including pain meds; procedures; as well as day-to-day needs such as meals and personal hygiene. While orders will come from medical staff, the patient's assigned nurse will always play a key role.

Obtaining orders from within the health care facility

There are a variety of ways for those who are affiliated with the health care institution, such as an employee,

---

Tip 11.2 Offer touch to everyone

Nurses, when asked for massage referrals, often try to second guess which of their patients would want one. Many times, I have been told that a certain patient wouldn't want a massage, only to receive an enthusiastic "Yes!" when asked. In gathering referrals from nurses, I now phrase the question in a few different ways:

- Do you have any patients that could use some extra attention today?
- Are there any patients today for whom pain or anxiety is a particular issue?
- Are any of your patients reporting insomnia?

Asking in this way shifts the nurse's focus to the medical condition and current side effects of the patients rather than perceived subjective considerations, such as the patient's age, gender, weight, or personality characteristics. Therapists, too, must never form a judgment about which people might say "Yes" when offered a massage. Loss of hair, loss of a body part, anxiety level, or prior experience cannot predict who will or won't want a massage. Offer touch to everyone!

Gayle MacDonald

---

independent contractor, or official volunteer, to procure orders for massage therapy service. More important than the method used, is the establishment of a system-wide protocol. Such a protocol will avoid confusion and speed up the process. The first two methods in the list below are generally the fastest and require the least amount of effort from the touch practitioner.

Types of orders

Standing orders

Standing orders give the nurse the discretion to decide who is appropriate to receive massage. Standing or Admitting orders are made when the person is admitted to the facility. With some prompting from the nurse,

orders for massage could be recorded at this time, saving the massage practitioner time and providing the patient fast access to the service.

Signed orders

Signed orders are routed to the hospital massage team at the same time as the referral.

Electronic health record orders

Electronic health record orders are placed by the physician, nurse practitioner, or nurse. There is no need for a paper copy or actual signature as it is included in the online process. Orders are viewable by everyone on the patient's health care team. (*Note*: Information Technology departments will need to give each manual therapist a log-in account with the appropriate authorization levels). The massage therapist will locate their referral list online and may print the list for convenience.

Initiating orders via text

The nurse places the order or makes the request for massage orders by contacting the MD/NP by text, email or pager. This does not always produce quick results. With EHR, however, the medical team can place orders from virtually any location.

Note in the medical chart

For organizations that are not yet converted to an EHR system, the touch therapist can leave a note for the medical provider in the chart requesting orders for massage therapy along with any pertinent instructions. In paper charts, the Physician's Orders section is a common place to attach the request. If possible, it is best to leave the note a day or two before the scheduled session. With an Electronic Health Record software system, a practitioner can use "staff messaging" to request orders be placed.

Combination of methods

At some hospitals, certain doctors allow standing orders while other doctors require their personal approval for each patient. This is a chaotic and frustrating system. Working with nurses familiar with physician protocols is a best practice.

Verbal orders

When orders are needed on the spur of the moment, the nurse can phone the patient's personal physician to obtain verbal orders. However, the return call may not be in time to provide the session during that shift. Another way to obtain orders on the spot is to phone the hospital's attending physician for verbal orders. The nurse or charge nurse would be the most appropriate member of staff to place these kinds of requests.

There are different protocols for recording the order. Some institutions allow the nurse to take verbal orders over the phone and record them in the chart. Other hospitals require the medical practitioner to personally place the order in the record. Important to the touch practitioner is insuring that the orders are in place before setting out to see the patient. This will save valuable time and can be done by checking orders in the EHR, or calling the nurses' station and confirming with the patient's nurse or the charge nurse. Without orders placed first, the session cannot be offered.

Tip 11.3 Getting new referrals

Medical centers can be very formal environments. I find it helpful to bring a sense of calm or even gentle humor to interactions with nurses. Sometimes when seeking additional referrals, I will say with a smile: "Give me your tired, your cranky, your huddled with anxiety..." It seems to lighten the conversation but also suggests additional reasons to refer their patients for massage therapy.

Carolyn Tague

The private practitioner

Patients or their families will sometimes make arrangements with an outside private massage therapist to come into a health care facility. Physician approval is generally appreciated within the facility before a private practitioner provides any integrative health services to patients in their care. However, patients have the right to invite whomever they wish into their room. In these cases, adequate consultation may not be available and may be a compelling reason to decline offering the service. Best practices would indicate requesting the patient to speak directly to their nurse or doctor to give permission for the touch therapist to be informed of all pertinent information regarding the patient's medical condition and specifically any contraindications for gentle massage therapy. This accomplishes three important things: first, the doctor and massage therapist have a chance to educate one another; second, it documents the therapist's attempt to practice safely; and third, it empowers clients to participate in their own healing process. The private practitioner planning to work with a medically complex client who is under direct medical care should seek approval from the client's doctor before initiating bodywork. Because of strict patient confidentiality regulations, they may request that their clients sign a Release of Information form so they can make health status inquiries. However, in reality, most bodyworkers don't carry a Release of Information form in their back pocket. An option here is for the patient to request the nurse accompany the practitioner to the patient's room, where with the patient's verbal consent, the nurse, therapist, and patient can confer about necessary adjustments.

Collecting patient data: The art of the intake

When massaging clients outside health care settings, bodyworkers gather the majority of health information directly from the clients themselves. With medically complex patients, especially those being cared for in medical facilities, this is not always possible or appropriate. Patients may be too sick to respond to intake questions; they may not actually be knowledgeable about all aspects of their condition; and certain questions would be inappropriate to ask a patient. Information, therefore, is usually gleaned from one or more of the following sources: 1) medical health record or chart; 2) nurse (or sometimes the doctor); 3) patient; and rarely 4) family.

It could be argued that the intake process is an important distinguishing factor of hospital-based work. How data is collected and the complexity of the information is unique from non-health care-specific settings. Patient safety requires that the massage therapist is well-informed about specific conditions and reasons for adjustments or contraindications. Treatment planning is dependent on informed assessments. As noted above, private practitioners without hospital affiliation are never permitted to look in the patient chart and must find other means of gathering patient data because of patient confidentiality regulations.

Consulting the medical health record

For those who have access to the medical records, the intake process opens up a vast array of information and history of the patient. A therapist could easily get lost for hours trying to read through and find the relevant information; knowing the organization of the data and what is relevant comes with focus and experience.

Tip 11.4 Important note: need to know

Orientation to hospital work usually includes a discussion of "need to know" principles and guidelines. Confidentiality regulations are also very clear. When accessing a patient's chart, there is no "need to know" anything financial, for example. So, accessing notes or tabs related to billing or insurance information needs to be avoided completely.

When using the medical record to gather information, apply strategies for efficient usage:

- Know what information and data you are looking for; Consultation Forms or templates help you organize.
- Read only the most recent notes.
- Look at latest labs for platelet counts and blood cultures which might indicate zero touch modalities for the day's session. Many hospital protocols will restrict bodywork for patients with platelet counts below 20,000 per microL (commonly referred to as '20') to biofield work only.

- *Clostridioides difficile* (C. diff) infections are also sometimes a contraindication as the therapist will be moving from room to room, putting themselves and compromised patients at risk of infection.
- Spiritual Care or Chaplain notes will often provide insights to how a patient is coping. The need to know here is related to the whole person who is in your hands, literally. This information may be very helpful in assessing the patient. Like any information, what is read in these notes should never be directly discussed with the patient or family. It is like any other data; it is reviewed to better understand the person being treated and help build the therapeutic relationship (see Chapter 4) and the best treatment plan.
- Once you review the medical record, it is imperative that you consult the patient's nurse or the charge nurse prior to seeing the patient. Much of the required information will not be included in the medical record as such. Questions about positioning restrictions, reasons for pressure adjustments or location of devices are best answered by the nurse. Perhaps even more importantly, the nurse is the patient's gate keeper, and will know the best timing for a touch session or if other therapies, tests, procedures, or physician visits are expected. It is important to know that many interventions such as Physical Therapy (PT), Occupational Therapy (OT) and many others are required or mandated by the patient's treatment plan, possibly affecting insurance reimbursements, each day or week of a patient's admission. For example, if the patient does not receive PT because the massage therapist started a session when PT was scheduled, both the patient and the hospital may be disadvantaged. There are very few "required" guidelines in health care-setting massage. Checking with the nurse prior to each session is one of them.

Consulting the medical health record versus the nurse

Some therapists who have chart privileges rely on the chart as the main source for their information about a patient and use the nurse sparingly. The advantages to this method are that the nurse is seemingly inconvenienced to a lesser degree and the therapist has access to a greater amount of information. However, while some patient information, such as age, gender, reason for admission, and vital signs, can easily be found in the chart, reading a medical chart requires specialized training, and the average massage therapist is neither trained nor experienced enough to find everything needed from the medical record. Another reason information may not be available from the chart is that providers sometimes wait until the end of the shift to record their notes. If charting is still done by hand rather than through an electronic health record, poor handwriting often hinders the reader's understanding of the chart notes. Therefore, consulting the chart takes a great deal of time and may not yield a complete picture of the patient's immediate health status.

Collecting intake information from the nurse

In light of the reasons presented above, a strong case can be made for relying on the nurse as the main source of information about a patient. Obtaining relevant patient data from the nurse is generally fast and therefore a better use of the practitioner's time – the therapist can then spend more time giving massage and less trying to navigate the health care record. This will translate into a safer massage session for both the patient and the touch therapist.

Hospital-affiliated therapists can procure information from nurses in one of two common ways: an intake form that the nurse fills out ahead of time, or a verbal interview. (An example of a completed form is shown in Figure 11.4). In Figure 11.2, the pressure/site/position framework forms the core. Whichever system is chosen will depend on staff preference and established policies and procedures. Both ways are useful; however, asking targeted questions will best utilize the consultation time for both the nurse and massage therapist.

For those without prior health care experience, approaching the nursing staff directly can be the most daunting part of hospital-based work. Nurses are almost always busy, and novice practitioners are uncertain when to wait for them to finish a task or when to gently break into their current activity. Only experience will teach the novice when to hold back and when to politely interrupt. Sometimes the intake interview will need to be conducted as the nurse walks to or from a patient's room or in common staff areas with many conversations happening all at once. If practitioners wait until the nurse "has a moment," they may be waiting all day.

Feeling like a burden to the nurses is one of the most common issues for touch therapists learning to work in health care settings. However, for the sake of patients' well-being, the sense of being a bother must not stop a massage therapist from getting all of the information needed to give a safe bodywork session. Eventually, practitioners will come to see the reality, which is that massage helps not only the patient, but nurses as well. By spending half an hour with one of their patients, the therapist frees up the nurse for that particular time and often, because the patient feels more relaxed, for an extended period afterward.

Figure 11.2 shows a sample form for collecting information from the chart, the nurse and the patient (the full form is discussed in Chapter 15).

When to get nurse input

Each time a massage is given to a patient, it is important to obtain an update about the patient's current status, even if the therapist has worked with that patient many times before. This is especially true in the acute care setting. Change occurs from hour to hour, let alone day to day or week to week. Libby, for example, was preparing to have a touch session with a patient she had massaged for a number of weeks in succession. The patient's nurse, however, was hurried and unreceptive toward the therapist. Since she had massaged the woman a number of times over the past month, Libby decided to sidestep the nurse and give the massage without updated information. However, the mental status of the patient had deteriorated since the last massage; the patient was confused, unsteady on her feet, and therefore had been rated as a fall precaution and was not allowed out of bed without staff assistance. To make matters worse, the patient

Massage Therapy Intake Form

Addressograph/medical records label

Massage referral from ☐ MD ☐ RN ☐ Patient ☐ Other

Part 1 – EHR and/or RN

Primary Dx   Secondary Dx

Communication challenges ☐ HOH ☐ Vision ☐ Speech ☐ Language, if not English speaking:

Pressure restrictions		Site restrictions	Position adjustments	Precautions
☐ DVT/PE	☐ Lymphedema	☐ Ostomy	☐ No walking	☐ Contact
☐ Blood thinners	☐ Edema	☐ IV/PICC _____	☐ Do not lie flat/back	☐ Droplet
☐ Low platelets <20	☐ Osteoporosis	☐ Shunt _____	☐ Do not lie flat/abdomen	☐ Airborne
☐ Clotting disorder	☐ Fractures _____	☐ Drain	☐ Sit up/HOB↑	☐ Enteric (C. diff)
☐ Blood transfusion	☐ Bone mets _____	☐ Open wound	☐ Do not lie on R side	
☐ Neutropenia	☐ Neuropathy	☐ Skin infection	☐ Do not lie on L side	Note
☐ Easy bruising	☐ Fragile skin	☐ Lymph node removed	☐ Incisions/wounds _____	
☐ Central line	☐ Fatigue	☐ Chest tube	☐ Log roll required (see RN)	

Gloving required? ☐ Yes ☐ No   NPO? ☐ Yes ☐ No   Allergies (lotion)

Check any that apply

☐ Received chemo in last 72 hours	☐ Hepatitis	☐ Fever
☐ Skin conditions/rash/cuts	☐ Radioactive implants or medications	☐ Paralysis
☐ Herpes	☐ Mentally disoriented or confused	☐ Fall risk
	☐ Other	

Part 2 – For patients with Hx of cancer

Type of cancer and location

Currently in Tx? ☐ Yes ☐ No   Date of last treatment:

Treatments ☐ Chemotherapy   Date of last treatment: ☐ Surgery   Date and location:
☐ Radiotherapy   Date of last treatment: ☐ Lymph nodes Bx/removed:

Part 3 – Goals for massage therapy (Check all that apply)

☐ General relaxation   ☐ Stress management   ☐ Pain management   ☐ Muscular/structural balancing

Pre-session scale   Fatigue   1 2 3 4 5 6 7 8 9 10   Pain location   NOTES
Anxiety   1 2 3 4 5 6 7 8 9 10
Pain   1 2 3 4 5 6 7 8 9 10

Signatures

MT name (print)	MD/RN (if required)	Date	Time
MT signature		Form #	Form date

FIGURE 11.2

Sample massage therapy intake form.

(Form created by Carolyn Tague. Reproduced with permission.)

had just been given furosemide (Lasix), a diuretic, and needed to use the commode 15 minutes into the massage session. Libby had left the room to give the patient privacy during this time. The nurse just happened to enter the room and found the patient naked on the commode with the massage therapist out of the room. To say that the nurse was irate would be an understatement.

Tip 11.5 Giving report

"Giving report" is a critical activity that happens at every shift change. Nurses from one shift will update the status of each of their patients to the oncoming nurse. This takes extra focus with the added pressure of very limited time. Manual therapists are best advised to avoid interrupting this activity.

Tip 11.6 Extra tip

Gather intake information for several patients to avoid down-time during a shift change and request the "okay" to offer the session during shift report times.

Skillful interviewing

The importance of skillful interviewing cannot be overemphasized. Aside from the knowledge of massage precautions and infection control practices, precise questioning of the nurse or doctor is the next most important ability for the massage practitioner who works in health care settings.

In the effort to be expeditious, it is sometimes tempting to ask the nurse open-ended questions such as: "Is there anything I need to know about the patient?", or: "Tell me how the patient is doing." However, these inquiries are too vague and will not elicit the information the touch practitioner needs to plan a safe session. One therapist who used this obscure line of questioning about a bone marrow transplant patient was cautioned only about the person's neutropenic status. However, when the therapist started conversing with the patient, she discovered that

the patient was being treated for a blood clot in the arm, most likely due to a peripherally inserted central catheter (PICC) line. If the bodywork practitioner had been more specific with the nurse, the nurse would likely have remembered to mention the blood clot.

It cannot be said too often or too emphatically that the question: "Is there anything I need to know about the patient?" is grossly insufficient when gathering data from nurses. This is also true when the session is going to be a 5-minute neck and shoulder massage for a patient's family member or one of the hospital staff. An intake always needs to be performed using specific questions. Tip 11.7 lists questions to ask when preparing to give a seated massage to staff or family.

Tip 11.7 General seated massage intake

As is true in any hands-on practice, the therapist needs to know basic health information prior to offering bodywork to anyone. This is certainly true for seated massage for family members or staff within a health care organization. Elderly patients are often accompanied by elderly spouses, and it is common to find the health of family members visiting the patient to be medically complex as well. Just as collecting information about admitted patients, questions should be specific, not vague. Remember it is the therapist's professional responsibility to obtain the information needed to provide a safe and effective touch session; it is not the responsibility of the client to guess what the practitioner needs to know.

Intake questions to include are:
- How are you feeling right now?
- How is your general energy level?
- Do you have any issues with your spine or neck? (or whichever area is to be treated)
- Are you being treated for any medical issues?
- Do you bruise easily?
- Are you pregnant? (when appropriate)
- Do you take any medications for pain or anti-inflammatories?
- Do you have any issues with your skin? (in the areas to be treated)
- Have you ever had any lymph nodes removed or treated?

Inpatient Massage Therapy	Addressograph/medical records label
Practitioner pre and post session intake	

Before session

PT presenting condition(s) *Low back pain; frustration   Primary Dx - renal failure*

☐ HOH   ☐ Vision   ☐ Speech   ☐ Interpreter required. Language _____   ☐ Paralysis

Precautions

☒ Fall precautions   ☐ Droplet   ☐ Airborne   ☐ Contact   ☐ C. diff = contraindications

Position precautions

☐ Head↑   ☐ Flat   ☐ No side-lying L/R   ☐ Other _____

Site precautions

☐ Wound   ☒ IV/PICC site ___ (R)   ☐ Skin *Fragile*
☐ Other _____

Platelet count _____   ☐ Chemo, last _____   ☐ DVT, Loc _____   ☐ Febrile   ☐ ↓WBC

Neuropathy? __X__   Location *Feet*

Lymphedema? _____   Present Hx (NA)   Nodes removed, Tx? Where _____

Current

	0	1	2	3	4	5	6	7	8	9	10
Pain	0	1	2	3	4	5	(6)	7	8	9	10
Fatigue	0	1	(2)	3	4	5	6	7	8	9	10
Nausea	(0)	1	2	3	4	5	6	7	8	9	10
Anxiety	0	(1)	2	3	4	5	6	7	8	9	10

FIGURE 11.3

Pre and post session intake form (partial).

(Courtesy of University of California, San Francisco.)

Nurses don't always know what information is important to a manual therapist, or they may need the practitioner's help in understanding the relevance of certain medications or conditions to the massage process. For example, despite knowing that people on heparin bruise easily, a nurse told a massage therapist that the patient had no pressure restrictions. When the therapist specifically asked if the patient was on heparin, the nurse suddenly realized the significance of the questioning and then agreed that the pressure should be moderated. A handful of very specific questions will speed up the process and ensure that the bodyworker has the necessary information.

Throughout the book, three categories have been the anchor points in working with people who are hospitalized or otherwise medically complex: pressure, site, and positioning adjustments. These classifications are also used in the collection of patient data. Figure 11.2 illustrates a sample consultation form used for patients in which the massage precautions are grouped by the three categories. This framework reminds bodyworkers of the questions they need to ask the nurse.

Either way, the simplicity of the pressure, site, and position framework is particularly useful for those unaccustomed to gathering information from health care staff. Three simple questions can be used as the centerpiece for the interview:

1. Are there any positioning restrictions?
2. Are there any sites to avoid?
3. Are there any conditions that require light pressure, such as risk for bleeding or bruising?

And relative to possible contraindications:

- Does the patient currently have a high fever?
- Are the patient's platelets above 20 (some services will set the limit for touch at 50)
- Has the patient ever had lymph nodes removed or biopsied? (History of cancer is just one potential cause of lymphedema; knowing the level of risk is what is being assessed with this question.)

Examples of skillful intake dialogue with nurses

Collecting patient data is seldom as linear and simplistic as the following two examples, especially once the

therapist is more experienced. However, when first learning to consult with the nurse, conversations may sound formal and rigid. As bodyworkers gain more expertise, they are able to be succinct and fluid.

Be mindful of confidentiality when speaking to the nurse about a patient, and move to a private area whenever possible. If nurses are too busy to step into a private or staff area, just show them the patient's name on the intake or referral form. In this way, if another patient or family overhears the nurse giving information to the touch practitioner, confidentiality about the patient's identity is not breached. If obtaining information over the phone, make the call from the nurses' station or other staff area, such as a charting room.

Example 1: Imagine that before contacting the nurse, the touch therapist was only able to discover some of the patient's basic information from the bedside chart: room number (355), gender (M), age (67), diagnosis (NHL), and most recent vital signs. The practitioner will then need to begin the conversation by asking about the reason for admission. The dialogue might sound something like this:

MT: I have a referral for your patient Mr James in room 355 for massage therapy. Is this a good time to get some information about him?

RN: Sure. What do you need to know?

MT: I saw that he has non-Hodgkin's lymphoma; what is he admitted for?

RN: He had his first cycle of allo-SCT and was discharged, but he was brought back because of a neutropenic fever.

MT: Does he still have fever? Would he be OK to receive some very gentle touch?

RN: Yes, no more fever. I'm sure he'd love a massage.

MT: Just a couple more questions. Are there any other issues, such as low platelets?

RN: His platelet count is a little low. I think it was 78 this morning. Light stroking is fine.

MT: Are there any sites you want me to avoid, such as a central line or skin problems?

RN: He has a Groshong on the right side of his chest. Check with him about the skin on his hands and feet. It was peeling after chemo and may still be sensitive. He also has sores in his mouth that are a bit uncomfortable.

MT: Does he have any positioning restrictions?

RN: Whatever is comfortable for him is fine. The mouth sores might make it difficult to lie on his face, but it's up to him.

MT: Few last questions: does Mr James have any sensory impairments? Translation needs? Extra precautions?

RN: Nope.

MT: Perfect, thanks for your time.

When seen in written form, the above conversation may appear to be lengthy and time consuming. However, it can be completed in just over a minute.

Example 2: Many institutions will provide cell phones to nurses. RNs will answer calls when possible even when away from the nurses' station. Having a prepared introduction and specific questions is essential for effective intake and keeping support for the service. Developing these skills takes practice but is well worth the effort. (See Figure 11.4)

MT: Hi Mark, this is Kumi, massage therapy. I have your patient Kozul in 55. Can I check in with you about her?

RN: Sure, she's really looking forward to seeing you. What do you need?

MT: I see she is admitted for a recent MI and had surgery. Can she lie flat yet?

RN: She has been advised to keep the head up, above heart, but she'll let you know what's comfortable.

MT: Great. Is she on any blood thinners or pain meds?

RN: Yep, heparin, and she is now just on Tylenol for pain. She says she doesn't like the morphine because of constipation.

MT: Ok, got it. I know she has a PICC line. Any other devices I should know about?

RN: No, I think that's it. She's going to be very happy to see you. Her spouse can't be here because of work, so she's been alone a lot.

MT: Good to know. Thanks so much. I'll let you know how it goes.

> ## Therapist's journal 11.1
> ### Touch for the family
>
> There are countless times when a family member has teased with something like, "Can I sneak my feet in there too?" I generally look to the patient for their reaction. This helps me assess how they are doing emotionally. Sometimes the patient responds with a laugh, sometimes it's a shake of the head and roll of the eye, or a response like, "No, you really don't want to be in my place." Sometimes it is, "Yes, can you please work on her, she needs it more than me!" I find it best to acknowledge the patient first then the companion. I generally offer positive encouragement for the guest to follow up with getting a massage session of their own. Knowing local sources for quality bodywork is also helpful.
>
> Carolyn Tague

Nurses will not be aware of all past health history, especially if the condition is unrelated to the patient's presenting symptoms and treatment. If the patient is coherent enough, the touch therapist should also ask him or her about previous health history. For example, prior musculoskeletal ailments, such as back surgery or a serious injury, or previous cancer treatment, will be relevant to the massage plan. History of lymphedema or risk of lymphedema should also be obtained. For example, if a patient is currently being treated for a hip replacement with instructions not to reposition, a practitioner may determine upper body work is indicated as it would not require moving. If not directly asked, this patient with lymphedema from injury to axillary lymph nodes during surgery may be treated with inappropriate massage strokes.

Medical and nursing staff don't always have a grasp of how potent bodywork can be. They frequently tell bodyworkers during data collection that the patient can have whatever he or she wants. If this occurs, the therapist needs to clarify exactly what that means. For nurses unfamiliar with the modality, ask to demonstrate on the nurse the amount of pressure that you expect to use. Manual therapists need to blend their own knowledge and experience with the nurse's instructions when planning the massage session.

Massage Therapy Intake Form

Kozel 67 yo F   Addressograph/medical records label

Massage referral from ☒ MD   ☐ RN   ☐ Patient   ☐ Other

Part 1 – EHR and/or RN

Primary Dx   MI surgery PO x 3 Stent placed   Secondary Dx

Communication challenges   ☐ HOH   ☐ Vision   ☐ Speech   ☐ Language, if not English speaking:

Pressure restrictions		Site restrictions	Position adjustments	Precautions
☐ DVT/PE	☐ Lymphedema	☐ Ostomy	☐ No walking	☐ Contact
☒ Blood thinners	☐ Edema	☒ IV/PICC _____	☐ Do not lie flat/back	☐ Droplet
☐ Low platelets <20	☐ Osteoporosis	☐ Shunt _____	☐ Do not lie flat/abdomen	☐ Airborne
☐ Clotting disorder	☐ Fractures _____	☐ Drain	☒ Sit up/HOB↑	☐ Enteric (C. diff)
☐ Blood transfusion	☐ Bone mets _____	☐ Open wound	☐ Do not lie on R side	
☐ Neutropenia	☐ Neuropathy	☐ Skin infection	☒ Do not lie on L side	Note
☐ Easy bruising	☐ Fragile skin	☐ Lymph node removed	☐ Incisions/wounds _____	
☐ Central line	☐ Fatigue	☐ Chest tube	☐ Log roll required (see RN)	

Gloving required? ☐ Yes ☒ No   NPO? ☐ Yes ☒ No   Allergies (lotion)   N/A

Check any that apply

☐ Received chemo in last 72 hours	☐ Hepatitis	☐ Fever
☐ Skin conditions/rash/cuts	☐ Radioactive implants or medications	☐ Paralysis
☐ Herpes	☐ Mentally disoriented or confused	☐ Fall risk
	☐ Other	

Part 2 – For patients with Hx of cancer

Type of cancer and location   N/A

Currently in Tx? ☐ Yes ☐ No   Date of last treatment:

Treatments ☐ Chemotherapy Date of last treatment: ☐ Surgery Date and location:

☐ Radiotherapy Date of last treatment: ☐ Lymph nodes Bx/removed:

Part 3 – Goals for massage therapy (Check all that apply)

☐ General relaxation   ☐ Stress management   ☒ Pain management   ☐ Muscular/structural balancing

Pre-session scale	Fatigue	1 2 3 4 ⑤ 6 7 8 9 10	Pain location Chest, shoulder	NOTES	PT notes her L arm and shoulder are sore post surgery
	Anxiety	1 2 3 ④ 5 6 7 8 9 10			
	Pain	1 2 3 4 ⑤ 6 7 8 9 10			

Signatures

MT name (print) KUMI YUMOTO	MD/RN (if required)	Date 5/16/20 Time 14:30
MT signature Kumi Yumoto		Form # Form date

FIGURE 11.4
Completed sample intake form for Patient Kozul.

To be sure, therapists should NEVER exceed the nurse's directions. They may, however, do far less if they feel, based on their education and experience, that the situation warrants it. For example, a nurse once told a therapist that she could give Swedish massage to the leg of a patient that contained a serious abscess. Based on her training, the therapist explained to the nurse she wasn't sure if that was a wise plan until the leg healed. Rather than performing Swedish massage, the practitioner chose to use static holds on the leg.

Intake taken directly with the patient

In many health center situations, the intake process happens directly with the patient. This is generally true in infusion centers or rehabilitation facilities. Here, the questioning requires additional effort. As in private practice, some clients are very private and may not understand the reasons for the direct medical questions. After introducing oneself and confirming consent for a touch therapy session, a few words of explanation go a long way in setting up a verbal intake. Remember, when working within a health care organization, the responsibility to the organization is also an important reason to be thorough with intake protocols. As Karen Armstrong, who teaches hospital-based massage therapy advises, when patients are hesitant to answer questions, explain to the patient: "I must know your health history to ensure safe treatment."

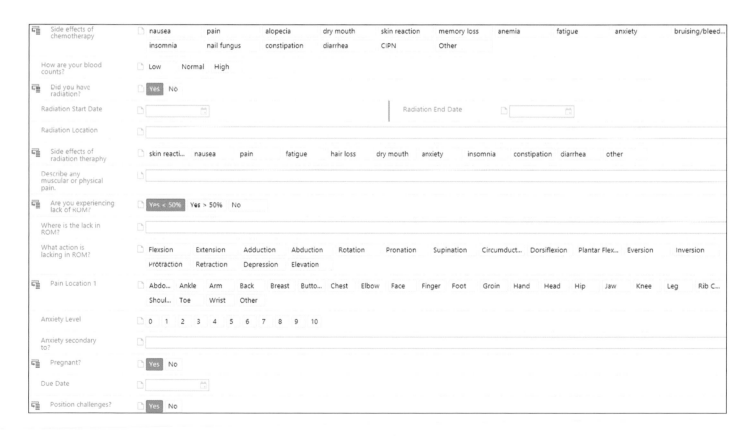

FIGURE 11.5

This is one screen of the intake EMR template used by massage therapists at Beaumont Hospital in Michigan, USA.

(Courtesy of Karen Armstrong, Beaumont Hospital, Michigan.)

Skillful questions for the patient

- I have just a few questions before we get started. Can you tell me if you currently have pain?
  - Many medical centers track "pain scale" before and after interventions, so you may want to collect a description or rate, such as "4 out of 10."
- How is your fatigue level?
- Do you have any swelling? Neuropathy? Nausea?
  - Many practitioners will use an intake form to collect data and to help remember what questions to ask.
- Have you had massage in the past?

The core principle here is to gather the important information needed to ensure a safe and appropriate massage for each and every patient, regardless of the setting.

In best practice, the intake is a three-stage process. First, consult the medical record if this is permitted. Second, have a conversation with the patient's nurse, however brief it might be. And lastly, always check in with the patient directly. Their direct, in-the-moment sharing of how they are feeling physically, mentally, and emotionally is obviously critical to the provider's assessment and treatment plan. New and experienced therapists alike are often amazed at how different a patient will present on paper as compared to who is before them in the room. Although the patient may appear physically strong and emotionally light hearted, if the medical record shows advanced disease or failing organs, be sure to adjust for the most compromised presenting conditions, whether on the note or in the room. Therapists will also experience patients that appear anxious and nervous, even when the chart suggests "improvement" and "discharge

plan". In these cases, too, touch practitioners adjust for the most challenging condition. Anxiety and stress are best acknowledged and addressed with gentle care.

Continuing the conversation with patients will be discussed in Chapter 12.

Contractors and third-party providers

For contractors or third-party massage therapy providers who do not have access to the medical records, creating a system of intake and notation is still highly recommended, and in some jurisdictions may be required. The Heart Touch Project team in Southern California, for example, developed a 13-page intake form with a patient waiver (see partial form in Figure 11.6). The form is quite detailed and will provide extensive information that would otherwise not be available. It is also bilingual which contributes to the length. In these situations, patients and their families would be responsible for providing the information.

Please see the Appendix for more sample intake forms.

Summary

Clear institutional protocols for referrals, orders, and intake tasks are best able to serve patients in a timely and safe manner. Touch therapists who have a system in place to utilize their time wisely, integrate into the health care team, and guarantee that legal protocols are observed, will find confidence and fulfillment in their work. Each session is a unique experience in which the therapist takes the information from the medical perspectives as well as the patient's story, and weaves them together.

Node irradiation involved? **YES / NO**   Location: neck   armpit   groin   other   don't know

¿Algún ganglio fue afectado? **SÍ / NO**   Dónde: cuello   axila   ingle   otro   No se

ADDITIONAL NON-ONCOLOGICAL SURGERY: (please list and explain)
CIRUGÍA ADICIONALES NO-ONCOLÓGICAS : (Por favor mencione y explique)

Procedure _____   Date _____

Procedimiento Fecha

Explain _____

Explique

Procedure _____   Date _____

Procedimiento Fecha

Explain _____

Explique

Procedure _____   Date _____

Procedimiento Fecha

Explain _____

Explique

MEDICAL DEVICES (check and explain all that apply)

Dispositivo médico: (marque y explique todos los que son aplicable)

Do you currently have any of the following? If yes, please notate **RIGHT** side / **LEFT** side / **BILATERAL**

¿Tiene usted actualmente algunos de los siguientes? Si es sí , por favor marque lado **DERECHO** / lado **IZQUIERDO** / **BILATERAL**

Mediport (reservorio venoso subcutáneo, RVS) :

Location (Ubicación) _____

FIGURE 11.6

Sample of one section of an extensive (bilingual) intake form.

(Courtesy of Shawnee Isaac Smith, Founder, Heart Touch Project, Santa Monica, California.)

Chapter ELEVEN

Test yourself

1. **Practicing with the massage therapy intake form**

   Instructions: Read the following case history. On a photocopy of the Massage Therapy Intake Form (Figure 11.2) or any of the sample forms in the Appendix, place the information from this patient's medical history. (See Figure 11.4 and the Appendix to review completed samples.)

   Your patient AB is a 53 yo F with multiple myeloma and is admitted for an autologous stem cell transplant. She has fatigue and hand/foot syndrome. Nausea is well controlled by Zofran. Her platelets are 38 today. She loves massage and requests shoulders and neck work because of soreness. Pain is 3/10. She has neuropathy in both feet since her previous cancer treatment 3 years ago. 15 nodes were removed from her neck, (R) side, during early adulthood due to severe infection unrelated to cancer.

2. **Intake practice**

   Instructions: Practice doing intake with a partner. One person plays the role of the massage therapist, the other plays the nurse. The nurse will use the following patient profile to answer the massage therapist's intake questions. Touch practitioners should make a copy of Figure 11.2, or use an intake form created by their instructor or the hospital, and practice recording the information given by the nurse.

   Patient profile (to be used by the person playing the nurse's role):

   GC is a 28 yo M with multiple fractures and internal injuries after an MVA, 10 days ago. He has an auto accident related TBI but is not showing any signs of cognitive impairment. GC's pain is rated as 7/10. The pain medication (Oxycodone) is causing constipation; he is given laxatives. He has a PICC line in his R forearm. He has a brace on his L leg and a cast on his L arm. His nurse reports he has been anxious and worried about missing work. His girlfriend is present. He has never had a massage before.

Reference

1. O'Donohue J. To Bless the Space Between Us. New York: Doubleday; 2008.

Additional resources

Adams CH, Jones P. Therapeutic Communication for Health Professionals (3rd edition). New York: McGraw Hill; 2011.

Thompson D. Hands Heal: Communication, Documentation, and Insurance Billing for Manual Therapists (5th edition). Baltimore: Wolters Kluwer; 2019.

One on one: The massage therapy session

Every cell in the human body has consciousness, and therefore needs to be treated with the utmost respect and dignity. Everything about you is touching the person: your eyes, voice, thought, feelings, breath, and hands.

Irene Smith, Everflowing[1]

Here it is: finally approaching the patient for the face to face work of the touch session. Like any quality massage session, the time together is personal, unique and often sacred. However, unlike those given in wellness centers or private practice, the potential vulnerability, anxiety, pain and physiological complexity of the patient makes the health care-based session a more intricate dance. Once at this point, however, the session should be easeful, and the comfort and care nature of the work is the core gift to both the patient and the practitioner.

The components of the bodywork session and the steps leading up to and following it will implement the adjustments discussed in earlier chapters.

Before the session

The following tasks are usually performed in more or less the sequence listed:

1. On the way into the room, hang the "Massage in Session" sign on the door. This doesn't guarantee that there will be no interruptions, only that they might be made more gently.

2. The massage begins the moment the therapist enters the room. Movements should be calm, slow, and gentle as the practitioner steps through the door, moves hospital furniture, or adjusts the bedding. Tedi Dunn advises that therapists should: "Match your movements to the patient's energy level, which is generally slower than the world outside the room."[2]

3. Discuss with patients what massage options you are able to offer given the patient's specific circumstances, taking into account any instructions given by the nurse. Also inquire about health conditions unrelated to their present treatment. (See Figure 11.2 for review of intake practices and sample form used to discover risk factors for lymphedema, DVT or other complications.)

4. Identify all intravenous (IV) sites, dressings, open wounds, lesions, and sore and painful areas.

5. Arrange the room so there is a path around the bed. The session will flow better if the therapist doesn't have to stop in midstream to move furniture, IV poles, or cell phones on chargers. Gently move the bedside table or chairs away from the bed, and push the IV stand slightly up toward the head of the bed and away from the side rails.

Before	Patient assessment and treatment plan Check in with RN Universal precautions: Contact, Droplet, Airborne as indicated Gather materials such as towels, gloves, lotion Sign on the door; dialogue with patient; prepare room
During	Positioning patient for support, comfort and practitioner ergonomics Site adjustments and session modifications communicated Hands-on touch with modified pressure, pacing, and direction of stroke as indicated
After	Closure: assessment dialogue Reposition bed and/or patient; returning room to original organization Chart note and/or data reporting

FIGURE 12.1
Touch therapy session workflow at a glance.

6. Generally there will be sufficient pillows, linen, and bedding in the patient's room. If this is not the case, custodial staff or nursing assistants are helpful in finding additional items. One towel is also recommended to provide a defined work space between the practitioner and the patient or client.

7. Practitioners new to hospital work must release their expectations of establishing the perfect environment. As Tedi Dunn points out in *Massage Therapy Guidelines for Hospital and Home Care:* "The physical and emotional environments in which hospital-based massage is practiced are often antithetical to the quiet sanctuary. . .usually associate[d] with massage."[2] Controlling all of the noise and chaos is impossible. However, it is possible to help the patient create an atmosphere more conducive to relaxation. Suggest that the television be turned down or off and the phone be turned to vibrate or silent if no calls are expected. Dim the lights, but not so much that the person's condition cannot be easily assessed. If the light is too low, the therapist may miss areas of skin that are problematic, swollen or inflamed, or sites containing body fluids. Lower the shades or draw curtains as needed.

8. Close the privacy curtain if the patient is in a shared room. Before closing the curtain, acknowledge the roommates. Dunn points out that: "This supports privacy because when the roommates are acknowledged, included, and not ignored, they can more comfortably allow the patient and the massage therapist to be alone."[2]

9. Take time to help the patient position comfortably (refer to Chapter 6 for information on positioning). If patients need significant help with positioning, the therapist must ask the nursing staff for assistance. Moving patients is outside the massage therapist's scope of practice because it requires special training.

10. Lower the bedrails on the side where the practitioner will be working. IV tubing, surgical drains, or catheters are often in the vicinity of the bedrails. Be mindful when lowering or raising them so as not to catch the tubing, thereby occluding it or causing it to pull at the insertion site.

11. Raise the bed to a height that's comfortable for the therapist's back. Figures 5.2, 6.2, 12.7 and 12.11 give excellent examples of this.

Components of the massage session

Providing comfort is the primary goal of most hospital massage services, and there is more than one way to accomplish this. Comfort might come in the form of myofascial release to ease stiffness after surgery, stimulating acupressure points to relieve nausea, using shiatsu to increase energy, or employing the repetitious rhythm of lomi lomi massage to induce relaxation. *The important*

A patient's story 12.1 | The doctor becomes the patient

In the documentary "States of Grace", doctor Grace Dammann shares her unique experience and insights as a long-term critical care patient. After a head-on collision on the Golden Gate Bridge in San Francisco, California, Dr. Dammann began a year-long process of surgeries, rehabilitation and coming to terms with her new physical self. "Because I was so sensitized, I could feel the energy, mood, and state of being of those who came in to care for me. I "knew" if a nurse, CNA, housekeeper or anyone, was "off." Sometimes I would pretend to be asleep, pulling the sheet over my head to avoid them. What I learned as a patient and say to every health care worker interacting with the seriously ill is: don't come to work if you are unhappy. You've got to love what you do, and the clients and team you do it with. Change careers, if need be. What heals are love, optimism, and happiness. And, it is your real job to work on yourselves and help teammates to bring these qualities to those who have been entrusted to our care."[3]

Grace Dammann MD

point is not the bodywork technique, but the way in which the practitioner modifies it. The focus is on being restful, simple, and nurturing rather than forceful, heroic, and ambitious. In more scientific terms, the modified techniques are intended to induce the parasympathetic nervous system's response to restore and repair, thus avoiding any stressing techniques that would stimulate or aggravate sympathetic nervous system responses (often referred to as "fight, flight or freeze.")

The hallmark of a bedside massage therapy session with a person who is ill, frail, or experiencing significant stress, is: "less is better." The effort level is less, the length of the session is shorter, draping is simpler, and body mechanics are based on ease. The hands and very being of the hospital massage therapist are:

- Gentle
- Soothing
- Nurturing
- Comforting
- Undemanding
- Restful
- Calming
- Effortless
- Unambitious
- Simple
- Slow
- Nonjudgmental
- Spacious

The rhythm of the massage strokes is slower, more repetitious, and predictable. Generally, when using a stroking motion, direct the focus of the movement toward the center of the body. Being ill is a fragmenting experience; moving toward the torso of the body gives people a sense of being pieced back together. One exception to this is for cardiac conditions. Gentle holds without circulatory intent are indicated.

The hands make full, broad contact rather than pointed, digging contact or light, feathery touch with just the fingers. Many patients find light and feathery

pressure to be ticklish and annoying. Often, when therapists first encounter ill people, they become fearful and pull away causing part of the hand to rise off the body. Instead, allow the entire hand – fingers, thumb, and palm – to settle onto the patient's body. People report that this type of touch feels the most nurturing and secure and gives a sense of more pressure than is actually being provided. Try the touch exercise (Journaling exercise 12.1) to test the effect of various types of touch.

Tip 12.1 A taste of your own medicine

If you are new to the field or have not recently experienced a modified session, be sure to receive adjusted touch sessions for yourself. Quality medical centered education programs will offer opportunities to experience the work through trades and practice sessions. But, if you have not had that opportunity yet, make an appointment with a practitioner who performs this type of bodywork. Experience what it is you want to be offering, or have already been giving to patients and clients. It will reinforce and reaffirm the tremendous gift you are to others. Massage therapists who have never had a taste of their own medicine are stunned at how supportive and powerful gentle bodywork is.

Journaling exercise 12.1
Experimenting with levels of contact

With a partner, perform effleurage strokes, experimenting with the following three ways of making contact:
1) Full-finger contact with the palm slightly raised off the body.
2) Full-finger and palm contact with the thumb and fingertips slightly raised (something that therapists often do unconsciously).
3) Full-hand contact, with fingers, palms, and thumbs completely relaxed onto the partner's body.

Chapter TWELVE

Starting the session

Therapists commonly ask: "Which part of the body do I start with?" There is no one right answer or exact formula. One good place to start is with the shoulder. The idea behind this is that in most cultures, the shoulders are a commonly touched place in daily contact, so would be a generally familiar experience for the body. For example, the session could start with the therapist resting her hands on the patient's shoulder and the two of them becoming aware of their next three breaths together. Be mindful that not all patients should be directed to take deep breaths if presenting with acute lung or heart conditions, but becoming aware and attentive to whatever breath is happening is generally calming.

It is also an appropriate option to start with the back because it is a place that commonly becomes painful when in bed for extended periods. Another wonderful place to start and may be the focus for the entire session, is the feet. Drawing on theories of reflexology, the practitioner may address the entire body through the feet. This is especially appropriate for patients who have very low platelet counts and are at risk for bruising and internal bleeding. Just as with healthy clients, there are several good ways to start.

Perhaps more important than asking, "Where do I start?", the therapist could ask, "How does the patient

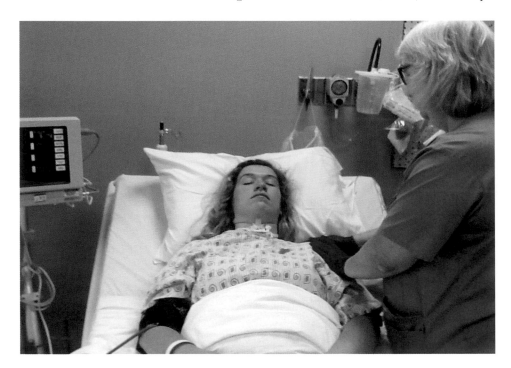

FIGURE 12.2
Starting bodywork at the shoulder is a common practice. Extra care is taken with central lines in the neck or chest ports.

(Photo by Cathrine Weaver, Baptist Health, Lexington, Kentucky.)

want to end?" Touch therapy often puts people to sleep or prepares them for a nap. If they want to continue to sleep, it makes sense to end in the position people prefer for sleeping. If they want to end on their side, then the session could start in supine position and end by massaging the back from the side-lying position. Patients who prefer to sleep on their back could be started side-lying or sometimes prone.

Skillful communications when starting the session

While it is tempting to ask very open questions such as "Where would you like me to massage?", it is more often the case that only a few options are available. It is most skillful to describe the choices and then ask which would be best for the patient. Here are two examples:

1. "So, in order to get to your back, we have a couple of options. Because we want to be careful with your PICC line, I could have you side-lying on the opposite side and I can massage your back and neck; or, you can stay on your back and I can offer you gentle touch by going under the sheet to get to your back."

If not able to visually check the client's back, it is important to confirm there is no damage to the skin and no medical devices implanted or medicine patches in the area before offering massage. It is crucial to stay gentle. By pressing wrists and arms into the bedding the therapist can reposition the hands and not move the client's tissue except for the gentle pumping or slight circles of the massage. Being under the sheet also helps keep the drag on gowns or soft tissue at a minimum.

2. "I understand you are pretty tired right now, so how about we keep you comfortable in bed as you are. I can offer you a really nice foot massage with some gentle reflexology or I can work your shoulders, neck and scalp, or both. What sounds best for you?"

Of course, these are dialogue examples that may work for some, but each therapist will find their own voice in asking questions and communicating with patients. The core principle here is to set appropriate expectations and still offer choice.

Closing a session

Ending in a similar way to how the session began brings closure and completeness to the session and indicates to the patient that the massage is over. The therapist may end by repeating the initial hold to the shoulder, or if a gentle breath was invited to begin, it could be repeated

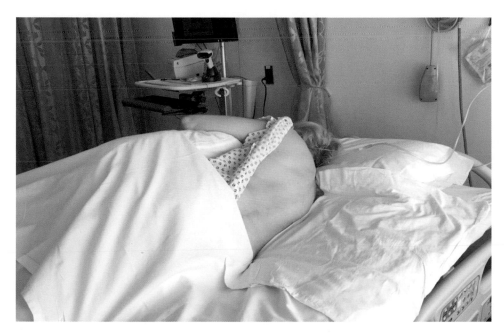

FIGURE 12.3
Side-lying patient. Notice pillow at chest for support and extra pillow case over the sheet to both protect the sheet from lotion and to be lifted on to the patient's back to remove excess lotion, and pat dry.

(Photo by Carolyn Tague.)

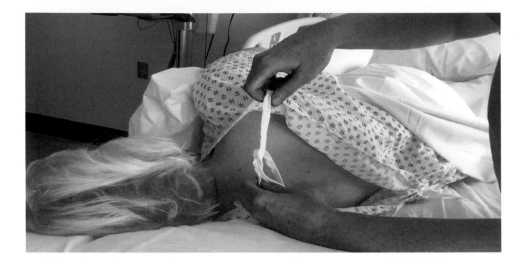

FIGURE 12.4
Simply untie the gown. Many gowns will have two ties to undo.

(Photo by Carolyn Tague.)

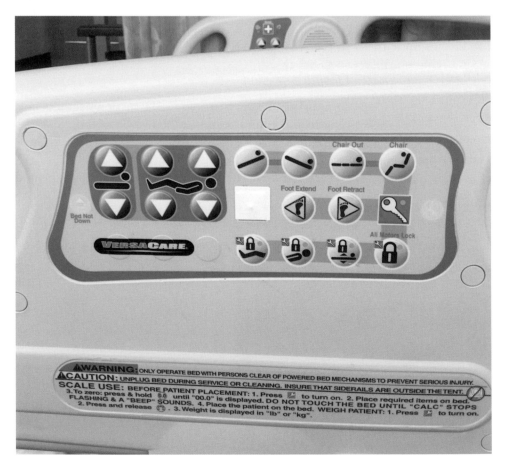

FIGURE 12.5
Typical hospital bed control panel. Look for bed alarm lights: if on, the bed will notify the nurses, station if a patient gets up from the bed. Alarms can also be set off if the bed is moved.

(Photo by Carolyn Tague.)

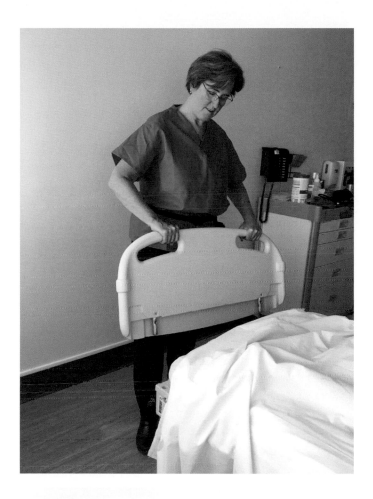

FIGURE 12.6
Patients are frequently amazed to see how easy it is to lift and remove the foot rail. It is can be easily leaned against a wall during a foot massage or reflexology session.

(Photo by Barbara Gideon.)

to close. It is generally appropriate in all bodywork sessions to remove the hands first, then verbally inform the client the session is over and request post-session feedback or "pain scale" report. If the person has fallen asleep, therapists may incorrectly suppose that the patient is no longer able to hear them. However, since hearing may be active, practitioners should assume that the patient can hear at some level and tell them, after the hands are slowly removed from the body, that the session has ended.

Massage lotions

For several reasons, massage lotion is preferable to oil when working with people who are in acute care settings. Petroleum-based products clog the pores of the skin, thereby inhibiting elimination through this route. Lotion absorbs more fully than oil, so patients aren't left with the sense of needing to shower away the greasy residue. Additionally, oil causes both latex and vinyl gloves to stretch grossly out of proportion, which decreases their protective capacity and makes it difficult to perform a smooth massage. Logistically, lotion also has the advantage of being easier to control, resulting in fewer spills and greasy fingerprints in the patient's room and minimal staining to the bedding. Unfortunately, some lotions supplied by hospitals lack good glide and are frustrating to use. When this is the case, the massage strokes can easily be performed without lubricant over the sheets or clothing so that the massage is smooth and flowing. A few basic guidelines should be observed with all patients regarding the use of lotion:

1. Describe the lubricant so that patients can approve or decline if they have allergies or personal preferences.[2]

2. If therapists are using a multiuse container of lotion, the bottle and top must be washed with antiseptic soap for 30 seconds between each client. In the hospital setting, if possible, it is recommended that a new container of lotion be used for each patient. The unused portion can be left with the patient.

3. Use unscented products. Illness and its treatments can trigger a sensitivity to odors.

Chapter TWELVE

I kept thinking, God must have been a massage therapist, because the laying on of hands allows true healing.

Feedback from an oncology patient,
San Francisco, California

Draping

By gently pulling the bedding out from the foot of the bed, draping can be performed in much the same way as when working with a client on a massage table. One of the differences is in how the sheet is secured. Rather than lifting limbs to tuck in the drape or firmly pushing the drape under the body, simply lay the bedding aside without tucking it in (see Figure 12.3). People who have just had surgery, are in pain, or are feeling fragile do not want to be handled in a rough manner. If necessary, push and tuck into the bed placing any pressure below the body to limit tissue movement.

Hospital patients invariably lose much of their modesty after the myriad procedures in which the body is exposed. This does not mean normal draping procedures should be abandoned. Just as in other massage settings, only expose the part of the body being massaged. An exception to this would be patients who are overly warm and have been lying on top of the bed in their gown. Proceed with the massage, moving the gown aside when necessary. Some patients who have been in hospital for weeks prefer to wear personal clothing, such as a T-shirt and pajama bottoms. Undressing for a massage can be difficult because of IV tubes threaded into the arm or neck of the garment. It is often easier in these situations to administer bodywork over the clothing.

Body mechanics

Although giving massage to a patient in a hospital bed is less strenuous than giving a deep tissue massage in a

---

Therapist's journal 12.2
Alone in the room

I've been a hospital-based massage therapist for over 13 years. When I first started hospital-based work, cell phones were simply phones. Patients and visitors would take calls which kept them reachable by doctors, family or for work obligations. When the call was over, typically I would observe the intimate connections with the visiting dyads of spouses, sisters, parents and adult children. Small talk was common and I was often invited into the exchange.

In the last several years, I've noticed a significant change. Today, it feels like an 80% chance that whomever else is in the room is on their smartphone, tablet or other device. In an entire 30–45 minutes that I am present, there can be literally no exchange between the hospitalized patient and their visitor. My heart breaks a little every time I see a patient staring off, glancing every once in a while, at their husband or daughter who is totally immersed in some social media world or streaming movie.

My hands do what they can to connect. My eyes attempt reassurance, but my heart does break a little.

Carolyn Tague CMT

---

leisure setting, working on people in the hospital environment forces the therapist to learn a whole new system of body mechanics. The following suggestions, combined with those generally taught to bodyworkers, such as do not bend and twist simultaneously, will help the therapist's physical comfort.

- Raise the bed, so that the therapist's stance is fully upright. Many bodyworkers are accustomed to setting their massage tables lower to gain leverage. Leverage is not helpful at the bedside, as the desired pressure is usually gentle. Raising the bed will not only ensure that the pressure is lighter, but it will also be comfortable for the practitioner's back, head, and shoulders. The therapist in Figure 12.7 demonstrates good body mechanics. For her own comfort, the bed is raised, and she can move around the bed when massaging different parts of the body.

- Therapists should stop and readjust the bed if the height is incorrectly set rather than continuing on in discomfort. Patients will not mind, and they will be glad for the therapist to take care of themselves. This way too, the touch practitioner can remain grounded, at ease, and truly focus on the patient in their care.

- Lower the bedrails on the side being massaged to avoid lifting the shoulders in order to reach over. Be sure to bring rails back up when complete and before moving to the other side.

- The footboards on many beds can be easily removed (see Figure 12.6), which will decrease shoulder strain caused by reaching over the board.

Massage the feet from the side if the footboard cannot be removed.

- Headboards, too, sometimes can be removed, which allows the practitioner a comfortable position from which to massage the face and head. If the headboard is permanently attached to the bed or there is insufficient room to get behind the bed, massage the face and head from the patient's side.

- Practitioners should place their body close to the bed so as to avoid reaching. Do not hesitate to ask patients to move closer to the side of the bed if they are able. If they are unable to move without minimal assistance or without causing pain, work with them where they are. Sometimes sitting on a chair or stool will put the therapist in closer proximity to the patient (Figure 12.8).

- With permission, the therapist may sit on the bed. This can be a comfortable way for some touch practitioners to work, especially when massaging the hands. Place a clean towel to sit or kneel on to main-

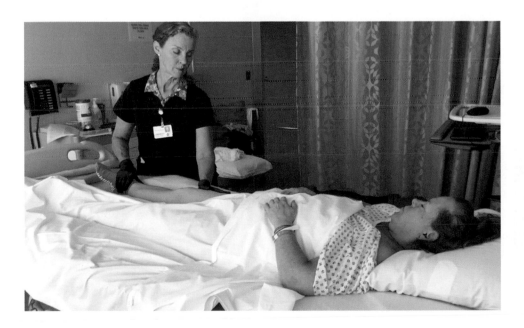

FIGURE 12.7
The MT is demonstrating good ergonomics. Simply raising the bed helps considerably. Lowering the head of the bed for the patient's comfort is also recommended for side-lying.

(Photo by Carolyn Tague.)

tain the "clean to clean" protocol. A second towel under the patient's hand and arm is also a preferred practice as it provides a defined workspace and a sense of safe boundary between patient and therapist (Figure 12.9).

- Use the bed for support by leaning against it. Be mindful never to allow body parts of the practitioner, such as stomach or chest to touch the patient. Be extremely careful to avoid crimping any tubing or wires that are in the area.

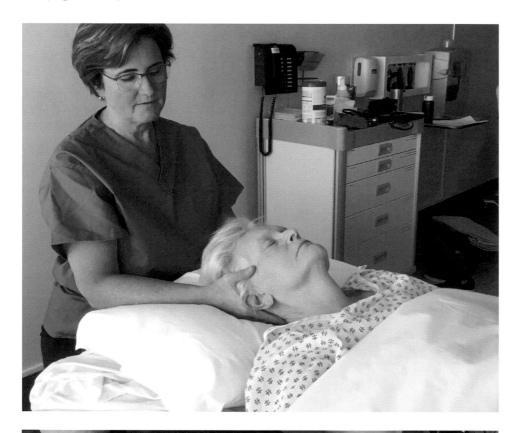

FIGURE 12.8
Craniosacral therapy and other touch modalities can be offered to the head, neck and shoulders by positioning the patient with their head at the foot of the bed.

(Photo by Barbara Gideon.)

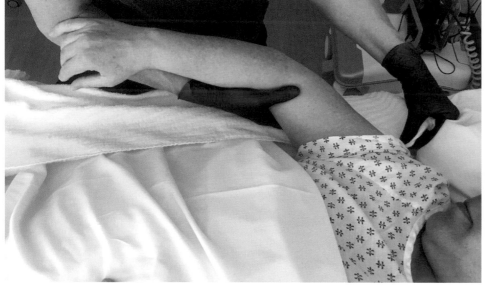

FIGURE 12.9
A skillful way to help a patient reposition an arm. This also allows a towel to be placed under the arm for keeping lotion off the bed sheets, and to be able to pat dry the arm as part of the touch therapy.

(Photo by Carolyn Tague.)

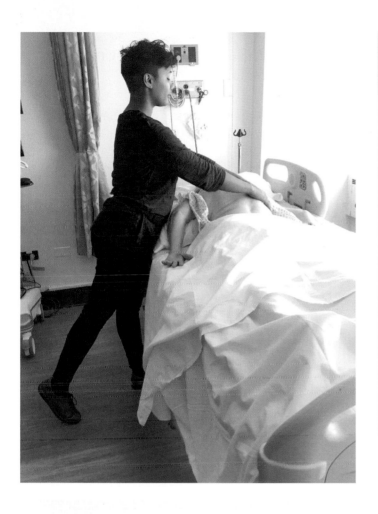

FIGURE 12.10
Here the MT is demonstrating how to keep the back straight by extending one leg back for a period of time. Switching legs is helpful in keeping comfortable and extending the time at the bedside.

(Photo by Barbara Gideon.)

- When massaging at the bedside, therapists will find themselves standing in one place more often. Shifting body weight and repositioning one's stance will help sustain the practitioner during the session. Elevating the bed or sitting in a chair will help keep hand pressure light on the client's body. Another useful stance is to extend one leg straight back with weight on the other leg (Figure 12.10).

Therapist's journal 12.3
I always forget the height of the bed

I always forget the bed height. Last week when I was working, I just rushed in and started the treatment with all kinds of awkward positions and then that night, my lower back was so sore and painful that I need my personal massage therapist (my husband) to fix it.

The most painful/awkward position is standing in the small space between the bed and the headboard when I offer head or face massage. I have to squeeze myself into that narrow gap, so every time I remind myself to work out much harder to keep my body slim so that I can squeeze into that. (Getting into that gap is even more challenging than getting the certification for massage therapist). Sometimes I am standing on only one leg for 5 to 10 minutes to finish the head massage – you can imagine how crazy it is. And I still don't know how to fix it except by moving the bed, but most of the time it is not possible.

Anonymous and slightly embarrassed MT

This angle helps the back stay straight. Switch legs often.

Touch modalities for the medically complex patient

A handful of bodywork techniques are commonly used in massaging people in acute care settings: gentle effleurage and petrissage, as well as modalities such as Reiki, Therapeutic Touch, Craniosacral therapies, or Jin Shin Jyutsu®. With the proper adjustments, almost any therapy can be administered. By using a broad hand, shiatsu could be applied along meridian lines; Trager Psychosocial Integration® could be used for some patients by decreasing the vigorousness of the jostling motion; and trigger-point or myofascial release therapies could be used by decreasing the effort and shortening the time applied.

Chapter TWELVE

The following lists of techniques are grouped into two categories. Info Box 12.1 presents examples of modalities that can be administered without pressure modification. However, care should still be taken when employing them: despite being gentle, they are also potent. Info Box 12.2 lists therapies that can be used if the appropriate pressure adjustments are made.

The need for bodywork that is undemanding cannot be overemphasized. Often a traditional massage session feels good in the moment, but later that night or the following day, the patient will feel unwell, often for several days. The person may feel fatigued, nauseous, chilled, sore, or fevered.

Biofield therapies

Both ancient and newly discovered bodywork modalities that intend to work with the body's energy system are termed by the National Institutes of Health (NIH) as "biofield therapies." Physics now states that, at the most fundamental levels of any physical form, is the reality of its energy composition. This science has made significant discoveries in the last few decades. Health care in general is slowly integrating the science into practice. This integration can take the form of high-tech treatments that use low frequency energy patterns such as low frequency sound stimulation (LFSS)[4] or low-frequency repetitive transcranial magnetic stimulation (rTMS).[5] Some health care centers are incorporating ancient practices such as traditional Chinese medicine (TCM) or energy medicine by a myriad different names such as Reiki, Pranic healing, or laying on of hands. Few medical centers currently promote biofield therapies, presumably because of lack of evidence. If not promoted as a cure but as a supportive, non-invasive, non-pharmacological service with no adverse side effects, such offerings may be tolerated, if not overtly welcomed. According to Shamini Jain, PhD, of the Consciousness and Healing Initiative (CHI): "Recent empirical advances in bioelectromagnetics suggest that perturbation of electromagnetic aspects of the biofield (involving very weak physical energies) can substantially impact health processes."[6] As with any modality or treatment, it must be patient centered and patient approved. Follow the lead of the organization and the patient if offering biofield therapy.

Info Box 12.1 Techniques requiring no pressure modification

The following are examples of techniques that can be administered with no pressure modification. They may be particularly good for the seriously ill patient. However, they can be very potent, and care should still be taken not to create a demand on the patient.

- Bowen Technique
- Compassionate Touch®
- Craniosacral therapies
- Healing Touch
- Jin Shin Jyutsu®
- Polarity therapy
- Reiki
- Rosen Method
- Shen
- Therapeutic Touch

Info Box 12.2 Techniques requiring pressure adjustments

The following are examples of techniques that nearly always require pressure modification from their typical use, but can be administered if the level of pressure and demand on the body is reduced.

- Acupressure
- Anma (or Amma)
- Bindegewebsmassage (connective tissue massage)
- Esalen Massage
- Jin Shin Do
- Kripalu Bodywork
- Lomi lomi (gentle aspects only)
- Myofascial release
- Neuromuscular therapy
- Reflexology
- Shiatsu
- Swedish massage
- Trager Psychosocial Integration®
- Trigger-point therapy
- Zero Balancing®

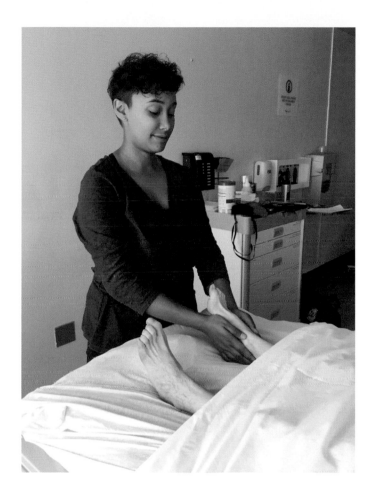

FIGURE 12.11
Foot massage and reflexology are often appropriate touch modalities for very compromised patients or those who intend to sleep after the session.

(Photo by Barbara Gideon.)

Using head and heart

Bodyworkers often believe that intention and intuition provide sufficient guidance toward performance of safe touch therapy sessions, but patients have stories to the contrary. When working with medically complex clients in whatever setting, intention and intuition must be combined with knowledge and skill. Heart and head are required when working with physically compromised individuals. Caution should always win out in cases of indecision.

It is not always prudent to depend solely on patients' feedback. A massage can feel wonderful in the moment, only to leave the person feeling worse later in the day. One therapist reports a new patient declining a second session because he became nauseous within a few hours after his last session. Healthier clients, too, may be sore the day following a massage. But this is less of a concern than with people who are ill. Patients in compromised health are already feeling vulnerable and are in pain or discomfort; the confidence in their body may be low. If a therapy such as massage makes them feel worse, they will abandon it more readily than healthy people, which means the opportunity to support them and ease their way is lost.

Length of the session

Sessions given in medical settings or with those feeling poorly at the time of the session tend to be shorter. Even if patients have a long history of receiving massage before their illness, there is no way for them to predict how they will respond to bodywork during an episode of illness. It is prudent to modify the length of the session at the start to assess patients' reactions. If they respond well to that amount of time and want to increase it for the next session, the practitioner should make a cautious increase.

Info Box 12.3 The pause

Being in a culture conditioned to high speed, the concept of an exhale that does not have an action or verbal information along with it may seem unfamiliar and even strange. However, personal reflection, listening to the texture of the body, and responding to the emotion of bonding, all require us as practitioners to be quiet, breathe, and listen to ourselves. The Pause. This process also allows the patient a moment to fully receive the previous action. The pause is the space where trust deepens; the space where bonding takes place; the place of observation and integration for both practitioner and patient. This is the empty space in a tea cup; the space that allows the cup to be filled. The empty space is in fact the most valuable space for without it there are no possibilities.[7]

Irene Smith, *Everflowing*

Chapter TWELVE

Inching forward, rather than taking leaps and bounds, is the best approach. Many hospitals will recommend 20–30-minute sessions. Interruptions and nursing activities are likely to happen in any given hour. In settings where the session is likely to be a one-time offering, the opportunity to inch forward is not possible. This should only confirm the practice of being cautious and focusing on the intention of comfort and care.

How to handle interruptions

As discussed in previous chapters, if a clinician enters the room during a session, it is best practice to ask the patient first whether they would like the therapist to stay and continue or to step out, and then also look to the clinician for confirmation.

Encourage a sense of teamwork and inclusion if staff members come in to take vital signs or deliver a meal tray. Everyone representing the medical center is part of that patient's health care team.

Press the call button right away if there is beeping or alarms going off. Carry on with the session to reassure the patient of the routine nature of the sounds and lights that might otherwise feel stressful. Sometimes a massage will be interrupted by a medical technician needing to perform a scan or by a phlebotomist who has come to draw blood for lab work.

When required to leave a session early because of a procedure or visitor, make sure to close the session with your client. Getting a post session report or quote is best practice, however, a quick "How are you feeling?" and a simple "thank you" can be enough.

A few general suggestions for the touch session

1. Evenings are a better time for hospital patients to receive massage. The day shift in a hospital often requires navigating patient schedules that will include physical therapy, tests and procedures away from the room, and important visits from the medical team. Bodywork sessions may be cut short, interrupted, late in starting, or unable to be scheduled at all because of these and other routine events in the day in the life of a patient. Not only are there fewer intrusions in the evening, but it helps the patient to relax before going to sleep. Although patients tend to have more visitors in the evening, this can be viewed as an opportunity to teach family and friends how to give attentive touch. If evenings do not fit for the service for whatever reason, simply adjust expectations to accommodate the inevitable scheduling challenges. Know that the stress-relieving touch will be appreciated whenever it is received.

2. Allow patients to do as much for themselves as they show an interest in. In sessions with healthier individuals, therapists usually encourage them to completely relax and be pampered. However, people who have had long-term health problems often get out of the

---

Therapist's journal 12.4
Sanctuary

A woman who had multiple bone metastases on her spine was lying in discomfort in her hospital bed. She said she'd been looking forward to her massage all day. She had multiple lines and tubes connecting her thin, pale body to bags and plugs and ports in the wall. I cautiously raised the bed, watching to make sure none of the tubes caught on anything on the way up. Then I gingerly stepped next to the bed, positioning myself in such a way I would not tangle myself in any of her hardware. After all this, I found a comfortable posture for myself and then, finally, connected with the impatient patient. She sighed, and as I focused on connection, all the hospital-standard beeps and clatter faded away. Her shoulders eased, her breathing slowed to a light snore. In the middle of the cacophony and bustle of the hospital floor, for even just a few minutes, her bed became a sanctuary.

Christine Knapp CMT
Hospital-Based Massage Therapist, Heart Touch Project

habit of doing for themselves or commonly, may feel guilty about the number of daily tasks that must be done for them. If patients show an interest in adjusting the bed or helping during draping, allow them to assist in these ways.

3. Encourage patients to move as much as possible. This may mean moving their slippers out of the practitioner's way or scooting closer to the provider while side-lying. Nurses appreciate the reinforcement of their requests for patients to move and keep up their strength and abilities. Muscle wasting happens in as little as three days of complete bedrest.

4. When speaking to patients who are in bed, stand in front of them where they don't need to strain to see or hear. This angle creates a more comfortable line of sight. When speaking, talk a bit more slowly, distinctly, and in short statements. People on medication or coming out of anesthesia can be temporarily confused or unalert.

5. Talking with patients and family members is a dance: they lead, the therapist follows. But, when it comes to the hands-on session, it is imperative that the therapist leads. Bodyworkers should communicate clearly before the session about how the touch will be adjusted for the patient's unique situation. Setting appropriate expectations is key: many people have specific expectations for massage and can easily be disappointed if the touch practitioner does not clearly describe what is actually being offered. Therapists are wise to explain to the patient what they are doing just before the fact, such as leaving the room to speak to the nurse, raising the bed, undraping the body, or clearing a space around the room. Explain briefly why these actions are being taken.

6. Most patients are able to carry on a conversation with their care team. Conversations are generally much like those with any other individual. In Western cultures, topics such as children, pets, the garden, and occupations are common subjects of discussion. In many Asian countries, personal topics such as family or professions would not likely be appropriate.

7. In many cultures, patients will avoid discussing serious diagnoses with family or friends. In some cultures, disclosing a life-threatening diagnosis with the patient is not acceptable. For all these various situations, "therapist follows" in the conversation dance is vitally important. Some patients openly talk about their illness, but many do not. Everyone wants to be understood. The goal is not to fix or solve problems but to appreciate what the patient is experiencing.

8. Report any findings to the nurse such as an unreported skin conditions, bruises, or swelling. Modify the session accordingly. Explain changes to the patient when appropriate, meaning at the time the patient is alert or after the session if resting during the touch therapy.

Group treatment

While this chapter is titled "One on one", there are many examples of touch sessions provided in clinics or care facilities where there are a group of clients and practitioners working together at the same time. Researchers from the University of Massachusetts Medical School and the Osher Center for Integrative Medicine, UCSF looked at group treatments and found: "Integrative group medical visits are an innovative model to improve access to non-pharmacological approaches to chronic illness care and health promotion. They may advance health equity by serving patients negatively impacted by health and health care disparities."[8]

Patient safety

It could be said that this entire book focuses on patient safety. This brief section, however, brings several other specific safety issues to the practitioner's attention.

- In an emergency, press the nurse's call button and quickly secure the patient, bedrails up and bed down. Pressing the call button many not get an immediate response: step out into the hall and call loudly to whichever staff member is nearby. Patients may need immediate attention if they are having difficulty breathing or they become unsteady and fall. All health care facilities will have a process for cardiac arrest. "Code blue" protocols should be understood, memorized and followed in the case of a patient who stops breathing.

Therapist's journal 12.5
Group treatments in our pain clinic

We provide group treatments where 8–10 residents, usually in wheelchairs, sit in a circle, and we work on them in rotation. Some of the services we provide are medical and nursing assessments, massage therapy, acupuncture, music therapy, acutonics, and medical Qi Gong. Additionally, the residents and staff participate in a guided group meditation for approximately 20 minutes generally halfway through each clinical session.

Our procedure is that the first practitioner who works on a resident starts with a pain assessment. Then a treatment is provided, and then various practitioners rotate around the room performing treatments that the resident would like to have. After all treatments have been completed, we ask them: "How do you feel now compared to when you first came in?" We have found that they typically answer that they feel much better at the end of a session.

One patient I worked with had Lou Gehrig's disease (ALS) with progressive muscle weakness and severe pain in her feet. As I provided massage therapy to her shoulders, neck and arms, she started to weep. At the end of the session she shared that during the treatment she felt like she: "had been transported to another realm that was beautiful and peaceful and free of pain." She continued to come to the clinic and she shared with us that during the group sessions she found tranquility and relief from her symptoms.

Sharon Brahms RN, CMT

- Patients may be at risk for falling and therefore listed as a "fall precaution." Look for signs and codes on patient doors and above beds. Weakness, disorientation, the side effects of medication, partial paralysis, poor balance due to deteriorating eyesight, dizziness, pain, or neuropathy are some of the reasons a person may be assigned this status. Actions taken to prevent them from falling include:
  - Allowing these patients out of bed only with the assistance of the nursing staff. The hospital will want only those with special training to provide this assistance.
  - Returning the bed to the lowest position with the top side rails up following the massage. (Unless specifically indicated, lower side rails should be left down.)
  - **Never leaving the bedside with the person unattended if the bed is elevated.**
  - Place skid free socks on patient before leaving if lotion was applied to feet.

After the session: important tasks

The following tasks are usually performed more or less in the sequence listed:

1. Lower the bed.
2. Raise the bedrails to their original position. These first two tasks MUST be done, even if the patient is asleep! Failing to perform these two tasks places patients in immediate and significant danger. **A patient falling from an elevated bed is absolutely unacceptable.** This error could easily lead to dismissal or probation of the therapist. (Note an exception: In the ICU many patients are significantly sedated or otherwise impaired from moving. Staff there will often keep beds elevated for better

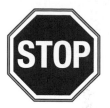
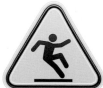
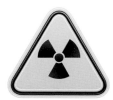
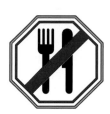

FIGURE 12.12
Common warning signs used in health care settings: stop; fall risk; x-ray or scan in progress (via mobile machine); food restriction – In and Out measuring, NPO.

access to patients for frequent tests and procedures. When attending patients in the ICU, leave the bed height as it was found.)

3. Bring side tables back to original placement; ensure the call button and telephone are within reach.

4. Tidy the patient's bed.

5. Ask if the patient needs anything before you leave.

6. Have a closing dialogue with the patient each time. Consider each session a one-time window of opportunity to be with that person. It is natural to say, "See you next week." However, there may not be a next week.

Patients may be discharged, they may take a turn for the worse and be transferred to intensive care, or they may die. Instead, one could say, "It was great to work with you," or "Thank you. It was great to meet you." Use whatever language is authentic. The main point is to be appreciative of the current exchange, and not over-promise any commitment regarding the future.

7. Remove the massage sign from the patient's door.

8. Thoroughly wash hands and forearms with soap and water after leaving the patient's room.

9. Report and document.

Case history 12.1	Exercise

Instructions

Part 1: On a piece of paper, make three columns: pressure, site, and position. List the conditions that apply to each category for the below case.

Part 2: Write a sample narrative with a treatment plan for a 30-minute touch session for the following patient using the bodywork modalities that you are trained in. Starting from the referral or request, write a description of an entire patient or client experience. In the narrative, include the following items:

- The imaginary intake conversation you would have with the nurse.
- The way in which you opened and closed the session with the patient.
- A description of the bodywork performed with the patient, including the adjustments.

Hope is a 47-year-old female who presented to the ER with stabbing pain in the chest and swelling in both lower extremities. Serious infection was found around the heart and lungs. Hope was admitted to a general medicine unit. She has been hospitalized for 23 days with no discharge date scheduled. She appears in good spirits but rates fatigue at 7/10 and is unable to take walks as the staff encourage her to do. She has an IV catheter on her right forearm. There is pitting edema in both lower extremities. The nurse has given the OK for Hope to receive massage therapy and identifies the upper torso as an area to avoid as the infection has not yet been completely resolved.

Chapter TWELVE

Summary

It is a calm moment; a moment of complete trust; a shared sacred space when a skilled massage therapist and their patient are connected by touch. The sessions will have a typical workflow that fits the needs of the client and the medical environment. The protocols are in place to keep everyone safe and supported. With focus and experience, the touch practitioner's anxieties about the care facility's culture and layers of information will become the music that invites the dance. Massage can bridge the gap between doing and being and help family, friends, and caregivers enter into the world of the person who is negotiating the gap. Through massage, the one who is sick and the one who is well can simultaneously come together, engaged in an experience that encompasses both "doing" and "being."

This chapter in particular has been about how to choreograph touch sessions for the care and comfort of each patient. One last suggestion: wear comfortable shoes!

Test yourself

True or False: Place a "T" next to all of the true statements and an "F" next to the false ones. Rewrite the false statements so they are true. There is usually more than one correct way to rewrite the false statements. For extra credit, explain why true statements are true.

1. Never leave the bedside with the person unattended if the bed is elevated.

2. Acknowledge others in the room: visitors or other patients.

3. Lower all of the bedrails prior to starting the massage so that there are no interruptions in the middle of the session.

4. Most patients prefer a feathery stroke using the fingertips.

5. Lotion is preferred over oil for massage in medical settings.

6. Rather than disturbing the patient with undraping and draping, reach under the linen when giving Swedish massage.

7. The bed should be raised high enough so that the therapist does not need to lean.

8. Clinical knowledge is more important to the massage therapist than intuition.

9. Ask patients to do as much as possible for themselves.

10. When a patient who is a fall precaution needs to move from the bed to the commode, the massage practitioner should lower the bed and side rails to make it easy for the person to get up out of the bed on their own.

References

1. Smith I. Bodywork for HIV Infected Persons. San Francisco: Everflowing Handbooks; 1994.

2. Dunn T, Williams M. Massage Therapy Guidelines for Hospital and Home Care (4th edition). Olympia: Information for People; 2000.

3. Dammann G. Personal communication, 10 September 2019.

4. Naghdi L, Ahonen H, Macario P, Bartel L. The effect of low-frequency sound stimulation on patients with fibromyalgia: a clinical study. Pain Res Manag. 2015; 20(1):e21–e27. doi:10.1155/2015/375174.

5. Berlim M, Van den Eynde F, Daskalakis, ZJ. Clinically meaningful efficacy and acceptability of low-frequency repetitive transcranial magnetic stimulation (rTMS) for treating primary major depression: a meta-analysis of randomized, double-blind and sham-controlled trials. Neuropsychopharmacol. 2013; 38;543–51. doi:10.1038/npp.2012.237.

6. Jain S, Ives J, Jonas W, et al. Biofield science and healing: an emerging frontier in medicine. Global Adv Health Med. 2015; 4(suppl):5-7. Available from: https://www.chi.is/biofield-science-and-healing-special-issue/?utm_source=CHI+COMMUNITY&utm_campaign=09f8ffcd8c-&utm_medium=email&utm_term=0_a80f47d270-09f8ffcd8c-162312093.

7. Smith I. Personal communication, 11 April 2019.

8. Thompson-Lastad A, Gardiner P, Chao M. Integrative group medical visits: a national scoping survey of safety-net clinics. Health Equity. 2018; 3.1. Available from: http://online.liebertpub.com/doi/10.1089/heq.2018.0081.

Additional resources

Adams R, White B, Beckette C. The Effects of massage Therapy on pain management in the acute care setting. Int J Ther Massage Bodywork. 2010; 3(1):4-11.

Benjamin B, Sohnen-Moe C. The Ethics of Touch (2nd edition). Arizona: Sohnen-Moe Associates; 2014.

Bohrer K. Integrative health care and massage therapy. 2019. Available from: https://www.amtamassage.org/articles/3/MTJ/detail/3920/integrative-health-care-massage-therapy.

The Farewell (movie). 2019. Recommended for a depiction of Chinese and American perspectives on communicating with patients.

Haun JN, Paykel J, Alman AC, et al. A complementary and integrative health group-based program pilot demonstrates positive health outcomes with female Veterans. New York: Explore; 2019. Available from: https://www-ncbi-nlm-nih-gov.ucsf.idm.oclc.org/pubmed/?term=31477475 [accessed 12 Aug 2019].

Kliegel E. Holistic Reflexology: Essential Oils, Crystal Massage in Reflex Zone Therapy. New York: Healing Arts Press; 2018.

Vallet M. A soft touch: massage and palliative care. 2017. Available from: https://www.amtamassage.org/articles/3/MTJ/detail/3746/a-soft-touch-massage-palliative-care.

Zagozdon R. Inpatient hospital-based massage therapy. 2017. Available from: https://www.amtamassage.org/articles/3/MTJ/detail/3776/inpatient-hospital-based-massage-therapy.

Beyond touch: Aromatherapy massage sessions in health care

Healing begins with an aromatic bath and daily massage.

Hippocrates

This chapter provides an overview of aromatherapy and its benefits, and offers practical advice on ways it can be used by qualified practitioners in health care settings. Aromatherapy is a vast and complex subject. This chapter touches lightly on some aspects, aiming to lay a groundwork of understanding and to inspire practitioners to see the benefits and to undertake further study and training in the discipline, with a view to integrating it into their practice.

History

Plants have been utilized for thousands of years for their fragrance, flavors, and as medicines. Their use as medicines predates written human history. For example, an archaeological investigation of a 60,000-year-old Neanderthal burial site found a large quantity of pollen from plants that are known to have been used in later times in herbal remedies.[1] Herbs were found in the personal effects of Ötzi, the iceman whose body was frozen in the Ötztal Alps for more than 5000 years. These herbs are thought to have been used to treat the parasites that were found in his intestines.[2]

In India, medicinal plants have been a core element in the Ayurvedic health care system for centuries dating back at least 4,000 years and are still used today. Surviving Sanskrit texts from between 1500 BC and 500 BC detail the use of hundreds of herbs and aromatics for religious and therapeutic purposes. Around 3500 BC, the Egyptians were using plants for perfumery, medicine, pharmacy, cosmetics, and in religious practice.

The Chinese medical text *Pen T'Sao*, believed to have been written by Emperor Shen Nung around 2500 BC, contains information on the medicinal use of over 350 plants. Emperor Shen Nung is said to have discovered tea and to be the father of Traditional Chinese Medicine.[3] The Greek and Persian contribution to plant medicine is also immense. Hippocrates (459–370 BC) classified over 300 medicinal plants by their physiological action and the Greek physician, Pedanius Dioscorides (40–90 AD) wrote *De Materia Medica* which details over 650 medicines derived from plants. In Persia, Ibn Sena, also known as Avicenna (980–1037 AD), is credited with the development of steam distillation to extract and concentrate volatile compounds from plants, which became the most widespread method of producing essential oils (EOs).[4]

Info Box 13.1 Rose otto

The essential oil called Rose otto, is made from rose petals by steam distillation. To create 1 ml (20 drops) requires around 3 kg (6 lb 9½ oz) of rose petals.[5]

The ancient knowledge of plant therapy has evolved into modern-day usage in conventional medicine. Aspirin is a case in point. The chemical name for aspirin is acetylsalicylic acid. Salicylic acid has been used as a remedy throughout the ages: "Medicines made from willow and other salicylate-rich plants appear in clay tablets from ancient Sumer as well as the Ebers Papyrus from ancient Egypt. Hippocrates referred to their use of salicylic tea to reduce fevers around 400 BC, and were part of the pharmacopoeia of Western medicine in classical antiquity and the Middle Ages."[6] In the 1700s, willow bark extract was used for its effects on fever, pain, and inflammation and in the 1800s, pharmacists were experimenting with and prescribing medicines taken from salicin, the active component of willow extract.[6] Many other modern medicines have their origins in plants, such as the heart drug digitalis (foxglove) and the chemotherapy drug Taxol (Pacific yew).

The roots of aromatherapy can be traced back to the ancient use of plants as medicines, however, essential oils have only been produced in the last 1,000 years or so. They consist of a concentration of only some of the chemical compounds that are present in the raw plant. The pharmacological properties and effects of the essential oils and the raw plants from which they are made can differ markedly. For example, essential oils extracted from citrus plants by expression contain non-volatile furocoumarin compounds, which can cause photosensitivity, whereas citrus oils produced by steam distillation do not contain furocoumarins. This is significant for patients who are on a medication regimen that can make their skin more photosensitive.[7] It serves to illustrate that it must not be assumed because a plant, or some part of it, has certain therapeutic effects, that the essential oils from that plant will have the same effects.

Aromatherapy and health care

From its inception, the term aromatherapy has been associated with health care. It was first coined in 1937 by Rene-Maurice Gattefosse, a French chemist, who after severely burning his hand in an explosion at his laboratory, discovered the benefits of lavender (*Lavandula angustifolia*) essential oil in stopping infection, healing his burns, and preventing scarring. This was followed by a pioneering career and lifelong investigation into the therapeutic use of EOs.

Many people contributed to the early development of aromatherapy, including Jean Valnet, an army physician and surgeon, who used essential oils in treating battle injuries and later in civilian medical practice. Marguerite Maury, an Austrian-born biochemist who was also a nurse and surgical assistant, established the first aromatherapy clinics in France, Great Britain, and Switzerland. In 1995, Jane Buckle, a nurse, established the first clinical aromatherapy course for nurses and doctors in the US. This course has been taught in 27 states.[8] Countless others have contributed to the development of the discipline, and references to some are included at the end of the chapter.

What is aromatherapy?

Aromatherapy is the use of volatile compounds extracted from plants to promote health and well-being through the means of inhalation or application to the skin. These phytochemical compounds are called essential oils (EOs), implying that they contain the very essence of the plant. Hundreds of essential oils are produced from plants all over the world using a range of techniques such as steam distillation, expression, and solvent and CO_2 extraction. EOs can be extracted from the various parts of plants (see Appendix 13.1 at the end of this chapter for examples). The top two major producers are China and India, followed by Indonesia, Sri Lanka, and Vietnam. A variety of African countries, North America, Mexico, Argentina, Paraguay, Uruguay, Guatemala, and Haiti are also major growers of plants and manufacturers of essential oils.[9]

Aromatherapy is sometimes used as an alternative therapy instead of mainstream medical treatment, and sometimes as a complementary therapy, alongside mainstream medicine. This is a significant distinction. It is important to be clear with patients and medical staff about the way aromatherapy is being used. With patients in medical settings, aromatherapy should never be undertaken without the knowledge and agreement of medical staff.

The ideal approach to health care involves consideration of the whole person. It should seek to promote well-being by understanding and treating symptoms and the underlying conditions that give rise to them in the context of the particular person's life. Within such an integrated, multidisciplinary approach, aromatherapy should be seen as part of an overall treatment plan. A study in 2016 in ten hospitals in Minnesota showed the feasibility of this approach: over two years, 3,357 nurses were trained and provided 10,372 interventions to patients, which helped in decreasing pain, nausea, and anxiety when provided as an adjunct to standard medical care. This had the benefits of being safe, low-cost, and non-pharmacological. Nurses reported ease of use, patient empowerment, patient satisfaction, and symptom reduction. One nurse said: "The ability to offer aromatherapy as an adjunct to medication in the perioperative area greatly enhances patient satisfaction. I have seen a decrease in pre-op anxiety and less anti-nausea medication being used postoperatively. The patients love it."[10]

Health care systems around the world are increasingly looking to integrate complementary therapies into their services as safe, low-cost, non-pharmacological ways to improve patient outcomes and satisfaction. One of the recommendations in a report by the UK government's All-Party Parliamentary Group for Integrated Healthcare (PGIH) in 2018 was that: "Every cancer patient and their families should be offered complementary therapies as part of their treatment package to support them in their cancer journey."[11] And in 2005, the Committee on the Use of Complementary and Alternative Medicine by the American Public wrote: "The committee believes that the goal should be to provide comprehensive care that is based on the 10 rules outlined in the Institute of Medicine report *Crossing the Quality Chasm* (IOM, 2001). A comprehensive system uses the best available scientific evidence on benefits and harm, recognizes the importance of compassion and caring, encourages patients to share in decision-making about their therapeutic options, and promotes choices in care that can include CAM therapies when appropriate."[12]

The World Health Organization (WHO) laid out three strategic objectives in its *Traditional Medicine Strategy (T&CM) 2014–2023*:

1. To build the knowledge base for active management of T&CM (traditional and complementary medicine) through appropriate national policies.

2. To strengthen the quality assurance, safety, proper use and effectiveness of T&CM by regulating products, practices and practitioners.

3. To promote universal health coverage by integrating T&CM services into health care service delivery and self-health care.[13]

Traditional medicine refers to the knowledge, skills, and practices based on the beliefs and experiences indigenous to different cultures.[14] The WHO *Global Report on Traditional and Complementary Medicine 2019* states that: "Traditional and complementary medicine (T&CM) is an important and often underestimated health resource with many applications, especially in the prevention and management of lifestyle-related chronic diseases, and in meeting the health needs of ageing populations."[15]

Ideally, in a people-centered health system, traditional and complementary medicine would work with mainstream medicine to help solve the health challenges of the 21st century.

Setting up an aromatherapy service

Primum non nocere, "first do no harm", is part of the Hippocratic oath which physicians swear. Although there is no requirement for a therapist to swear the Hippocratic oath, this principle is the first thing that should be considered in all aromatherapy practice. Patient safety is of prime importance, but so is that of staff as well as the reputation of the aromatherapy service. The following points provide a foundation for establishing a safe aromatherapy service:

- Define the service to be provided and the way it will operate, including the methods and materials that will be used.

- Establish a list of approved essential oils with their common name, botanical (Latin) name, specific benefits, contraindications and research evidence of effectiveness and safety (see Info Box 13.2). The same applies for carrier oils, such as grapeseed, sweet almond, or sesame. Such guidelines should be reviewed regularly.

- Develop an education program to introduce the service to clinical staff; this will help nurses, medics and clinical managers understand how aromatherapy can be integrated into their patients' care and how to refer appropriately. It may involve formal teaching sessions, talks/workshops, attendance at unit meetings, treatments for staff, and brief conversations in the course of the day. A member of the committee of the Royal College of Physicians (RCP), commented that: "Doctors need training to have the knowledge and confidence to discuss complementary therapies with their patients".[16]

- Ensure that therapists have strong qualifications, are members of a professional body, undertake continuing professional development, have completed adaptive training for working in a health care setting, and have their own professional insurance.

Chapter THIRTEEN

- Aromatherapists must practice only within the bounds of their own expertise and knowledge.

- Aromatherapists must adhere to the policies of the health care facility where they work. This may require working with the nursing and medical staff to establish agreed procedures for the use of aromatherapy in their particular area. These procedures should then be incorporated into the overall service documentation. Consideration needs to be given to medical conditions, e.g. cancer, dementia, gynecological, respiratory, and the treatment setting, e.g. hospital ward, single room, chemo-infusion suite, ICU.

- Undertake on-going evaluation and review of the service.

Info Box 13.2 Examples of entries for an approved essential oils list

Beragamot FCF *(Citrus bergamia)*
Has a relaxing, sedative effect[17] and has been used in the treatment of depression,[18] also in treating the symptoms of cancer pain, mood disorders and stress-induced anxiety.[19] Rectified bergamot oil is furanocoumarin free (FCF). This oil, unlike unrectified bergamot, is not phototoxic.[20]

Black pepper *(Piper nigrum)*
Mildly analgesic [21] and useful in the treatment of pain.[22] Has antiviral and bactericidal properties, is a good expectorant and stimulating to the nervous system.[23] Inhaled black pepper EO through a hollow plastic tube helped with smoking cessation by significantly reducing cravings at 3-hour sessions.[24]
No irritation or sensitizing at 4% dilution when tested on humans.[21]

Treatment process

Aromatherapy must not be used without the explicit, informed consent of the patient. When patients arrive at a health care facility, many decisions are made for them: when they will have meals, medications, blood draws, observations taken, procedures, and scans. They are away from their loved ones, friends, work and hobbies. Although most patients are very grateful for the care they receive, they can find it difficult not having control of their lives. Aromatherapy gives patients some control.

In a hospital setting aromatherapy treatment should broadly follow the sequence below.

- Referral by a health professional.

- Offer the patient the choice of receiving aromatherapy or not. Continue to offer choices throughout the process.

- Access medical notes, either paper or electronic.

- Consultation with the patient and with others responsible for, or involved in, the patient's care (medics, ward staff, relatives).

- Assessment of physical, emotional, psychological, medical history/conditions/ongoing treatments.

- Filling out an assessment form should lead on to a discussion about what symptoms the patient would like the essential oils to help them with, such as pain, nausea, breathlessness, low mood, anxiety, or a combination of these. Consider the context: area in hospital, time of day and what else is going on. Assess the working space around the patient.

- Offer appropriate essential oils on smelling strips for the patient to select.

- Decide with the patient how to use the oils. For example, they could be added to a carrier oil for a massage, used undiluted in an aroma diffuser, on a tissue, cotton ball, nasal stick inhaler, or aroma-patch for inhalation during a massage session. Aromatherapy treatment should be individually tailored for the particular person in the particular setting.

- Obtain the patient's written consent to treatment.

- Provide treatments, observing and adapting as necessary.

- Seek feedback/evaluation at the time or later as appropriate.

- Document the session.

- Report any observations or concerns to medical staff.

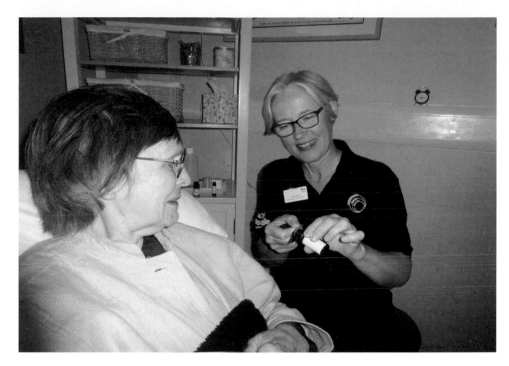

FIGURE 13.1
Therapist prepares a test strip for a patient to sample.

(Photo by Angela Secretan.)

Therapists should routinely record feedback on the outcomes of the treatments they provide, and where possible a systematic approach to this should be incorporated into practice. Data gathered in such a way allows on-going analysis and evaluation of the service.

One tool that therapists can use is the Measure Yourself Medical Outcome Profile (MYMOP).[25] It is designed to measure the outcomes most important to the patient. Measure Yourself Concerns and Wellbeing (MYCaW) is an adaptation specifically for patients receiving complementary therapies in cancer care settings. It provides a way to gather and summarize quantitative and qualitative data for research and evaluation. Links to these are provided in the Reference section at the end of the chapter.

Chemistry and essential oil safety

Essential oils must be handled with care. They are powerful chemical compounds that can be harmful if used incorrectly. Also, their beneficial properties can be degraded if not stored appropriately. It is important to be aware that not all EOs are safe for clinical use. Essential oils for aromatherapy constitute only a small part of the world market. The perfumery and food sectors are the largest users. Oils marketed for these other purposes may be adulterated or of a lower quality than necessary for use in aromatherapy. Only high-quality oils should be used in the health care setting.

The properties of an EO depend upon its chemical constituents and their respective proportions. For example, an essential oil from organically grown lavender consists of a mixture of up to 300 different chemical compounds.[26] However, the chemical composition of essential oils from the same genus and species of plant can vary depending on growing conditions, extraction methods, and other factors. Furthermore, some plants have variants, referred to as chemotypes, which have a consistently distinct chemical profile. The essential oils from different chemotypes of the same genus and species will contain different proportions of their constituents. A chemotype ("ct.") is usually denoted by the most distinct component. For example, one type of thyme (*Thymus vulgaris ct. thymol*) contains a high proportion of thymol whereas another type of thyme (*Thymus vulgaris ct. linalool*) contains a higher proportion of linalool. These two EOs have different properties and therapeutic effects.

Chapter THIRTEEN

In order to use an EO in the safest and most effective ways it is necessary to know its composition and to understand the properties of its different components. Gas chromatography–mass spectrometry (GC–MS) is the most frequently used technique to analyze the composition of EOs. It provides a list of the compounds in the oils and the percentage of each. This can help confirm that there are no additives and is useful in selecting the best oils for a particular purpose.

There is no regulated grading standard for essential oils, though some companies use terms like "therapeutic grade" implying that their oil is better than others. This is a marketing tool, not a regulated standard. It is important that EOs for aromatherapy in a health care setting be sourced from reputable suppliers who can provide a GC–MS analysis and a Material Safety Data Sheet. Their labels should have the following information:

- Botanical (Latin) name of the plant.
- Part(s) of the plant used.
- Chemotype if applicable – not all plants have different chemotypes.
- Production batch number.
- Expiry date.
- Any cautions specific to this oil.

EOs should be stored in airtight, dark glass bottles to prevent loss through evaporation and to protect from the damaging effects of sunlight (photochemical reaction), and oxidization, which alter their chemical composition and therapeutic properties. For example, alcohols can react with oxygen to become aldehydes,[27] which can have toxic effects.

Store EOs in a lockable cool cupboard or refrigerator, as heat can speed up chemical reactions. It is more important to keep the top note essential oils in a refrigerator: EOs are volatile, and top notes evaporate most readily.[26] Frequent changes of temperature can have detrimental effects on EOs, so once taken out of the refrigerator and transferred to your working box, they can be kept at room temperature.

Do not use out-of-date oils. It is advisable to maintain an inventory of oils with their expiry dates, and ensure labelling is intact and legible. When making blends these

---

Info Box 13.3 Fragrance notes

In the 19th century, GW Septimus Piesse, an English chemist and perfumer, is credited with classifying fragrances like notes on a musical scale. Thus, a fragrant compound can be described as a top (head), middle (heart) or base note depending on its position on the scale. This categorisation is subjective, but it broadly correlates with volatility (the rate of evaporation).

Top note EOs, such as lemon, niaouli and sage, are generally the first to be noticed and will fade the soonest; they are often described as light, sharp, or fresh. Middle note EOs such as geranium, marjoram and chamomile take a little time to come to the fore and will last longer; they may be characterised as warm, mellow, or smooth. Base note EOs such as cedarwood, patchouli and vetiver are the slowest to be perceived and longest lasting; they are typically considered heavy, rich, or earthy. This way of thinking about fragrances can be helpful when blending EOs.

---

must be clearly labelled with the patient's name, DOB, ingredients, expiry date, and instructions for use. This information should also be recorded in the patient's notes.

Be clear about actions that should be taken in the event of possible accidents such as getting oils in the eyes or swallowing them and adverse reactions to EOs or carriers. For example, if an essential oil causes dermal irritation, apply a small amount of vegetable oil or cream to the area affected and discontinue use of the EO or product that has caused irritation. File a report of any adverse reactions to aromatherapy treatments through the standard route for the hospital. It is advisable to carry a blank reporting form in your working folder while on the wards. An example of the IFPA's Adverse Reactions Form can be found at: https://ifparoma.org/wp-content/uploads/2019/07/Adverse-Reaction-Report.pdf.[28]

The International Federation of Professional Aromatherapists (IFPA) states that it: "does not endorse the use of essential oils internally or by neat application unless carried out by a practitioner trained and qualified at the appropriate level [training includes advanced chemistry, formulation training and safety aspects alongside the study of human anatomy and physiology] and who holds indemnity insurance to cover their practice, or working with a doctor or clinician who remains in charge of the patient's treatment and is clinically accountable for the care offered by an IFPA member."[29]

Before using on the skin, blend essential oils with an appropriate carrier oil. Prior to all treatments, patch testing is advisable, especially if the patient is known to have skin sensitivity. Do not apply EOs over irradiated skin: the skin will be more sensitive, and they may cause irritation, which could delay someone's daily radiotherapy treatment plan. Essential oils can interact adversely with other medication. For example, wintergreen EO contains methyl salicylate. "As methyl salicylate is converted into salicylic acid in the body, this essential oil is contraindicated in persons sensitive to aspirin (particularly asthmatics)."[30] Another example is when patients are receiving chemotherapy. They may have allergic reactions due to the cancer medication, therefore it is best to keep things simple and not add EOs into the mix during this time. EOs can be used between treatments to help with possible side effects.

Carrier oils

For application to the skin, EOs should be blended with a carrier oil, which can itself have useful properties. For example, grapeseed oil (*Vitis vinifera*) is one of the most popular base oils in massage and aromatherapy. It leaves the skin with a smooth satin finish without being greasy, has no known contraindications and is non-toxic.[30,31] Another example is jojoba (*Semmondsia chinensis*), which is a liquid wax. Its chemical structure resembles sebum, making it useful in cases of acne and other skin conditions. It also has anti-inflammatory properties, which could be useful for rheumatism and arthritis. Tisserand and Balacs suggest in their book *Essential Oil Safety* that: "Whilst in hospital, lining the inside of the nostrils with a little jojoba, with a clean fingertip or cotton bud, may discourage multiplication of bacteria."[20]

Therapeutic action of essential oils

Research shows that essential oils have chemical properties that can reduce pain[32–38]; nausea[39]; anxiety[35,37,40–42];

> ### Tip 13.1 Working with people at the end of life
>
> When working with people at the end of life, the therapist must be very mindful that patients' senses are often heightened: this includes touch, smell, taste, vision and hearing. For this reason, it is better to massage with a fragrance-free carrier oil, using the essential oil blend on a tissue or patch, that can be removed easily if found overpowering.

headaches[37]; stress[37,40]; fatigue[37,42]; depression[35,37]; and improve sleep[40–42] and the general feeling of well-being.[35]

Aromatherapy works by the application of essential oils, most often through inhalation or application to the skin. Compounds in the oils can have direct physiological effects – on the skin itself or if they enter the body via the skin or mucous membranes. Essential oils can directly affect micro-organisms on the skin. Tea tree oil, for example, has been shown to have anti-allergic, anti-inflammatory and anti-microbial properties.[43]

When inhaled, the fragrant molecules from the oils trigger scent receptor cells in the nasal membranes. People differ in the number, types, and distribution of scent receptors in the nose and nasal passages, so some can detect a much greater range of smells than others, and some can detect smells at much lower concentrations than others. The signals from the scent receptors are processed in the olfactory areas of the brain which link directly with structures of the limbic system involved in mood, emotion, alertness, cognition and memory. Smells can have strong associations to past experiences and can evoke intense memories and emotions in some people.

The way a patient experiences a fragrance is partly a function of that person's particular physiological make-up, but psychological processes also play a major role. Each person has a unique individual history. Life experiences, feelings, thoughts, beliefs, and expectations mold the way people respond to things. The context of a previous encounter with a particular fragrance, how the patient was feeling at the time, what was happening and what happened next can also strongly influence the way they react to a subsequent exposure to the same or a similar fragrance. Feelings and thoughts can have diffuse effects throughout the body via the endocrine and autonomic nervous systems; signals from the body in turn affect feelings and thoughts. Mind and body are intimately interconnected.

Responses to the same fragrances can be different at different times of day and in different settings. Do not presume that a previous preference of EOs will still apply, and always offer the patient choices. Also, the way essential oils are delivered will influence their effects: whether singly or in combination; in a carrier oil or neat; along with other treatments such as massage or alone.

Essential oils can have a synergistic effect: two essential oils mixed together can have a better therapeutic effect than a single oil. For example, when supporting respiration, a blend of frankincense (*Boswellia carterii*) and eucalyptus (*Eucalyptus radiatia*) is usually effective; when addressing nausea, peppermint (*Menta piperita*) and spearmint (*Menta viridis*) work well together. Using a blend of EOs rather than using them singly may also help prevent the aroma becoming associated with the hospital experience and potentially causing distress later on when exposed to the same aroma.

How the therapist engages with the patient will make a difference to the effectiveness of the treatment. For instance, when explaining the benefits of the EOs, some people will engage through the facts about the oils (botanical detail, place of origin) and others will connect on an emotional level (personal associations; see example in Figure 13.8 below). This is hardly surprising given the psychological mechanisms involved.

Ways to use essential oils in the health care setting

Essential oils can be used in a variety of ways. As well as being used for patients they can also be helpful for professional caregivers and family.

Massage blend

In the hospital setting, typically the dilution is 1%, which would be 1 drop of EO in 5ml (1/6 oz) of carrier oil. The dilution may be increased at the qualified aromatherapist's discretion, such as 5 drops in 5 ml for local application in pain control, for a limited period of time.

> ### Tip 13.2 Naming blends
>
> A client is given a blend of EOs on a tissue to inhale during a massage session to help relieve feelings of nausea. They find the feeling of nausea is reduced, so you both agree a nasal inhaler stick with the same EO blend would be helpful for them. Labeling the stick "Nausea Blend" will remind them of feeling nauseous. It would be better to strengthen the association between the oils and the positive outcomes from the treatment session. Ask how they feel after the treatment, for example, "I feel much more settled and relaxed". Use this to label the nasal inhaler stick "Settling and Relaxing Blend," so strengthening the psychological association between the EO blend and the emotional/physiological benefits experienced.

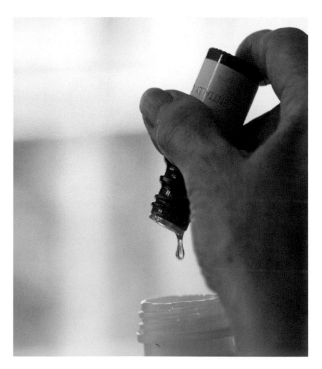

FIGURE 13.2
Dropping essential oil into the carrier oil.

(Photo by Sheila Scott.)

TABLE 13.1 Example of dilution ratio of carrier oil to essential oil

There are approximately 20 drops in 1 ml (1/30 oz) of essential oil.

Carrier oil volume		Essential oil dilution				
ml	USA fluid oz	1% Dilution	2% Dilution	3% Dilution	4% Dilution	5% Dilution
5 ml	1/6 oz	1 drop	2 drops	3 drops	4 drops	5 drops
10 ml	1/3 oz	2 drops	4 drops	6 drops	8 drops	10 drops
15 ml	1/2 oz	3 drops	6 drops	9 drops	12 drops	15 drops
20 ml	2/3 oz	4 drops	8 drops	12 drops	16 drops	20 drops
25 ml	5/6 oz	5 drops	10 drops	15 drops	20 drops	25 drops
30 ml	1 oz	6 drops	12 drops	18 drops	24 drops	30 drops
50 ml	1 2/3 oz	10 drops	20 drops	30 drops	40 drops	50 drops
100 ml	3 1/3 oz	20 drops	40 drops	60 drops	80 drops	100 drops

Dropper sizes can vary, so use a consistent dropper where possible.

Greater accuracy can be achieved by weighing the oils but the most common practice is to work with drops.

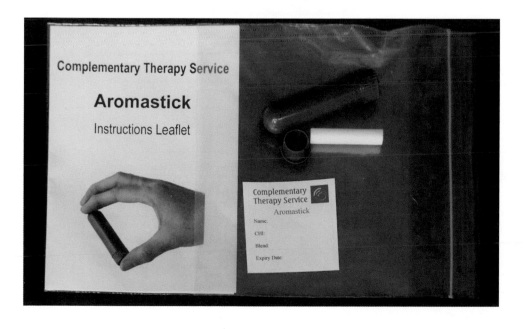

FIGURE 13.3
Aromastick kit (NIAS).

(Photo by Andrew Secretan.)

Nasal inhaler aromastick (NIAS)

One big advantage of NIAS is their low cost because one inhaler can be used for months. Saturate the cotton core of the stick with 10–20 drops of EO or blend. NIAS are used routinely to help patients achieve and sustain a calm state when undergoing stressful procedures, e.g. scans, cannulation (catheterization), radiotherapy (especially for patients with head and neck cancers), and to assist in smoking cessation.[44] They can also help with sleep, nausea, breathlessness, fatigue and anxiety. One patient remarked that the NIAS was: "Very good for relieving instant tension and then using every ten minutes until anxiety had lifted. My anxiety is caused by my illness, so overall I feel it definitely helps".[45]

Rhiannon Lewis advises reducing the dilution by half (5–10 drops) for patients with nausea and for palliative care patients. For nausea it is more effective to use the aroma for short periods of time at regular intervals.[46] Dyer et al. report that using a NIAS helped patients to recall benefits received during aromatherapy massage.[45] This associative effect may help to prolong treatment effectiveness.

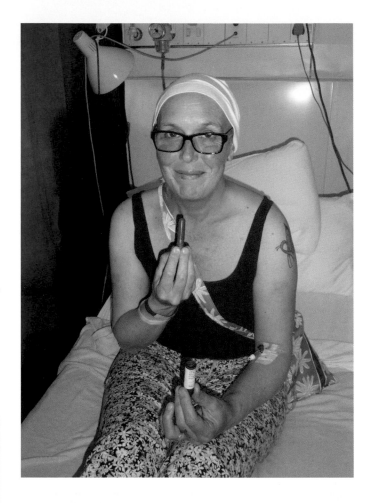

FIGURE 13.4
Patient using an aromastick prepared by the therapist.

(Photo by Angela Secretan.)

Info Box 13.4 Sample nausea blend

Note: blend may not be suitable for every individual.

50%	*Citrus limon*	(Lemon)
20%	*Mentha spicata*	(Spearmint)
20%	*Zingiber officinale*	(Ginger)
10%	*Pelargonium x asperum*	(Rose geranium)

Tip 13.3 Asthma or breathing difficulties

Patients with asthma or other breathing difficulties should not use a NIAS prior to, or immediately after, the use of nebulized or inhaler-delivered drugs.[45]

Aromapatch

Add 1–2 drops on the blank patch and stick onto chest area. They can be worn for 2–8 hours. These are designed so that the EOs enter the body through inhalation rather than being absorbed through the skin like a pain-relief patch.

Aroma diffusers

Suitable for use in single bedded rooms and shared spaces in which all of the patients give their consent. Use 2–4 drops of EOs, can be renewed every 2–3 hours subject to review/assessment.[20]

Room spray/spritzer

Hydrosols (aromatic waters) can be used in a clean spray bottle or EOs can be added to sterilized water. EOs don't dissolve in water, so shake the spray bottle vigorously every time before use. Spray as high as possible in the room to avoid spraying eyes or skin. The spray droplets will fall to the floor drawing down odor molecules and bacteria.[19]

Tissues/cotton ball

Place 2–4 drops on a tissue or cotton ball. The patient can either hold the tissue and inhale, or it can be put into a pajama pocket or inside a pillowcase.

Info Box 13.5 Blend for malodor

Offer several different pre-blended EOs for the patient to select fom. This can be added to a room spray, NIAS, or tissues, and can also be offered to nursing staff and relatives. With aroma diffusers, use 3–4 drops of EO blend. Can be renewed every 2–3 hours subject to review/assessment.[47]

10%	*Cymbopogon citratus; Cymbopogon flexuosus*	(Lemongrass)
30%	*Pogostemon cablin*	(Patchouli)
60%	*Citrus sinensis*	(Sweet orange)

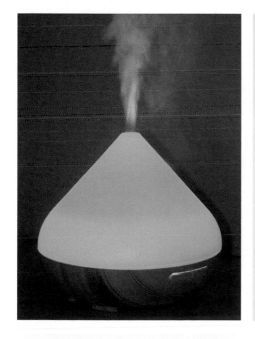

FIGURE 13.5
Aroma diffuser.

(Photo by Andrew Secretan.)

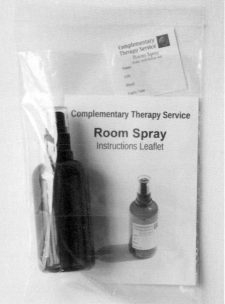

FIGURE 13.6
A room spray pack with bottle, label, and information leaflet.

(Photo by Andrew Secretan.)

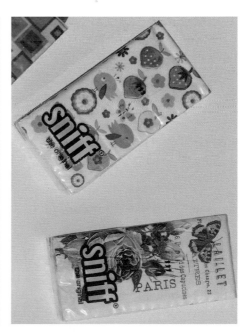

FIGURE 13.7
High quality, decorative tissue selection.

(Photo by Andrew Secretan.)

Chapter THIRTEEN

Jane, a lady in her 70s, was admitted to the palliative care unit for end-of-life care. She had advanced metastatic disease resulting from breast cancer that was treated 15 years prior. During the admission, one of Jane's sons disclosed that the family (husband and four sons), had only recently become aware of her diagnosis and prognosis.

The day after Jane's admission, I received her referral for complementary therapy. When I went to see Jane and introduce the complementary therapy service, her husband and son who were visiting were keen for her to receive massage. As she was so frail and had never received massage before, I suggested HEARTS (an acronym for a therapeutic process: **H**ands on, **E**mpathy, **A**romas, **R**elaxation, **T**extures, **S**ound.) I asked Jane if she liked any particular aromas. She told me she liked the smell of flowers, so I used a couple of drops of rose geranium and bergamot essential oils on a tissue and placed it on her bed. While she enjoyed the aromas, I gave her a short, comfort-oriented session incorporating gentle touch techniques over her clothing and bedding.

Her husband and son stayed in the room during the session. And as it happened, her son was happy to join in during the session by holding his mum's hand and gently copying the strokes on her arm that I was doing on her legs through the texture of the soft blanket. Jane said it felt lovely, and she rested during the 20-minute session. Her husband and son were so grateful that she had "the massage".

On my next visit with Jane, a week later, she was very weak and verbally unresponsive. Her family was standing vigil by the bedside and asked if she could have "the massage" again. While I was with her, Jane's family chose to go to the restaurant for coffee. I selected the oils she had chosen previously and placed the tissue on her bed. Resting my hand on Jane's, I noted it was cool to touch. I covered her hand with the soft blanket and spoke gently to her while stroking her arm. Jane's breathing began to change after a few minutes, so I beckoned the staff nurse to call back the family. They arrived just before Jane took her last breaths. Her family, all men, were visibly upset. I offered my sympathy and left them to be with their mum. Before I left, Jane's family expressed how pleased they were with the care and were comforted to see that she was at peace in her passing. The staff nurse also commented on how peaceful it was coming back into Jane's room; it was a lovely experience for her to witness.

Ann Marie McGrath RGN, BSc
Complementary Therapist, Dublin, Ireland

Settings

Aromatherapy options will vary depending on location in the hospital. There may be specific protocols for some areas. One area where EOs should not be used is a chemotherapy unit, due to the possibility of the aroma becoming associated with the chemotherapy and its side effects. These units also tend to be shared areas and it is difficult to get consent from all. In other shared spaces, such as a ward or four-bedded room, the presence of other patients will affect the acceptability of using essential oils in some ways. For example, a room diffuser should not be used unless suitable for and agreed on by everyone; a particular blend may not be helpful for all patients in that area or at that particular time. However, an aroma NIAS and EOs in a massage oil may be fine.

Ideally, health care facilities will have a dedicated Complementary Therapy room. This provides a space in which the aromatherapist can offer patients multiple ways to use the oils with fewer constraints.

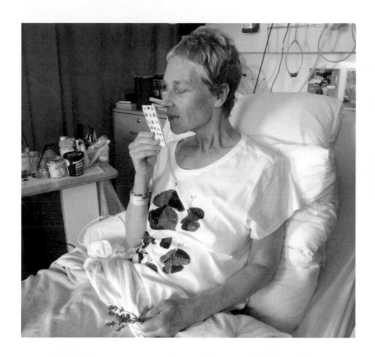

FIGURE 13.8
Delivering EOs on a tissue. A few minutes before we arrived to offer a session to this patient, the sister of a fellow patient brought in a sprig of lavender for her, which she is holding in the photograph. The previous day they had discussed how much the patient loved lavender. She was very touched by this kindness. We also noticed that the patient was wearing a butterfly top that her niece had hand-painted for her. Therefore, when offering her a choice of tissues we included ones with butterflies as an option, to carry on the theme. We also offered her lavender essential oil as part of the EO choices, which she did in fact choose. She was delighted how it had all come together and she felt very cared for. Picking up on cues and tapping into what is happening for the patient in the moment can help to enhance their healing experience.

(Photo by Angela Secretan.)

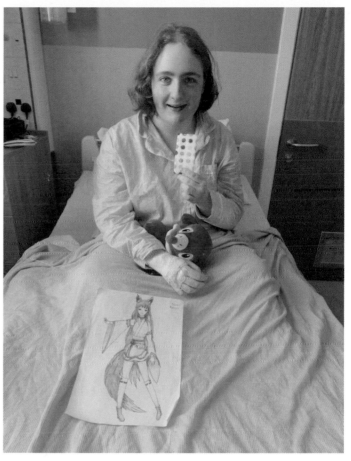

FIGURE 13.9
A drawing, plush toy, a smile, and aromatherapy tissue. This patient found aromatherapy sessions very relaxing and helpful, especially with the side effects of her chemotherapy treatment.

(Photo by Angela Secretan.)

Summary

Aromatherapy is a vast topic involving plant biology, chemistry, human physiology and psychology, amongst other disciplines. It offers exciting possibilities to improve outcomes for patients and the treatment experience as a whole. Although aromatherapy has been used within some mainstream health care and hospital settings over the past 30 years, it is still just starting its journey to become more broadly accepted and fully integrated into holistic patient care.

Test yourself

Multiple choice: Circle all of the correct answers. There may be more than one.

1. Which of the following is true about essential oils?

   A   The majority are created for the food and perfume sectors.
   B   They should never be used when taking other medications.
   C   They come from distillation of the root of the plant.
   D   They are natural and can do no harm.

2. Name two chemical compounds in EOs.

   A   1,8-Cineole.
   B   Copper oxide.
   C   Linalool.
   D   Bisodol.

3. Which department of the hospital typically should not use EOs?

   A   General medicine.
   B   Chemotherapy infusion.
   C   Cardiology.
   D   Palliative care.

4. Which of the following items should be on an EO bottle label?

   A   The chemotype, if applicable.
   B   The Greek name of the plant.
   C   Expiration date.
   D   Batch number.

5. Which of the following might alter the chemical composition of EOs?

   A   Heat.
   B   The carrier oil used to blend with the EO.
   C   The expectations of the therapist.
   D   Storage in a clear container.

6. The recommended ways for a therapist to use EOs is via:

   A   Blending with a massage carrier oil.
   B   Direct application of the EO to the skin.
   C   Room spray/spritzer.
   D   Application to the cervical, axillary, and inguinal areas of the body.

7. Which of the following oils is helpful for nausea?

   A   Rosemary.
   B   Siberian ginseng.
   C   Lemon.
   D   Eucalyptus.

8. Which of the following oils is helpful for malodor?

   A   Sweet orange.
   B   Eucalyptus.
   C   Ginger.
   D   Olive.

9. Which of the following are advantages to using an EO in a nasal inhaler aroma stick (NIAS)?

   A   The scent expands to fill the entire room.
   B   The patient can control the usage.
   C   The scent is more confined and better for shared settings.
   D   They last a long time.

10. Which of the following are true about essential oils?

   A   The pharmacological properties and effects can differ from plant to plant.
   B   EOs are regulated globally by the Council of Traditional Medicine.
   C   Essential oils should be stored in a cool, dark cupboard.
   D   Reputable suppliers of EOs can provide a gas chromatography–massage spectrometry report and a Material Safety Data Sheet.

References

1. Boyce R. Data indicate Neanderthal man used herbs for healing 60,000 years ago. The New York Times, 26 Nov 1975.

2. University of Virginia. A brief history of herbalism. 2007. Available from: http://exhibits.hsl.virginia.edu/herbs/brief-history/

3. Battaglia S. The Complete Guide to Aromatherapy. Virginia Q, Australia: The Perfect Potion (Aust) Pty Ltd; 1995.

4. Holmyard EJ. Alchemy. Mineola: Dover Publications; 1990.

5. Whitehead N. Essential oil profiles: how to choose a rose oil. 2014. Available from: https://www.oshadhi.co.uk/blog/essential-oil-profiles-how-to-choose-a-rose-oil/

6. Connelly D. The history of aspirin. 2014. Available from: https://www.pharmaceutical-journal.com/news-and-analysis/infographics/a-history-of-aspirin/20066661.article?firstPass=false

7. Shutes J. National Association of Holistic Aromatherapy: How Are Essential Oils Extracted? Available from: https://naha.org/explore-aromatherapy/about-aromatherapy/how-are-essential-oils-extracted

8. Buckle J. Clinical Aromatherapy Essential Oils in Healthcare (3rd edition). St Louis: Elsevier; 2015.

9. Barbieri C, Borsotto P. Essential oils: market and legislation. 2018. Available from: https://www.intechopen.com/books/potential-of-essential-oils/essential-oils-market-and-legislation

10. Johnson JR, Rivard RL, Griffin KH, et al. The effectiveness of nurse-delivered aromatherapy in an acute care setting. Complement Ther Med. 2016; 25:164–9.

11. All-Party Parliamentary Group for Integrated Healthcare (PGIH). Integrated Healthcare: Putting the pieces together. 2018. Available from: https://www.cnhc.org.uk/sites/default/files/Downloads/PGIH-Report.pdf

12. Committee on the Use of Complementary and Alternative Medicine by the American Public. Complementary and alternative medicine in the United States. Washington: The National Academies Press; 2005.

13. WHO. WHO Traditional Medicine Strategy 2014–2023. 2013. Available from: https://www.who.int/medicines/publications/traditional/trm_strategy14_23/en/

14. WHO Africa. Traditional Medicine. Available from: https://www.afro.who.int/health-topics/traditional-medicine

15. WHO. Global Report on Traditional and Complementary Medicine 2019. 2019. Available from: https://www.who.int/traditional-complementary-integrative-medicine/en/

16. Kohn M. Complementary therapies in cancer care: abridged report of a study produced for Macmillan Cancer Relief. 1999. Available from: https://www.bradfordvts.co.uk/wp-content/onlineresources/clinical-knowledge/complementary-medicine/complementary%20therapies%20in%20cancer%20care.pdf

17. Manley CH. Psychophysiological effect of odour. Critical Reviews in Food Science and Nutrition 1993; 33(1):57–62.

18. Komori T, Fujiwara R, Tanida M, et al. Effects of citrus fragrance on immune function and depressive states. Neuroimmunomodulation. 1995; 2:174–80.

19. Bagetta G, Morrone LA, Rombolà L, et al. Neuropharmacology of the essential oil of bergamot. Fitoterapia, 2010; 81(6): 453–61.

20. Tisserand, R, Balacs T. Essential Oil Safety. New York: Churchill Livingstone; 1995.

21. Price S, Price L. Aromatherapy for Health Professionals. New York: Churchill Livingstone; 1995.

22. Buckle J. Clinical Aromatherapy in Nursing. Arnold, MI: Singular Publishing Group, 1997.

23. Caddy R. Essential Oils in Colour. Rochester: Amberwood Publishing Ltd; 2000.

24. Kitikannakorn N, Chaiyakunapruk N, Nimpitakpong N, et al. An overview of the evidences of herbals for smoking cessation. Complement Ther Med. 2013; 21:557–64.

25. University of Bristol. Measure Yourself Medical Outcome Profile. Available from: http://www.bris.ac.uk/primaryhealthcare/resources/mymop/

26. Clarke S. Essential Chemistry for Safe Aromatherapy. London: Churchill Livingstone; 2002.

27. Bowles EJ. The Basic Chemistry of Aromatherapeutic Essential Oils. Crows Nest, NSW, Australia: Allen and Unwin; 2003.

28. International Federation of Professional Aromatherapists. Suspected Adverse Reaction to Aromatherapy Treatment. 2010. Available from: https://ifparoma.org/wp-content/uploads/2019/07/Adverse-Reaction-Report.pdf

29. International Federation of Professional Aromatherapists. IFPA Statement on Internal and Neat Use of Essential Oils. 2017. Available from: https://ifparoma.org/wp-content/uploads/2019/07/Statement-on-Internal-Neat-Use-of-Essential-Oils.pdf

30. Price L, Smith I, Price S. Carrier Oils for Aromatherapy and Massage. Stratford-upon-Avon: Riverhead; 1999.

31. Percival A. Aromatherapy: A Nurse's Guide. Christchurch: Amberwood Publishing Ltd; 1995.

32. Lakhan SE, Sheafer H, Tepper D. The effectiveness of aromatherapy in reducing pain: a systematic review and meta-analysis. Pain Research and Treatment 2016; 7:1–13.

33. Ganji R. Aromatherapy massage: a promising non-pharmacological adjuvant treatment for osteoarthritis knee pain. Korean J Pain 2019; 32(2): 133–4.

34. Martin GN. The effect of exposure to odor on the perception of pain. Psychosomatic Medicine 2006; 68(4):613–6.

35. Louis M, Kowalski SD. Use of aromatherapy with hospice patients to decrease pain, anxiety, and depression and to promote an increased sense of well-being. The American Journal of Hospice & Palliative Care 2002;19(6):381–6.

36. Bagheri-Nesami M, Espahbodi F, Nikkhah A, et al. The effects of lavender aromatherapy on pain following needle insertion into a fistula in hemodialysis patients. Complement Ther Clin Pract 2014; 20(1):1–4.

37. Bouya S, Ahmadidarehsima S, Badakhsh M, et al. Effect of aromatherapy interventions on hemodialysis complications: a systematic review. Complementary Therapies in Clinical Practice 2018; 32:130–8.

38. Seyyed-Rasoolia A, Salehib F, Mohammadpooraslc A, et al. Comparing the effects of aromatherapy massage and inhalation aromatherapy on anxiety and pain in burn patients: a single-blind randomized clinical trial. Burns 2016; 42:(8): 1774–80.

39. Fearrington MA, Qualls BW, Carey MG. Essential oils to reduce postoperative nausea and vomiting. J Perianesthia Nursing 2019; 34(5):1047–53.

40. Cho EH, Lee MY, Hur MH. The effects of aromatherapy on intensive care unit patients' stress and sleep quality: a nonrandomised controlled trial. 2017. Available from: https://www.ncbi.nlm.nih.gov/pmc/articles/PMC5742427/

41. Ayik C, Ozden D. The effects of preoperative aromatherapy massage on anxiety and sleep quality of colorectal surgery patients: A randomized controlled study. Complementary Therapies in Medicine 2018; 36:93–9.

42. Muz G, Tasci S. Effect of aromatherapy via inhalation on the sleep quality and fatigue level in people undergoing hemodialysis. Applied Nursing Research 2017; 37: 28–35.

43. Peace Rhind J. Aromatherapeutic Blending: Essential Oils in Synergy. London: Singing Dragon; 2016.

44. Carter A, Maycock P, Mackereth P. Aromasticks in clinical practice. In Essence 2011; 10:16–19.

45. Dyer J, McNeil S, Ragsdale-Lowe M, Tratt L. A snap-shot of current practice: the use of aromasticks in symptom management. International Journal of Clinical Aromatherapy 2008; 5(2): 17–21.

46. Lewis R. Clinical Aromatherapy Challenges in Cancer and Palliative Care. Essential Oil Resource Consultants course notes. Strathcarron Hospice (Scotland), March 2009.

47. Tavares M. Integrating Clinical Aromatherapy in Specialist Palliative Care: The Use of Oils for Symptom Management. Canada: 80Print; 2011.

Additional resources

Collinge and Associates. Touch, Caring & Cancer: Simple Instruction for Family and Friends. Maine: Collinge and Associates; 2009.

Conrad P. Women's Health Aromatherapy. London: Singing Dragon; 2019.

Godfrey H. Essential Oils for Mindfulness and Meditation. Rochester: Inner Traditions Bear & Company; 2018.

Kerkhof M. Complementary Nursing in End of Life Care. Wernhout: Kicozo; 2015.

Kerkhof M. CO_2 Extracts in Aromatherapy: 50+ Extracts for Clinical Applications. Wernhout: Kicozo; 2018.

Ratajc P. Botanical names and chemotypes: do you know what's in your bottle. 2017. Available from: https://phytovolatilome.com/botanical-names-and-chemotypes/

Tisserand R, Young R. Essential Oil Safety (2nd edition). Churchill Livingstone: London; 2014.

Journals

Aromatherapy Today. https://www.aromatherapytoday.com/

Aromatika. www.aromatika.hu

International Journal of Aromatherapy. Co-editors: Robert Tisserand and Bob Harris.

International Journal of Clinical Aromatherapy. Editor: Rhiannon Lewis; Associate editor: Gabriel Mojay.

The International Journal of Professional Holistic Aromatherapy. Editor: Lora Cantele.

Perfect Potion. Editor: Salvatore Battaglia.

Conferences

(AIA) International Aromatherapy Conference and Wellness Expo

Aromatica: https://www.aromaticaaustralia.com/

Botanica: http://botanica2020.com

International Conference on Botanical Medicine and Aromatherapy: https://waset.org/conference/2019/06/copenhagen/ICBMA

(NAHA) Aromatherapy Conference: http://www.nahaconference.com

The Essence of Clinical Aromatherapy: https://www.royalmarsden.nhs.uk/essence-clinical-aromatherapy

Websites

Aromatherapy Trade Council: www.a-t-c.org.uk

Australian Research Centre in Complementary and Integrative Medicine: www.uts.edu.au/research-and-teaching/our-research/complementary-and-integrative-medicine

Dropsmith Aromatherapy: https://dropsmith.com

Essential Oil Resource Consultants: www.essentialorc.com

National Centre for Complementary & Integrative Health (NCCIH): https://nccih.nih.gov

United Nations Industrial Development Organization: https://www.unido.org/

Professional bodies

In many parts of the world, aromatherapy is unregulated and unlicensed. Many CAM bodies have voluntary registers or professional associations that practitioners can join if they choose. Usually, these associations or registers require that practitioners have completed relevant training or hold certain qualifications and agree to uphold professional Codes of Conduct, Ethics and Performance. Examples are given below.

AIA	Alliance of International Aromatherapists (AIA): www.alliance-aromatherapists.org
BCAOA	British Columbia Alliance Of Aromatherapy: https://bcaoa.org/
CFA	Canadian Federation of Aromatherapists: www.cfacanada.com
CNHC	Complementary & Natural Healthcare Council: https://www.cnhc.org.uk (In the UK many NHS jobs and opportunities for working with integrated health care require CNHC registration.)
FHT	Federation of Holistic Therapists: https://www.fht.org.uk
HKAA	Hong Kong Aromatherapy Association: www.aahk.com.hk
IFA	International Federation of Aromatherapists: https://ifaroma.org
IFPA	International Federation of Professional Aromatherapists: www.ifparoma.org
JSA	Japanese Society of Aromatherapy: www.aroma-jsa.jp
NAHA	National Association for Holistic Aromatherapy: www.naha.org
NZROHA	New Zealand Registrar of Holistic Aromatherapists: http://www.aromatherapy.org.nz
PIA	The Pacific Institute of Aromatherapy: www.pacificinstituteofaromatherapy.com

Chapter THIRTEEN

APPENDIX 13.1 Examples of essential oils extracted from different plant parts

Part used	Essential oils, *Latin names,* (botanical family name)	Some essential oil properties	Typical chemical constituents
Roots	Ginger *Zingiber officinale* (Zingiberaceae)	Analgesic, anti-inflammatory, anti-emetic, antiseptic, antispasmodic, bactericidal, carminative.	α-Pinene (trace–0.5%), camphene (0.1–2.1%), β-pinene (trace–2.0%), 1,8-cineole (4.1–11.2%), linalool (0.8–2.7%), borneol (0.5–2.2%), γ-terpineol (0.4–2.4%), nerol (0.1–2.8%), neral (8.1–27.4), geraniol (3.1–23.0%), geranial (12.7–35.8%), geranyl acetate (trace–29.4%), β-bisabolene (0.9–2.9%), zingiberene (1.8–13.7%).
Resin	Frankincense *Boswellia carterii* (Burseraceae)	Analgesic, antibacterial, anticatarrhal, antidepressive, anti-infectious, astringent, balsamic, calmative, carminative, cicatrisant, expectorant, immune tonic, stomachic, vulnerary.	α-Pinene (4.6%), camphene (1.1%), octanol (8.0%), linalool (2.5%), octyl acetate (52.0%), bornyl acetate (1.0%), incensole (2.4%), incensyl acetate (3.4%).
Wood	Cedarwood, Atlas *Cedrus atlantica* (Pinaceae)	Analgesic, anti-inflammatory, antiseptic, antispasmodic, astringent, diuretic, expectorant, insecticide, sedative.	α-,β- and γ-Himalchenes (70%), α- and γ-atlantone isomers (10–15%), himachalol (2–4%), δ-cadinene, γ-curcumene.
Leaves	Eucalyptus, blue gum *Eucalyptus globulus var. globulus* (Myrtaceae)	Analgesic, antibacterial, anti-inflammatory, antineuralgic, antirheumatic, antispasmodic, antiviral, astringent, balsamic, cicatrisant, decongestant, deodorant, diuretic, expectorant, febrifuge, hypoglycemic, rubefacient, stimulant, vermifuge, vulnerary.	α-Pinene (10.66%), β-pinene (0.18%), α-phellandrene (0.09%), 1,8-cineole (69.10%), limonene (3.29%), terpinen-4-ol (0.22%), aromadendrene (1.63%), epiglobulol (0.80%), piperitone (0.1%), globulol (5.33%).
Seeds	Cardomon *Elettaria cardamomum* (Zingiberaceae)	Antiseptic, antispasmodic, carminative, cephalic, digestive, diuretic, expectorant, stimulant, stomachic, tonic.	α-Pinene (1.5%), β-pinene (0.2%), sabinene (2.8%), myrcene (1.6%), α-phellandrene (0.2%), limonene (11.6%), 1,8-cineole (36.3%), γ-terpinene (0.7%), p-cymene (0.1%), terpinolene (0.5%), linalool (3.0%), linalyl acetate (2.5%), terpinen-4-ol (0.9%), α-terpineol (2.6%), α-terpinyl acetate (31.3%), citronellol (0.3%), nerol (0.5%), geraniol (0.5%), methyl eugenol (0.2%), trans-nerolidol (2.7%).
Berries	Juniper *Juniperus communis* (Cupressaceae)	Antirheumatic, antiseptic, antispasmodic, antitoxic, astringent, carminative, cicatrisant, depurative, diuretic, emmenagogue, nervine, rubefacient, stimulating, stomachic, sudorific, tonic, vulnerary.	α-Pinene (25-55%), sabinene (up to 30%), β-myrcene (up to 25%), terpinen-4-ol (up to 18%), ι-limonene (up to 10%), γ-terpinene, δ-3-carene, *para*-cymene, β-caryophyllene, α-terpineol.

continued

APPENDIX 13.1 Examples of essential oils extracted from different plant parts *continued*

Part used	Essential oils, *Latin names,* (botanical family name)	Some essential oil properties	Typical chemical constituents
Flowers	Rose *Rosa damascena* (Rosaceae)	Analgesic, anti-asthmatic, antidepressant, anti-inflammatory, antiphlogistic, antioxidant, antiseptic, antispasmodic, antiviral, aphrodisiac, astringent, bronchodilator, bactericidal, choleretic, cicatrisant, depurative, emmenagogue, hemostatic, hepatic, laxative, sedative, stomachic, tonic.	Citronellol (34–55%), geraniol and nerol (30–40%), stearopten (16–22%), phenyl ethanol (1.5–3%), farnesol (0.2–2%).
Needles & twigs	Cypress *Cupressus sempervirens* Cupressaceae	Antibacterial, anti-infectious, antirheumatic, antispasmodic, antisudorific, astringent, calmative, deodorant, diuretic (mild), lymphatic decongestant, neurotonic, phlebotonic, prostatic decongestant.	α-Pinene (49%), δ-3-carene (22%), limonene (5%), α-terpinolene (5%), myrcene (4%), α-cedrol (3.5%), β-pinene (2.5%), germacrene D (1.5%), sabinene (1%), γ-terpinene (1%).
Leaves & twigs	Petitgrain *Citrus aurantium var. amara* (Rutaceae)	Antiseptic, antispasmodic, deodorant, digestive stimulant, nervine stimulant, stomachic, tonic.	Esters (40–80%), mainly linalyl acetate and geranyl acetate, also linalol, nerol, terpineol, geraniol, nerolidol, farnesol, limonene, and others.
Blossoms	Neroli *Citrus aurantium var. amara* (Rutaceae)	Antibacterial, antidepressive, anti-infectious, antiparasitic, astringent, calmative, digestive stimulant, phlebotonic.	Linalol (34%), linalyl acetate (6–17%), limonene (15%), pinene, nerolidol, geraniol, nerol, methyl anthranilate, indole, citral, jasmone, others.
Fruit	Orange, bitter *Citrus aurantium var. amara* (Rutaceae)	Anti-inflammatory, antiseptic, astringent, bactericidal, carminative, choleretic, fungicidal, sedative, stomachic (mild), tonic.	Monoterpenes (90+%) mainly limonene, myrcene, camphene, pinene, ocimene, cymene and small amounts of alcohols, aldehydes and ketones.

The last 3 EOs listed above all come from the same tree. Different parts of the tree at different times of the year are used to make different EOs. They have similar properties, but different chemical composition and therapeutic uses.

While the goal of most hospitalization is to save lives, people do sometimes die in health care settings. This can occur unexpectedly due to post-surgical complications, or in the course of treating almost any serious illness. Even when death is expected and planned for by signing on to hospice or terminal care services, an inpatient environment is sometimes needed to cope with symptoms. This chapter is dedicated to the end of life in health care settings, including hospitals, skilled nursing homes, and assisted living facilities, and the role that massage therapists can play in supporting this experience. As the title of this chapter suggests, death and dying involve deep mystery for all concerned – patients, their loved ones, and their caregivers. Therapists will be affected and changed by their encounters with people during this very challenging, sacred time.

Dying in the hospital

According to numerous studies, most people say they want to die at home. Yet in many countries, the majority of expected deaths (60–75%) occur in the hospital.[1,2] Hospital deaths present a challenge in that many elements of care that dying people say are important to them a sense of control and person-centered care, for example – are hard to achieve in settings designed to treat the physical body, even at the expense of the patient's mental and emotional well-being. In an effort to address this problem, many hospitals around the world now feature palliative care departments, with multidisciplinary teams to address the physical, psychological, social and spiritual needs of patients and their families. Designed to reduce symptoms of disease and side effects of treatment, palliative care can exist alongside curative treatment, beginning at diagnosis with any serious illness.

Palliative care is not synonymous with hospice care, though the two are often confused. Both palliative care and hospice care focus on holistic support to reduce suffering and enhance quality of life. However, hospice is considered to be end-of-life care, which is exclusively comfort-focused. In order for patients to qualify for hospice services, they must stop curative treatment for the terminal illness. A common misconception is to equate hospice with "no care," which is grossly inaccurate. Hospice treats symptoms, aggressively if necessary, so that patients can live their remaining days to the fullest.

In the US, a patient can begin hospice when two physicians certify that the person has a likely six-month prognosis. In the Netherlands, the time frame is three months, while Australia defines end-of-life care as that which occurs in the last 12 months of life.[3] Prognosis is, of course, an inexact science. When patients outlive their projected lifespans, they may request to be recertified for hospice services. Some countries refer to hospice as end-of-life care, or terminal care, and this is typically provided where the patient lives, e.g. at home or residential care facility. If symptoms cannot be managed at home, a more aggressive approach to achieving patient comfort is provided in designated inpatient environments. These may be freestanding facilities, or a delegated area of an existing hospital.

Massage therapists may find themselves providing services in any of the environments described above, hospitals, residential care facilities, or hospice inpatient units. It is important for therapists to be informed about the environments in which they work. But it is also important for therapists to be aware of the ways that the dying process is impacted by the context in which it occurs. Patients and their loved ones are affected by the presence or absence of rules governing who can visit and when, whether pets are allowed, support or lack thereof for visitors, including furniture for them to sit or sleep on, lighting, whether privacy is available, whether food preferences are honored, and even what the patient wears. While a hospital gown allows easy access for care of the physical body, some patients report feeling disempowered and "stripped" of their identities when they wear a gown instead of clothing.[4] Even the story of how a person arrives at the inpatient environment is relevant.

The intent of this chapter is to prepare massage therapists with information that will help them provide skilled, compassionate care that fosters choice, dignity, safety and peace. This care extends to the significant others who are impacted by the patient's illness. Clinical considerations in this chapter therefore include care for the loved ones that therapists will encounter at the bedside.

Chapter FOURTEEN

Some patients arrive at our hospice inpatient unit by car, but most come by ambulance. They come in crisis, exhausted and frightened, as are their loved ones. Some are transferred to our care from the hospital after it becomes clear that treatment is not working, or the side effects of treatment have become too much to bear. For these patients, the referral to hospice is new, and they are still absorbing the impact of their situation. Regardless of their stories, patients come to us with some degree of trauma.

I was thinking about this one day when I arrived at work and saw an ambulance in our driveway. The EMTs were brisk and efficient, unloading the patient and getting him into the elevator before his eyes could adjust to the changes in light. I found myself looking into his eyes, which were very wide and jaundiced. Resisting my brain's urge to guess his terminal diagnosis, I checked in with my heart and felt a surge of com passion and protectiveness toward this scared, sick person. Because the elevator was small, I stood very close to him. "Welcome," I said. "We're going to take good care of you." The man nodded, but said nothing.

Later in the day after he had been assessed by the medical team, I visited this same patient to offer him massage. His room was full of family, but my eye contact was with him. "Hello, I'm not sure if you remember meeting me from this morning," I began. But he quickly said "Yes," and just as quickly said yes, he would like a massage. I worked in silence on his hands, arms, shoulders, neck, legs and feet. His family visited with one another and occasionally checked in with him. "How are you doing, Dad? Does that feel good, Dad?" The patient did not say a word, just nodded his head. I could see that he was tired, but he remained vigilant and alert. He'd only been with us a few hours, and it would likely take more time for him to feel relief from his symptoms.

I finished up and lowered the patient's hospital bed so that his family would be at eye level while sitting next to him. I straightened his covers and was about to leave the room when the patient put his hand on my arm. "You all sure know how to take care of people," he said. I smiled and replied, "That's good to hear." Though it was likely too soon for his actual symptoms to be improved, I realized this patient already felt better. He felt better because he felt safe.

Cindy Spence LMT
Dallas, Texas

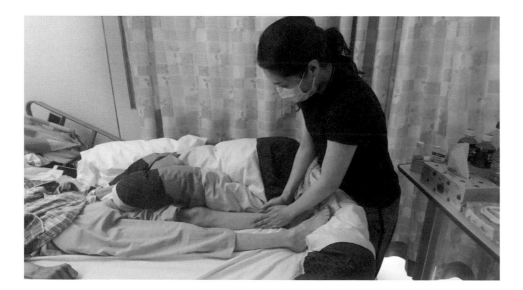

FIGURE 14.1
Massage can soften the clinical setting of a hospital, allowing the patient to experience transcendent moments of pleasure.

(Photo by Alfred Kwok.)

Adapting massage for the end of life

Massage can offer moments of comfort, well-being and beauty that honor the dying person up until and even beyond the last breath. Benefits of end-of-life massage include decreased anxiety and fear, decreased pain, improved relaxation and sleep, enhanced lubrication of distressed skin, and reduced feelings of isolation. Therapists who work with this population report that the benefits of massage extend to loved ones who are comforted by the sessions, both because they provide relief to the dying person, and because they are relaxing to observe. A caregiver in Dallas wrote, "My husband died of prostate cancer at the hospice unit last year. The staff gave him wonderful care, but I think the thing he appreciated most was the gentle and loving touch he received from the massage therapist. I could tell it calmed his nerves, and it calmed mine too, knowing he enjoyed it so much." Another benefit is that massage therapists can serve as role models and teachers for loved ones who wish to remain connected to the dying person through gentle touch.

Because the goal of care is shifting from focus on cure to focus on comfort, the massage therapist's role at the end of life is not to "fix" or treat. It can be difficult for result-oriented therapists to make this shift. But any agenda to change outcome can create expectation that is not helpful to the dying person. The massage therapy session that aspires to nothing more than caring presence can offer rest in the midst of turmoil, uncertainty and grief. This is not to say that hope is lost when treatment has failed to achieve the desired results. People at the end of life still hope for many things. They may hope for time to reach a particular milestone, a good night's sleep, a bowel movement, or to feel well enough to enjoy a loved one's visit. It can be helpful for the massage therapist to ask, "What are you hoping for today?" so that the intention of each massage session can be geared to the patient's changing goals and realities.[5]

All of the modifications described in Chapter 6 – pressure, site and position – apply to working with people at the end of life. As dying demands more energy and symptoms become more severe, the massage session must adapt to these changes by dialing back. A 60-minute session, considered by many to be standard, is typically too long. The length of the session should match the energy level of the recipient, becoming shorter over time as the patient declines. At the very end of life, the session might be only 10 minutes in length. It is sometimes necessary or preferable to work over clothing or bed linen. Potential reasons for this include the demands of undressing and dressing, lack of privacy, cultural norms regarding modesty, and warmth for the patient.

Site restrictions for end-of-life massage mirror those mentioned elsewhere in this book (see Common site restrictions, Chapter 6). Compromised areas of the body – extremities with edema, for example – may be touched gently with resting hands or a light stroke. Some terminal patients experience such intolerable pain in an area of the body that they do not want that area touched, even lightly. Other localized site restrictions include fractures and open skin from falls; bedsores, cellulitis, fungating tumors and other areas of skin breakdown; and indwelling medical devices or pain patches. It would be difficult to list all of the potential end-of-life scenarios that might require site restrictions. It is incumbent on massage therapists working in inpatient environments to utilize the patient chart or information from medical team members to determine a safe approach to the touch session.

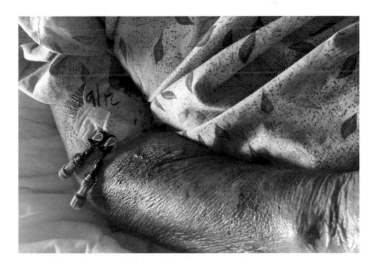

FIGURE 14.2
This photo demonstrates several common scenarios at the end of life, which indicate site restrictions. The double-lumen PICC line is to be avoided, as is the scabbed skin just distal to the elbow. Gentle holds could be applied to the lower arm, while the hand and shoulder would likely tolerate light lotioning.

(Photo by Cindy Spence.)

Chapter FOURTEEN

Positioning adjustments for the end of life likewise follow the information offered in Chapter 6. Common end-of-life conditions requiring positioning adjustments include ascites, dyspnea, edema or lymphedema, fractures, heart conditions, and broken skin. In early decline, patients may still tolerate a range of positions, including side-lying or seated, which both give excellent access to the back. In later decline, patients spend more time in bed where the most commonly tolerated position is supine with the head of the bed elevated. A true side-lying position may become difficult, though staff will often place a thin pillow under a hip, creating a side-leaning supine position; this allows pressure to be periodically shifted off the sacrum. Patients typically provide information, verbal or nonverbal, to indicate their preferred positions. The patient's favored sleeping position can be a nice option for massage, given the likelihood of falling asleep during the session.

The most important adaptation to be made for massage at the end of life is the adjustment of pressure. Advanced disease and dying place great demands on every organ system. Some of these demands are obvious, and others are hidden below the surface of the skin. Deep pressure to even a small area of the body can cause damage to fragile tissues and bone. Therapists who have been trained to fix problems are at risk of overtreating and causing unintended harm to their patients. In terms of pressure, less is *always* more when working with end-of-life patients. Deep presence can be communicated by leaning in (energetically, rather than physically), by using full-handed contact, and listening with *all* of the senses such that the rest of the world falls away for the duration of the session. The depth of this focus is safer and far more powerful than deep pressure.

As mentioned previously in this book, there is no person who is too medically fragile to receive some type of skilled touch. The Pressure Scale (Table 6.1) is a helpful gauge for therapists working with hospital patients and other compromised clients. Level 2 pressure (light contact with superficial muscle) is appropriate for most conditions and most areas of the body at the end of life, though some conditions or sites require level 1 pressure

(light lotioning). During active dying, as discussed later in this chapter, level 1 pressure is indicated. Therapists working with people at the end of life would do well to seek training in a variety of soft-touch modalities, including Reiki or Therapeutic Touch.

Tip 14.1 When patients request deep pressure

Even patients at the end of life sometimes request deep massage pressure, requiring the therapist to balance confidence in his or her knowledge with the expressed desire of the dying patient. Communication, concise education, and finesse can go a long way in reassuring the patient that the therapist is hearing the request. Promising "focused attention" on the area of concern is one approach. Another is to provide slightly firmer pressure on a safe area of the body. An example of this might be the plantar aspect of the feet in a patient who is still ambulatory. Most patients (indeed most therapists) are surprised to discover how effective light pressure can be, when provided with focused, caring attention.

Common symptoms at the end of life

Death and dying involve many of the same conditions and symptoms discussed in Chapter 8. However, some are presented again in this chapter because the causes, significance, progression, and appropriate responses to these symptoms are unique during the dying process. Symptoms are often linked, one causing or exacerbating another, as systems of the body slow down and eventually stop. A symptom that might be considered an emergency at any other time in the life cycle may indicate the normal process of dying. The patient's terminal diagnosis, comorbidities, age, degree of social support, culture, religion, beliefs about death, and general coping style all play a role in the presentation of symptoms at the end of life. Those same factors, combined with the goals of the patient and his or her appointed decision-makers, guide the end-of-life care plan.

Anorexia and cachexia

One of the first signs of decline in a terminal patient is loss of appetite, or anorexia. Anorexia is a natural end-of-life symptom as the body loses its capacity to make use of food and water. The stages of the digestive process (chewing, swallowing, moving food and fluids through the digestive tract, breaking food down and eliminating waste) all require energy. As the efficiency of this system declines, a number of factors contribute to impaired food intake, including fatigue, early satiety, nausea with or without vomiting, and difficulty swallowing. End-of-life nutrition can be further complicated for some patients by poverty, inadequate caregiver support, depression, dementia, poor oral health, pain, and dyspnea.

Cachexia refers to the extreme wasting of muscle that results from anorexia. Often associated with advanced cancers, cachexia can accompany almost any terminal diagnosis, including cancer, AIDS, renal disease, congestive heart failure (CHF), chronic obstructive pulmonary disease (COPD) and aging. Anorexia and cachexia involve systemic inflammation and release of cytokines, which interfere with the absorption and synthesis of nutrients. Even if the dying person could consume enough calories to sustain life, the body would be unable to break down and use those calories. For this reason, artificial nutrition and hydration are rarely worth the serious problems they can cause, including increased congestion, edema, infection, aspiration of food into the lungs, and subsequent pneumonia. Corticosteroids may be used on a short-term basis to temporarily increase appetite, but side effects can likewise outweigh benefits.

The symptoms of anorexia and cachexia can be extremely hard for loved ones to accept, as eating is associated with will to live and rituals that bind people together. Families often say, "If he would just eat something," indicating grief, frustration and misunderstanding about the role of anorexia in the dying process. It is not uncommon for conflicts about food to arise between patients and their loved ones, who may have difficulty understanding why the medical team is not taking a more aggressive approach toward nutrition and hydration. Hospice philosophy is to support patient comfort throughout the natural dying process, including the body's release of pain-relieving endorphins as the patient becomes unable to eat and drink. Pleasure feedings are provided as desired and tolerated by the patient, along with education and compassionate support for patients and families to make their own decisions. These measures include education, bereavement services, and encouragement to explore connections with the patient that don't involve food. Spouses, partners, parents, siblings, and friends, even very young children, can be taught to provide gentle touch as a means to "nourish" the dying person.

Clinical considerations: Anorexia and cachexia

Pressure:

- Level 2 pressure for mild to moderate cachexia.
- Level 1 pressure for severe cachexia (indicated by temporal wasting).

Site:

- Bony prominences may be especially sensitive.

Positioning:

- Bony prominences are at risk of skin breakdown. "Floating" both heels (see Figure 6.3) and shifting the patient to left- or right-leaning supine can protect the heels and sacrum.
- Extra propping with pillows or rolled towels to fill hollow spaces will provide a sensation of support.

Other:

- Length of massage session should be shortened to reduce demands on the body.

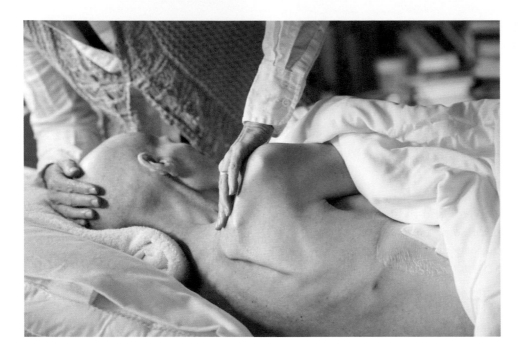

FIGURE 14.3
A rolled washcloth fills the hollow space between the patient's neck and the pillow below. Supporting these spaces helps the patient to feel grounded and safe.

(Photo by Candice White.)

Anxiety

The human brain is hard-wired for survival. Sensing danger, the primitive brainstem activates the sympathetic nervous system for fight or flight. Neurochemicals, such as cortisol and norepinephrine, are released into the body, triggering sensations that range from a vague sense of unease to full-blown panic. Dying typically involves some degree of anxiety, as the body's survival is literally at risk. Loss of control, fear of the unknown, pain and other symptoms, pending separation from loved ones, and worry about family and finances are just a few of the factors which contribute to end-of-life anxiety. Anxiety in turn can negatively impact other symptoms, including pain and shortness of breath. While medication is often needed to help patients manage this symptom, nonpharmacological approaches can play a helpful role. Massage therapy can help shift the body out of "fight or flight" and into "rest and digest," also known as the parasympathetic nervous system.

Science suggests that nerve fibers in the skin known as CT afferent fibers, or "pleasant touch fibers," respond most favorably to slow, gentle movement, specifically, gliding touch at a speed of five centimeters, or two inches, per second.[6] Slowing down is reported by patients and families to be very calming, both on and off the body.

A therapist who is mindful of the speed with which they move, speak, initiate contact, conduct the touch session and exit the room creates a very different energy than a therapist who is not mindful of these things. Irene Smith, a pioneer of end-of-life massage, urges therapists to "pause, listen, and observe" the feelings and dynamics already present in the client's space.[7] Moving slowly and gently, a sense of grounding, and attending to one's own breath, especially the exhalation, can help therapists who aspire to be the calm one in the room. Calm, caring presence in the face of anxiety and fear may be the biggest gift we have to offer people and their loved ones at the end of life.

Of note, anxiety in patients with dementia or nonverbal patients may present as extreme restlessness, including inability to be still, attempting to get out of bed for no known reason, or insistence on looking for "lost" items. The reactions of these patients must be closely monitored to assess whether massage is making things better or worse. Even patients who have previously enjoyed massage may reach a point, temporarily or permanently, when they do not wish to be touched. Assessment for changes in response to massage should be ongoing, providing patients with choice and control.

Clinical considerations: Anxiety

Pressure:

- Full-handed level 2 pressure (holds, gentle compression or slow gliding).

Site:

- Discuss any area the patient protects or wishes not to be touched.
- Simply holding the patient's hand can be soothing, but hold from underneath rather than on top.

Positioning:

- Support patient preference, offering propping for comfort and security.

Tip 14.2 Propping to reduce anxiety

Anxious patients, both those who do not tolerate touch and those who do, will benefit from attentive propping. Pillows and other soft materials, such as rolled towels, washcloths, blankets, and pieces of foam, can be used to create contours that conform to, cradle and hold the patient's body. One example of this is placing pillows beneath each arm when the patient is in high Fowler's, or semi-seated in bed, a common "vigilant" position for anxious patients (see Figure 14.4).

Apnea

Apnea is defined as the temporary cessation of breathing. Unlike sleep apnea, which is generally a treatable condition in a healthy person, end-of-life apnea is a natural and progressive process, which takes place as the respiratory system begins to shut down. Respirations may be fast, slow, shallow, deep, or any combination of those features, punctuated by periods of no breathing at all. This variable pattern, known as Cheyne–Stokes breathing, is a hallmark of active dying. As the ability to swallow is lost, secretions gather at the back of the throat. This congestion is audible as a crackling sound, historically known as the "death rattle." There may be loud gurgling, snoring, or soft moaning with each exhalation. As active dying progresses, periods of apnea may increase up to a minute or longer, with lots of waiting in between.

One example of matching the massage session to the patient's energy level can be for the therapist to stop moving during an episode of apnea, simply resting the hands

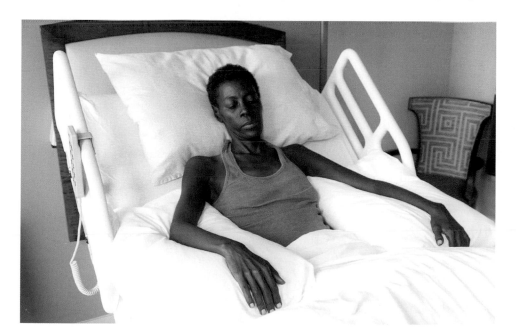

FIGURE 14.4
Pillows under the arms give the upper extremities something to rest on, conveying a sense of security and support. Good propping can communicate to the nervous system that it is safe to let go.

(Photo by Candice White.)

on the patient's body. This also provides the opportunity for the therapist to monitor the duration of apnea for charting or reporting to the medical team. It is not unusual, as the patient relaxes, for periods of apnea to grow longer during a massage session.

Clinical considerations: Apnea

Pressure:

- Apnea signals that the patient is in the active stage of dying. Level 1 pressure or holds are indicated.

Positioning:

- Generally, by the time a patient has apnea, he or she will be in a supine position.

Confusion, agitation and restlessness

Confusion may be part of a terminal disease process, such as dementia, renal failure, liver failure, brain cancer, or cancers that metastasize to the brain. Some medications can cause confusion, such as steroids and opioids. It can also be triggered by infections, particularly urinary tract infections, as well as dehydration, electrolyte disturbance, the urge to urinate or defecate, fecal impaction, hip fracture, hypoxia, acidosis, lung disease, or diabetic ketoacidosis. The accumulation of opioid metabolites in the body, once urination ceases, is an additional cause.

Confusion ranges from mild and benign to severe and disturbing. It may manifest as a disturbance of the wake-sleep cycle, or a phenomenon known as "near death awareness," when patients seem to have access to another dimension in which deceased loved ones visit the bedside. Another common presentation is terminal restlessness, characterized by picking at bedclothes, random or repetitive hand motions, or attempting to get out of bed. In severe cases, known as terminal delirium, the patient may hallucinate, cry out, or become combative.

If the source of confusion seems clear, such as with fecal impaction, infection, or low oxygen level, the care team will attempt to treat the cause. But if death appears to be imminent, it is sometimes necessary to provide support for confusion, without determining or addressing the cause. Sedation and around-the-clock observation may be required. Sometimes confusion is helped by the presence of familiar loved ones. At other times, visitors seem to be a complicating factor. Reducing stimuli, such as lighting, noise and activity, is generally helpful. For some patients, slow, grounding touch by a massage therapist or family member may be soothing. For others, touch is a source of stimulation that causes arousal rather than comfort. Massage therapists working in the inpatient environment should check with nursing staff prior to visiting patients with agitation. If staff members have worked hard to get a restless patient settled, they may not want that patient to be touched.

Clinical considerations: Confusion, agitation, and restlessness

Pressure:

- Level 2 holds may provide a sense of grounding.

Site:

- If holding the patient's hand, hold from underneath rather than on top so as not to convey a sense of confinement.

Positioning:

- Defer to patient preference, or rely on family or staff.
- A slight change in position or gentle range of motion can sometimes help with agitation.

Other:

- Create a calm, quiet environment with low light.
- Presence of familiar people.
- Reorientation without contradiction.
- Visual and hearing aids, if worn, can help.
- If the patient is fearful, stay calm and present.
- Monitor reactions to massage closely to ensure that touch is helping rather than making the problem worse.

Constipation

The body continues to produce stool up until the very end of life, even after eating has stopped. But numerous factors can interfere with the ability to produce bowel movements. Narcotics are the number one cause of constipation at the end of life. Decreased consumption of food and fluids, reduced activity level, decreased efficiency of the digestive system, and lack of privacy all interfere with normal habits of elimination. Certain conditions, such as Parkinson's disease, cerebral infarction, multiple sclerosis, and abdominal malignancies, to name a few, are associated with higher risk of constipation.[8]

Persistent constipation over a prolonged period of time can cause changes in mental status, including confusion and decreased level of consciousness. Pain, fever, abdominal distention, nausea, vomiting, and intermittent diarrhea can also occur. The care team will typically initiate a "bowel regimen" of stool softeners and laxatives when narcotics are used, using more aggressive measures when necessary, including digital extraction, to avoid painful fecal impaction and bowel obstruction. Though not a replacement for these measures, massage can be very effective for some patients, either as a means to induce relaxation, which facilitates digestion, or to provide direct stimulation for peristalsis through abdominal massage. Food moves up the ascending colon on the right side of the abdomen, across the transverse colon, then down the descending colon on the left side of the abdomen. Abdominal massage using a light effleurage or a gentle wavelike motion similar to that used in manual lymphatic drainage should be applied in a clockwise direction, with approval by the medical team and adjusted for patient comfort.

Clinical considerations: Constipation

Pressure:

- Level 1 or level 2 full body or abdominal massage in clockwise direction, to patient tolerance.

Site:

- Check with medical staff to rule out obstruction before providing abdominal massage.

Positioning:

- Most patients with constipation will not tolerate positioning other than supine or semi-reclining.

Other:

- Reflex points in the hands and feet to stimulate digestion.

Dyspnea

Patients can experience dyspnea as a result of cancer in the lungs, COPD, pulmonary fibrosis, CHF or amyotrophic lateral sclerosis (ALS). Dyspnea can also occur in advanced diseases that cause fluid to collect in the abdomen, such as renal or liver failure. During the dying process itself, the body's oxygen and carbon dioxide receptors begin to fail, which can result in shortness of breath. Respiratory distress is understandably a frightening symptom for patients and their loved ones. Air hunger leads to anxiety, and anxiety in turn increases the sensation of air hunger.

Dyspnea is addressed by the medical team with supplemental oxygen, bronchodilators and steroids to open the airway, and medications including morphine, which reduce the patient's perception of air hunger. While massage does not address any of the root causes of dyspnea, it does reduce anxiety and can therefore have a positive impact on this symptom. Massage can also provide relief to accessory muscles, which are working overtime in the dyspneic patient, including the intercostals, scalenes, sternocleidomastoid (SCM), pectoralis major and minor, serratus anterior and posterior, and latissimus dorsi.

Clinical considerations: Dyspnea

Pressure:

- Level 1 for extreme respiratory distress.
- Some patients are helped by gentle tapotement (no greater than level 2) applied over the posterior lungs.

continued

Site:

- Be sensitive to any pressure, even resting hands, over the chest, which may feel like constriction.

Positioning:

- Patients will be unable to lie flat. Seated or high Fowler's position will be most comfortable.

Other:

- Reflex points for the lungs in hands and feet.

Edema

Edema is a common and irreversible symptom for many end-stage diseases as the body loses its ability to process, absorb, and eliminate fluids. There are several types of edema. Peripheral edema often presents in one or both of the lower extremities, but may also occur in the upper extremities. Ascites, discussed in Chapter 8, is edema that occurs in the abdomen. In some patients, edema is generalized all over the body, a condition called anasarca. Lymphedema is another type of swelling, typically due to damage or removal of lymph nodes during cancer treatment (see Chapter 8) or because a tumor is blocking a lymphatic channel. Lymphedema occurs in the extremity and quadrant closest to the treated lymph nodes. All of these forms of fluid retention can be uncomfortable for the patient, causing discomfort or pain, and shortness of breath in the case of ascites. Edema and lymphedema, when severe, can cause weeping of fluids from the skin, which creates risk of infection. The medical team may treat edema with diuretics – diuretics are not effective for treating lymphedema. Guidelines for massaging edematous limbs can be found in the edema section of Chapter 8.

Clinical considerations: Edema

See Chapter 8: Ascites, Edema, and Lymphedema sections.

Tip 14.3 The role of MLD in hospice or palliative care

Therapists with training in manual lymphatic drainage can use this modality, when appropriate, at the end of life. Caution must be used, however, so as not to increase lymphatic return to the heart and kidneys if they are compromised, which is often the case with end-stage disease. It is not enough to know the terminal diagnosis – therapists must also be informed about comorbidities that would contraindicate or restrict the use of MLD. If determined to be safe, the length of the session should be adjusted to the patient's energy level, generally shorter than a full MLD treatment. The goal of the session is comfort and relaxation.

Fatigue

Given the significant demands that advanced disease and dying place on the body, fatigue is a normal part of the dying process. Patients at the end of life experience incremental loss of energy for activities they once took for granted: the ability to walk across a room, take a shower, dress by themselves, sit in a chair, have a conversation, or finish a meal. Some of the causes can be addressed, such as anemia, insomnia and infections, but the reality is that there is no medication to treat end-of-life fatigue. A major focus of the care team is to help patients and loved ones adjust their expectations to new realities. Dying people sleep more and need increasing assistance as they decline. Moments of wakefulness become a gift to be enjoyed to the fullest. The role of the massage therapist is to provide a session that is supportive and nurturing, never demanding. The pressure and duration of the massage, conversation during the session, undressing, and repositioning all require energy that is in short supply for the patient. Therapists must also be mindful of socializing with staff in areas where patients could be impacted by noise. A restful environment helps patients get the sleep they need, so that they can conserve energy for experiences that are meaningful to them.

Clinical considerations: Fatigue

See Chapter 8, Fatigue section.

Fractures and other injuries

Fractures and other acute injuries are common in terminal patients, due to diseases that compromise bone health and falls which occur from weakness, disorientation, and changes in gait. Injuries from falls and other causes may result in bruises, acute swelling, and/or cuts requiring bandaging or stitches. In the case of fractures, a decision must be made regarding repair. Surgery on hips and other long bones of the body have inherent risks and involve a long and difficult recovery. When a patient is dying, a more compassionate approach can be to stabilize the joint and to provide pain control while the body does whatever healing it can on its own. Factors to consider are anticipated life expectancy, overall bone health, and goals and wishes of the patient and family.

Clinical considerations: Fractures and other injuries

Pressure:

- Level 1 or 2 pressure overall.

Site:

- The affected area may tolerate a level 1 hold, or may be too tender for any type of touch.

Positioning:

- The injured area may need to be supported and protected.
- Consult with medical staff prior to repositioning patients with untreated fractures.

Loss of communication

The ability to communicate may be impacted by certain diseases at the end of life, including ALS, Parkinson's, dementia, and cancers of the head and neck. Communication issues also occur when the patient speaks a language that is different from the language of the care providers. In the end, all dying patients become impaired in their communication with others. They may remain verbal but unable to be understood. They may grow too weak to produce sound, even with great effort. Talk to the patient even if he or she is nonverbal. Ask loved ones what name the patient likes to be called and use the patient's name when communicating. If a translation service is used, look at and talk to the patient and family, rather than the translator.

A person who cannot communicate their needs is extremely vulnerable. Care providers, including massage therapists, must watch for nonverbal signs that a patient is in pain or other distress. A grimace or frown, rapid respirations, increased heart rate or blood pressure, sweating, writhing or shifting in bed, guarding a body part, reluctance to move, moaning, groaning, and drawing the legs up are examples of possible distress. Sometimes signs are more subtle and require a deeper kind of listening. The therapist's job, to the best of his or her ability, is to honor the patient's wishes and needs.

Clinical considerations: Loss of communication

Pressure:

- Level 1 for patients who are nonverbal.
- Watch closely for nonverbal feedback.

Site:

- Important to read the patient chart or communicate with staff or loved ones.

Positioning:

- Consult chart, staff or loved ones.

Other:

- While eye contact can be a means of communication, it is not respectful in all cultures.

Loss of mobility

Dying typically involves a transition from independent mobility to lack of mobility, with a number of possible steps in between. Some diseases, such as ALS and Parkinson's, actually target mobility; for those patients, loss of mobility may come early in the dying process. For others, there is a gradual decline in strength and stamina, which eventually requires the use of mobility aids and assistance from others. Regardless of terminal diagnosis, most are on a trajectory that ends with confinement to bed.

Loss of mobility at the end of life is a game changer, with profound physical, social and psychological ramifications. Dignity issues arise when the patient needs help with bathing and toileting. The patient's world likely becomes smaller, with an increasing sense of isolation. Physical complications of immobility include increased risk of constipation, deep vein thrombosis (DVT), pneumonia, urinary tract infections (UTIs), pressure injuries and contractures. Some patients are understandably resistant to giving up ambulation and become a fall risk.

Clinical considerations: Loss of mobility

- Slow the pace. Allow more time for everything.
- Allow more time for transfers, or work with the patient in situ. Ask staff for help rather than attempting to do a transfer without adequate training or assistance.
- Return the bed to a low, locked position at the end.
- Be aware that bed alarms and cameras are sometimes used to monitor patient safety.

Pain

Pain with terminal illness can be very complex. Dying doesn't in and of itself cause pain. Some patients have very little to no pain at the end of life, but most do, and most need pharmacological support to cope with pain at some point during the dying process. Pain can happen with any diagnosis, though some diagnoses are more associated with pain than others. An example of this is bone cancer or cancer that has metastasized to bones. The patient

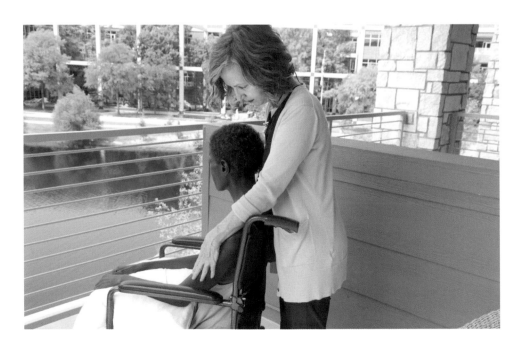

FIGURE 14.5
Loss of mobility presents the opportunity for the therapist to be flexible. A practical approach is to work on the patient wherever he or she happens to be. In this photo, the massage session is provided in a wheelchair on the patient's patio. A pillow is placed on the patient's lap to support the arms and shoulders.

(Photo by Candice White.)

may be asked to rank the pain, often using the Edmonton scale of zero to ten. Pain is treated according to severity, whether it is constant or intermittent, and type of pain (nociceptive or neuropathic). Nociceptive pain includes inflammation, tumor compression, and obstruction. Neuropathic pain results from nerve damage, such as from shingles or peripheral neuropathy as a result of diabetes or some chemotherapies. In addition to pain that can be caused by the terminal diagnosis, end-of-life pain may be related to inactivity, inadequate propping, old injuries, and arthritis.

Cicely Saunders, who is credited with the birth of the hospice movement, developed the concept of "total pain." Total pain refers to the fact that end-of-life pain is rarely just physical. In addition to physical pain, terminal patients experience psychological, social and spiritual pain related to grief, loss, fear, anger and isolation. The hospice team includes a variety of disciplines working in collaboration to address total pain, including doctors, nurses, social workers and chaplains. Massage therapists can be an excellent addition to this team approach, given that skilled human touch impacts the patient not just physically, but also psychologically, socially and even spiritually. Some massage sessions at the end of life are akin to a gentle anointing that can profoundly impact patients and their families on a spiritual level.

It is important for every member of the end-of-life care team, including massage therapists, to understand the patient's beliefs and goals related to pain control. Many people – patients, loved ones, even some medical professionals – are resistant to the use of narcotics to control pain. Fears about addiction are common, as are concerns about the development of drug tolerance, or the need for ever-increasing doses of medication that may eventually become ineffective. End-of-life experts agree that fears about long-term consequences are generally unfounded when life expectancy is short. While it is true that terminal patients often require higher doses of pain medication over time, this is likely due to disease progression rather than drug tolerance. The wish for the patient to remain awake and alert (either the patient's own wish

or that of their loved ones), can be another source of resistance to adequate pain control. This rationale does have some validity, as the medications used to control pain often cause drowsiness, especially during the first days of use. There are also patients with belief systems that find meaning and value in suffering; these patients may view pain as a means of redemption. Professional caregivers must work closely with patients and their loved ones in order to achieve a pain-control approach that best supports the patient's needs and desires.

Clinical considerations: Pain

Pressure:

- Level 1 or level 2, to patient tolerance.

Site:

- Allow the patient to report vulnerable and painful areas.

Positioning:

- Allow the patient to determine comfortable positioning.

Tip 14.4 Applying heat for pain

Heat can be very effective for mild to moderate pain. Some inpatient environments will require a prescription before allowing a patient to use a heating pad from home. Heating pads can be problematic at the end of life, since many patients are impaired in their ability to give feedback and burns can result. An alternative is a warm compress, which can be created by soaking a hand towel or wash cloth in hot water. Use a disposable, waterproof pad under the compress to keep the patient's bed dry. Another option is for the therapist to hold the painful area, creating a comforting sensation of heat with the hands.

Chapter FOURTEEN

Skin changes

The body's largest organ is vulnerable to a number of problems at the end of life, causing distress that ranges from mild irritation to intense and unremitting pain. Some conditions change the color of the skin, such as subcutaneous bleeding, and diseases of the liver, which can cause extreme jaundice. Itching is a common symptom which may be due to a temporary reaction to opioids, an allergic response, dry skin related to dehydration, end-stage liver or kidney disease, pancreatic cancer, lymphoma (especially Hodgkin's), leukemia, fungal infection, or a reaction to laundry detergents or soaps. Skin tears and wounds are also common from falls or friction. Prolonged immobility causes the well-known phenomenon of pressure ulcers, which commonly occur at bony prominences such as the heels, sacrum and shoulders. Standard protocol in many hospitals for at-risk patients is to reposition the patient every two hours. There are also malignancies that invade the skin, including skin cancer, fistulas, and fungating tumors. Any disruption of skin integrity creates risk of infection that can become systemic and hasten death.

Massage therapists have an important role in caring for the skin they touch, beginning with lubrication. Therapists generally have their favorite products, all of which are likely to be superior in quality to the lotions provided in hospitals and nursing homes. Lotions and creams tend to have a more hydrating effect on thirsty skin than oils. Unscented products are best for the hospital environment, given possible sensitivities in this population. Use of a one- or two-ounce container with a lid, often available in restaurant supply stores, is preferable to carrying the same lotion bottle between patients. A small disposable cup has the additional advantage of making it easy to leave a sample behind for family or aides to use with the patient. Patients and their families often express curiosity about the lubrication used for massage. The therapist should be prepared to speak knowledgeably about the products they use, including ingredients to which patients may be allergic. Some patients arrive at the hospital with their own preferred lotion. If the patient has positive associations with a particular product, it may be best to accommodate their preference.

Clinical considerations: Skin changes

Pressure:

- Level 1 or holds for fragile skin or pink areas at bony prominences.

Site:

- Skin that is not intact should be not be touched, with or without gloves.

Positioning:

- "Float" heels by placing a pillow under the lower legs (see Figure 6.3).
- Side-lying for short periods only. A side-lying position places pressure on the greater trochanter of the hip and should be avoided for extended periods at the end of life. A more comfortable position can be attained by using a right-leaning or left-leaning supine position. Tuck a pillow under the upper side of the pelvis to help the patient maintain the position. This also takes the pressure off the sacrum for a moment.

Stages of dying

Non-sudden death has a natural order as the functions of various systems shut down. The body begins to shift energy away from digestion and elimination, reserving a waning supply of energy for the brain, the lungs and the heart. The changes that take place make sense when viewed through this lens, but that doesn't mean the process is an easy one. Leaving the body often requires effort and may be associated with pain or other discomforts. The goal of end-of-life care, ideally, is to support rather than interfere with the natural process of dying, while assisting the dying person with physical, psychological, social and spiritual distress.

While dying involves a process with common patterns, it is important to remember that every death is unique. Just as some births are more difficult than others, death seems to come harder for some patients. Some deaths are prolonged in a way that we try to understand. But the truth is that we don't always know why some people linger, while others die suddenly from an "exit event" that catches everyone off guard. A person with cancer who is expected to live for weeks or months, for example, can die abruptly from a stroke, heart attack or blood clot. Any discussion of the stages of dying must be accompanied by a great deal of humility and tolerance for the unknown. Learning more about the process, however, can help massage therapists at the dying patient's bedside to be a calm, supportive presence. The following information on stages of dying is based on work by Valerie Hartman RN, LMT [9] and countless others.

Functional period (six to twelve months of life)

Many patients experience a period of transition from curative care to end-of-life care that is known as the "functional period," when life expectancy may be six to twelve months. Patients are likely to be experiencing one to three symptoms of disease at this point, such as insomnia, anxiety or pain, usually mild to moderate in severity, while coming to terms with a diagnosis that is likely to be terminal in the near future. They may be on palliative care to address symptoms or to address side effects of treatment. Treatment, which may involve a phase I, II or III clinical trial, is likely to have waning benefits with worsening side effects. Patients who stop treatment during the functional period may actually feel better for a time, as the side effects of treatment diminish. Functional patients may still be working or driving. They may be focused on legacy work, travel and other meaningful experiences.

Therapists may encounter functional clients while working in assisted-living facilities or during a hospital stay for an acute crisis. These patients and their loved ones need understanding and compassion as they adjust to a changing treatment plan with dwindling treatment options and the emerging reality of a limited lifespan. Common emotions for patient and family during this period include disbelief, denial, anger, fear, grief, and hope to "beat the odds." The patient may express any or all of these emotions, or none of them. Loved ones will also be experiencing a wide range of feelings, which may or may not correspond at any given time to what the patient is experiencing.

In adapting the massage session for a patient in the functional period, therapists must consider the terminal diagnosis, secondary or tertiary diagnoses, and side effects of treatment that warrant special care. This is a good time to build rapport and to discover the patient's preferences. Find out who the important people are in the patient's world, and how decisions are made regarding care. Focus on symptom relief and support for the patient's goals. The patient may desire as much normalcy as possible. They may tolerate being on a massage table for a 60-minute session, and are likely to tolerate level 2 pressure.

Early decline

During early decline, patients experience three to five symptoms, or an increase in severity of the previous one to three symptoms from the the functional period. This causes denial to wane, as the reality of the disease progression becomes more concrete. Anxiety increases during early decline, which may exacerbate other symptoms. Hospice care might be started, as this period marks an expected life span of six months or less. Unfortunately, most people wait much longer to take advantage of hospice services. The average stay on hospice in the US is 76 days, but more than half are enrolled for 30 days or fewer.[10] In the UK, the average length of hospice care is 91 days, with one third of people receiving care for less than two weeks.[11] Regardless of the timing, sign-on day is typically difficult for both patients and their families.

As symptom burden grows, the medical team may begin adding to or changing the patient's medications. Opioids may be started for pain, which can cause side effects as the patient adjusts. Families may misplace blame for decline on "too much medication" or other perceived problems with the care plan. Medical equipment may begin to enter the home, including a hospital bed, which can be a difficult transition for some people. Digestive issues, such as decreased appetite and constipation, are common.

The goals of massage during early decline are to provide support and reduce anxiety. The location of massage needs to be reevaluated for comfort and safety. Patients who have used a massage table previously may not be safe to do so as they decline. Listen and validate without judgment and resist the impulse to teach or "fix."

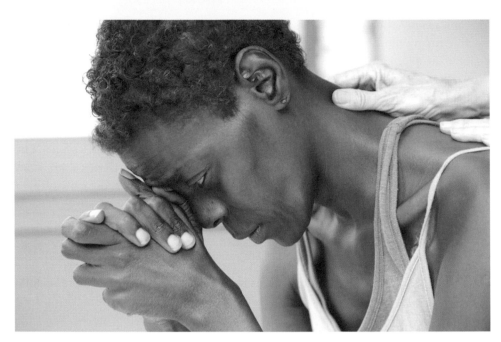

FIGURE 14.6
Each stage of dying involves loss and grief, as the patient and loved ones adapt to new realities of the disease process. Anxiety, fear, anger and sadness are all normal reactions. Acceptance for whatever arises during the massage session will help the patient feel heard and supported.

(Photo by Candice White.)

Create a calm oasis, even if it's just inside the patient's bed. Begin dialing back, with shorter sessions and slower strokes. The massage session might be 30 to 60 minutes in length, with pressure adjusted for the patient's declining condition. Pressure level 2 is generally safe. Use level 1 for patients with nausea, fever, edema or any other condition that makes them fragile.

Tip 14.5 Shall I wake you?

As patients decline, their waking hours decrease, making it likely that the therapist will at some point arrive to find the patient sleeping. It can be helpful early in the patient–therapist relationship to ask if the patient would prefer to remain sleeping or if they'd like to receive massage even if they're not awake. This exchange creates a dynamic in which the patient's choices are honored at each step of the dying process.

Late decline

During late decline, fatigue increases exponentially, causing the patient to sleep for longer periods, up to 16–20 hours per day. With increasing periods of sleep, the patient's reality begins to shift; it's as if the veil between two worlds grows thinner. Patients may see deceased loved ones. They may use symbolic language to describe their experiences. This language often reflects the patient's interests or how they spent their time. An architect, for example, might talk about "climbing stairs," while an accountant might speak of getting his numbers "in line."

As the digestive system slows down, the patient's appetite decreases drastically. Weight loss accelerates, unless the patient is retaining fluids due to cardiac problems or steroid medication. The patient becomes weaker, and may need assistance to walk, or may stop walking altogether. The risk of falling becomes greater. Swallowing may become difficult, resulting in dehydration. With dehydration and decreased circulation, skin becomes compromised, distressed and slow to heal.

The patient may become incontinent during late decline. Dignity issues surface when the patient must be helped to a bedside commode or wear diapers. Reduced kidney function may result in edema, often in one or both lower extremities. The patient may begin to need supplemental oxygen, as the lungs are working harder. Patients are often on opioids and antianxiety medications at this stage. The delivery system for these medicines will likely change over time, from oral to topical or sublingual. In hospital and inpatient environments, IVs may be used.

In late decline, the length of the massage session might be 20–40 minutes, using level 2 pressure. Level 1 pressure should be used for the conditions indicated in Table 6.1. Feelings of grief and fear may be strong, for both patients and families. Massage therapists are in a position to model calm support through quiet voice and gentle touch.

Pre-active dying (1–2 weeks)

During pre-active dying, the patient's level of consciousness and arousal begin to change. The patient becomes semi-responsive, waking for brief periods when their name is spoken, or when they experience pain. The eyes may be open or closed. When open, the patient may stare past people and objects, appearing to lose focus. The patient is withdrawing from the world, spending time in another space that the living do not comprehend. The patient has likely stopped eating. The body still produces fecal matter, and the care team will want the patient to have a bowel movement every third day or so to prevent impaction. The patient may still be able to use a bedside commode or bed pan but will need assistance.

Swallowing has become difficult, with risk of aspiration and pneumonia. The medication delivery system will change if it hasn't already, from oral to sublingual, topical or IV. Dehydration progresses, causing dry mouth, decreased urinary output, dark urine, dry skin, dizziness, and drowsiness. Blood flow and oxygen to the brain decrease, causing further disorientation and drowsiness. With growing weakness, the patient likely becomes bedbound, if they aren't already. Risk of skin breakdown increases. The patient may have terminal restlessness, pulling at bed linens, trying to get out of bed, or reaching for imaginary things. Patients who continue to ambulate are at extreme risk of falls and related injuries.

The body is still working to keep the airway open, but breathing begins to change. The body's oxygen and carbon dioxide receptors are no longer functioning well. The patient may begin to experience a pattern of shallow breathing with short periods of apnea. There may be edema in the lower extremities and sometimes throughout the body, which may be the body's way of storing fluids where they cause the least harm. Unless the patient has a vascular disease, the extremities are still warm during pre-active dying.

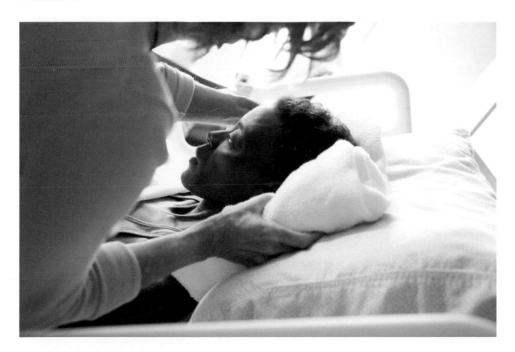

FIGURE 14.7

In pre-active and active dying, the patient's eyes may be open or half open, though the patient otherwise seems to be sleeping or unconscious. Here, the therapist uses a rolled towel to provide bilateral support to the head.

(Photo by Candice White.)

Chapter FOURTEEN

During pre-active dying, the therapist should prop as needed to support growing weakness (Figure 14.7). Continue the application of emollient cream for dry skin. A moistened washcloth can be applied to the lips, followed by lip balm. Provide a calm, supportive environment to accept whatever arises, without judgment. Speak quietly to the patient, telling

Tip 14.6 Offering massage during pre-active or active dying

The space around an imminently dying person is hallowed ground. The massage therapist who enters this space must be especially sensitive, particularly if it is a first encounter with the patient. Once a patient is no longer speaking for himself, a surrogate decision-maker will consent to or decline the massage session. Loved ones are understandably protective and may be resistant to massage for a number of reasons. They may feel it is "too late" for the patient to benefit. They may have preconceived notions regarding massage, which make them assume it would be painful or "too much." Or they may feel that their few remaining hours are too precious to share with anyone outside the patient's inner circle.

One tip for entering this delicate situation is to avoid use of the word "massage." Loved ones are generally more open to the idea of light lotioning to honor and care for dry skin. The therapist should assure the family that the patient does not need to be undressed or repositioned for the session and that the session will be brief and gentle. The family can be invited to assist the therapist in observing any response (furrowed brow, or increase in respirations) that indicates the patient does not wish to be touched. Loved ones sitting or standing close to the patient should be assured that they are not "in the way." The session should be fashioned in a way that accommodates their rightful presence at the bedside, either by confining massage to an area of the body that the therapist can reach without displacing family or by inviting the family member(s) to participate in the massage. In the event of an unfavorable response, the session should be dialed back or discontinued. An attitude of quiet humility can go a long way in assuring loved ones that their wishes and needs will be honored.

them who you are and what you're doing. Offer gentle and unconditional support to the family as their grief intensifies.

Active dying (2–4 days)

The final stage of the dying process is referred to as active dying, and an actively dying patient is referred to as *imminent*. While the difference between pre-active and active dying may seem subtle when described on paper, there is no mistaking this last phase. Family or staff will often say, "There's been a change." One of the most visible signs of active dying is color change to the skin, including mottling, a distinctive red or purple marbling that often begins on the lower extremities (Figure 14.8). Cyanosis of the upper extremities is also common, typically beginning with the fingernails. Mottling and cyanosis occur when the heart grows too weak to circulate blood to the extremities. Mottled and cyanotic extremities are cold to the touch, though the remainder of the body may be warm or even hot.

The second most obvious change that heralds active dying is a change in the patient's breathing pattern. Breathing may be rapid and shallow, with use of accessory muscles and lengthening periods of apnea. The sternocleidomastoid tightens, extending the head to keep

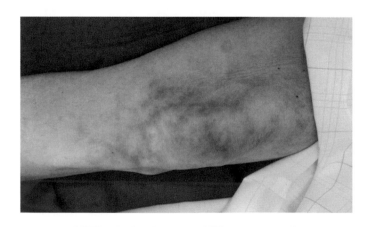

FIGURE 14.8
Mottling is red or purple discoloration, which often appears during active dying. The most common places for mottling to begin are the feet or the knees, followed by the hands. Mottling is typically progressive, but can come and go over a period of several days. Skin that is mottled will feel cool to the touch.

(Photo by Dr Alex Peralta.)

the airway open. With loss of the swallowing reflex and inability to cough, secretions gather in the throat, which can be heard in the patient's breathing. This sound can be very disturbing to loved ones at the bedside. The family may worry that the patient is "drowning" or struggling to breathe, but end-of-life experts agree that this is generally not the case. Care staff typically educate families to watch for facial grimace, restlessness or other signs of discomfort.

The imminent patient has likely not taken food or fluids in one or more days. The mouth can become very dry, due to dehydration, open-mouth breathing, and the drying effect of supplemental oxygen. Caregivers will use wet sponges to swab the mouth and apply lip balm for the patient's comfort. There is little to no urine output. Electrolyte disturbances occur with dehydration, producing a natural anesthetic in the body. When this happens, some patients seem more peaceful, though medication for pain and anxiety continues as needed. Once urination ceases, there is a risk of toxicity from opioid metabolites that are no longer being excreted. This can cause involuntary twitching called myoclonus. Opioid rotation can reduce this problem.

The patient's level of arousal during active dying is typically lower than previously. Imminent patients do not usually respond to their names, but may respond to pain by grimacing, moaning or crying out when being repositioned. An exception to this happens occasionally when a patient has a last short surge of energy. He or she may "wake up" and suddenly request a favorite meal, a visit with a certain person, or other desires seemingly out of nowhere. This surge may last minutes, hours or even a day or two, startling loved ones and creating the illusion that a miraculous recovery is underway. When this last surge of energy is complete, however, the end is often very near.

Clinical considerations: Pre- and active dying

Pressure:

- Level 1 pressure, holds or light caress.

Site:

- Focus on warm areas of the body. Limit or avoid massage to extremities that are mottled or cold.

Positioning:

- Do not reposition the patient for massage, unless family requests it.

Other:

- Massage of short duration (10–15 minutes) with focus on the upper body.
- Light energy work or holds.
- Emollient creams to "anoint" the upper body, including balm for dry lips.
- Essential oils if family desires and patient has liked them in the past.
- If fever or sweating are present, apply cool wet cloths to forehead, feet and/or back of the neck.
- Add or remove blankets as needed, but avoid electric blankets.
- Speak quietly to the patient, tell them who you are and what you're doing.
- Be sensitive to any change in desire to be touched (facial expression or breathing).
- Care and attention shifts to the family.

Therapist's journal 14.2
Supporting a peaceful sleep

The patient was 65 years old and had been diagnosed with kidney cancer two years previously. Before I met her, she had surgery to remove her right kidney, chemotherapy, immunotherapy, and radiotherapy. The tumor had spread to the lymph nodes around her neck and had become a bleeding wound, resulting in swelling, pain and numbness in her left arm and hand. She complained of sleep problems, lack of energy and loss of appetite. She was prescribed an antidepressant, anticonvulsants and laxatives.

On my first visit, the patient's daughter showed me an over-the-counter traditional Chinese oil which she was using to massage the patient's arm and hand to relieve pain. This oil is very popular among the elderly in Hong Kong for minor discomforts; it contains a high content of menthol, eucalyptus

continued

and wintergreen and is intended for use on a small area only. I advised the family to discontinue use of the Chinese oil and instead prepared a custom blend of essential oils inaloe vera gel for pain. I applied the mixture on her left arm and hand with light touch. With full hand contact, I massaged the patient's legs and right hand with jojoba oil and a second custom blend for relaxation and relief of muscle tension. The patient slept during the entire session. At the end of the session, I offered aroma patches with essential oils to increase appetite and promote sleep, which her family could apply whenever she needed it.

After two days, I followed up with the patient's family and was told that the massage had greatly improved their mother's sleep. I was able to provide four more sessions before she died. Sometimes I could only massage her legs as her body had medical devices, sometimes I only did foot massage because her limbs were so swollen.

The last time I saw the patient, her bed had been moved in front of the nursing station. Although she was not very conscious, the patient still recognized me when I spoke her name. I massaged her hands, arms, legs and head with a blend of lotus, sandalwood and lavender essential oils. Lotus, in our culture, is associated with purity, spiritual awakening and perfection, which can be very helpful in transition. Her daughter told me that after I left, her mother slept peacefully. She died the next day.

Kaman Cheung Massage and aroma therapist
Hong Kong

Self-care

Therapists who work with the dying will bear witness to extraordinary physical, mental and emotional suffering. People who are drawn to this work tend to be sensitive and empathic by nature, but few of us are prepared for the intensity of caring for people and their loved ones at the juncture of the dying process. Therapists must develop coping skills that allow them to move in and out of the dying world, without forsaking the living world. Good boundaries and role-shedding rituals are helpful; something as simple as removing one's name tag and leaving it in the car can signal an intention to leave the

work day behind. Self-care strategies are individual, but essential for longevity in end-of-life care. Finding a way to balance the emotional demands of this work with adequate rest and joy will increase both the tenure and effectiveness of the care we have to offer.

Summary

The inpatient environment can be a challenging but rewarding place to provide care that facilitates a peaceful, supported death. Massage therapists, working in collaboration with palliative and hospice care teams, can play an important role in reducing suffering for dying patients. All aspects of the massage session – duration, speed, positioning, and particularly pressure – should be matched to the patient's changing condition, with the goal of offering comfort and rest. While therapists will be helped by information about common symptoms and patterns at the end of life, it is important to remember that every patient's journey is unique. Symptoms can be managed but can't always be eradicated. Gentle touch, with no other agenda than caring presence, can be a profound comfort.

Test yourself

Multiple choice: Circle all of the correct answers. There may be more than one.

1. Which of the following terms describes comfort care that can be provided alongside curative treatment?

   A   Terminal care.
   B   Palliative care.
   C   Hospice care.
   D   Integrative care.

2. What is the most important adaptation to be made for end-of-life massage?

   A   Avoiding limbs with edema.
   B   Propping patients in a side-lying position.
   C   Decreasing the pressure.
   D   Beginning the massage stroke on the distal part of the extremity.

3. Which of the following would be most helpful for a patient with anxiety?

   A   Lying the patient supine so that he or she becomes sleepy.
   B   Continuing the massage long enough that the patient finally settles down.
   C   Deeper pressure to make the nervous system feel grounded.
   D   Placing pillows under the patient's arms.

4. What approaches would be most helpful for a patient with dyspnea?

   A   Side-lying position.
   B   High Fowler's position.
   C   Level 1 pressure for mild or severe dyspnea.
   D   Tapotement.

5. Which of the following are appropriate adjustments for an imminent patient?

   A   Repositioning the patient for massage.
   B   Level 2 pressure.
   C   Focus on cool areas of the body to warm them up.
   D   A 10-minute massage.

6. Cachexia:

   A   Occurs from the lack of water absorption in the small intestines.
   B   Calls for a level 1 pressure.
   C   Is a condition of extreme wasting that results from anorexia.
   D   Occurs in the final 3 days of life.

7. Science suggests that CT afferent nerve fibers in the skin respond most favorably to:

   A   Slow, gentle, gliding movement, at a speed of five centimeters or two inches per second.
   B   A circling pattern made with the thumbs.
   C   Compressive holds.
   D   Level 0 pressure.

8. Itching is a common skin condition for people at the end of life. It can occur because of:

   A   Hodgkin's disease.
   B   End-stage liver or kidney disease.
   C   Dehydration.
   D   Insomnia.

References

1. Broad J, Gott M, Kim H, et al. Where do people die? An international comparison of the percentage of deaths occurring in hospital and residential aged care settings in 45 populations. Int J Public Health 2013; 58(2):257–67.

2. Public Health England. End of Life Care Profiles. London: Public Health England; 2018. Available from: https://www.gov.uk/government/publications/end-of-life-care-profiles-february-2018-update/statistical-commentary-end-of-life-care-profiles-february-2018-update

3. Australian Government. Australia's Health. Canberra: Australian Institute of Health and Welfare; 2016. Available from: https://www.aihw.gov.au/getmedia/68ed1246-886e-43ff-af35-d52db9a9600c/ah16-6-18-end-of-life-care.pdf.aspx

4. Edvardsson D. Balancing between being a person and being a patient: a qualitative study of wearing patient clothing. Int J Nurs Stud 2009; 46(1):4–11.

5. Fanslow-Brunjes C. Using the Power of Hope to Cope with Dying: The Four Stages of Hope. Fresno: Quill Driver Books; 2008.

6. McGlone F, Wessberg J, Olausson H. Discriminative and affective touch: sensing and feeling. Neuron 2014; 82(4):737–55.

7. Smith I. How to be receptive to the physical and emotional challenges of hospice. Massage Magazine. 2017. Available from: https://www.massagemag.com/receptive-physical-emotional-challenges-hospice-44346/

8. Kinzbrunner B, McKinnis E. Gastrointestinal symptoms near the end of life. In: Kinzbrunner B, Policzer J. End-of-Life Care: A Practical Guide (2nd edition). New York: McGraw-Hill; 2011, p. 221.

9. Hartman V. Circle of life: hospice and palliative massage workshop. Dallas training notes, Concord training notes; 2012, 2009.

10. National Hospice and Palliative Care Organization. Facts and Figures. Alexandria: NHPCO; 2018. Available from: https://www.nhpco.org/nhpco-releases-updated-edition-of-hospice-facts-and-figures-report/

11. Caper K. Hospice care in the UK: scope, scale and opportunities. London: Hospice UK. Available from: https://www.hospiceuk.org/docs/default-source/What-We-Offer/publications-documents-and-files/hospice-care-in-the-uk-2016.pdf?sfvrsn=0

Chapter FOURTEEN

Additional resources

Callanan M, Kelley P. Final Gifts: Understanding the Special Awareness, Needs and Communications of the Dying. New York: Simon and Schuster; 1992.

Dunn H. Hard Choices for Loving People: CPR, Artificial Feeding, Comfort Care and the Patient with a Life-Threatening Illness. Lansdowne: A&A Publishers; 2009.

Halifax J. Being with Dying: Cultivating Compassion and Fearlessness in the Presence of Death. Boston: Shambhala; 2008.

Holecek A. Preparing to Die: Practical Advice and Spiritual Wisdom for the Tibetan Buddhist Tradition. Boston & London: Snow Lion; 2013.

McPhee S, Winker M, Rabow M, et al. Care at the Close of Life: Evidence and Experience. New York: McGraw-Hill; 2011.

Nelson D. From the Heart Through the Hands: The Power of Touch in Caregiving (2nd edition). Findhorn: Findhorn Press; 2006.

Warner F. Soul Midwives Handbook: The Holistic and Spiritual Care of the Dying. London: Hay House; 2013.

Focused on clear questions, bearing the goals of communication in mind, the therapist can guide a successful exchange that benefits the physician, the therapist, and, ultimately, the client who deserves the care.

Tracy Walton[1]

The health care session is not complete until the documentation is complete. Charting and other follow-up documentation is a valuable tool for practitioners and health care teams. The value of good quality chart notes to the individual patient is the most important aspect of documentation, as it directly helps to ensure quality care and clear communication between team members.

Documenting patient care fulfills the following purposes:

- Apprises team members of the actions and observations of all providers.
- Provides continuity of care to the patient, meaning multiple practitioners or sessions over time maintain cohesion and are provided in the context of an overall treatment plan.
- Fulfills legal obligations for documenting patient care. Requirements will vary widely.
- Provides a place to plan and organize patient care such as orders for physical therapy, lab tests, or diagnostic procedures.
- Allows for accurate treatment assessment.
- Provides practitioners with time to reflect on the care given and bring closure to the session.
- Provides an educational and research document: research is sometimes performed retrospectively, i.e. researchers obtain their data by reviewing the chart after the fact.

We will also briefly address patient feedback or evaluations. This step occurs after the session has completed and may involve nurses or other staff in collection. Analysis of data collected may serve many functions including support for additional funding.

Types of charts

Therapists working in health care facilities may encounter different charts, each with its own function: the kardex, the bedside chart, and/or the medical chart which may be paper or electronic.

The kardex

Nurses refer to the kardex as their "cheat sheet" because information for each patient is boiled down to just a few pages. Usually it comprises a single binder (or sometimes two), that contains basic data about all of the patients on a unit: the diagnosis, plan of care, family contact information, assessment of condition, and some lab results. The pages in this chart are not legal documents and are not part of the medical record. When the patient is discharged, kardex materials are shredded or permanently removed. Some medical centers will maintain an electronic kardex.

The bedside chart

Hospitals still transitioning to electronic health records may utilize some form of bedside chart. This binder may be found on the footboard of the patient's bed, just outside the patient's room in a wall frame, or in a designated place at the nurses' station. The forms enclosed in the bedside chart are usually for the purpose of tracking vital signs, instructions for activities of daily living, or in some cases daily lab results. Some hospitals will post much of this information for the patient to see on a wall white board. Goals, treatment plan, and blood counts may be included to help the patient be empowered and fully participate in their healing process. Confidentiality guidelines may limit the amount of information available in non-secure documentation.

Chapter FIFTEEN

The medical chart: paper

The medical chart is located at the nurses' station and contains doctors' orders, the medication administration record, progress notes, lab and procedure results, medical history, and personal information known as protected health information (PHI). It is the patient's legal medical record. Because of its legal status, some hospitals do not allow the massage team, particularly massage students or volunteers, to have access to it. Massage therapists who are employed will generally have full access to the chart.

The medical chart: electronic health record (EHR)

The electronic health record is an online portal with databases and user interfaces of forms or templates (screens) that house patient data and provide authorized access to medical information. The EHR (sometimes also referred to as the electronic medical record or EMR) is viewable by all providers with authorized permissions or rights. One of the initial motivations for the development of EHRs was to efficiently share patient medical records between providers and multiple health care centers across institutional lines. Portability and data sharing are expected to provide safer, more complete medical information.

An EHR is a digital version of a patient's paper chart. EHRs are real-time, patient-centered records that make information available instantly and securely to authorized users. While an EHR does contain the medical and treatment histories of patients, an EHR system is built to go beyond standard clinical data collected in a provider's office and can be inclusive of a broader view of a patient's care. EHRs are a vital part of health informational technology (IT) and can:

- Contain a patient's medical history, diagnoses, medications, treatment plans, immunization dates, allergies, radiology images, and laboratory and test results.
- Allow access to evidence-based tools that providers can use to make decisions about a patient's care.
- Automate and streamline provider workflow.

EHRs are built to share information with other health care providers and organizations – such as laboratories, specialists, medical imaging facilities, pharmacies, emergency facilities, and school and workplace clinics – so they contain information from all clinicians involved in a patient's care.[2]

Tip 15.1 Learning medical terminology

Community colleges offer courses in "Medical Terminology" and "Reading the Medical Record." Touch therapists new to health care should consider taking one of these courses as a way to speed up their learning process. Resources may be provided by the hospital free of charge.

Guidelines for charting in the medical record: Paper

The following charting policies are common to most health care facilities. Figure 15.1 illustrates the guidelines in use.

- Record legibly in black or blue permanent ink. Record the date and time care was given. Use military time, such as 8/30/2020; 13:30.
- Do not leave a space between entries. This ensures that nothing else can be inadvertently inserted into the space by another care provider.
- If a line is left partially filled, draw a line through the remainder of the unused space.
- If the entry must be continued onto another page, write the word "continued" at the end of the first page and again at the start of the second; continue with the note.
- If a new page is added to the chart, be certain that the patient's name is on it. This is usually done with a card stamp or a self-adhesive label printed with the patient's name, medical number, and other information.
- If an error is made, cross out the incorrect part of the entry with a single line, and write the word

PROGRESS NOTES			Place patient label here
Instructions Date and time for each entry Describe the significant findings and actions taken Sign each entry in full			
Time	Date	Note significant findings and actions taken	
15:20	11/16/19	Massage Note: Pt stated she has Ⓛ shoulder pain 5/10 and reports frequent headaches. Positioned Pt side-lying on Ⓡ with pillows for support. Gently lotioned full back, neck with focus on shoulder. 30 min session. Pt's husband was present. Pt stated "I'm so relaxed." Further massage is indicated. Report given to Cheryl, RN. —— Carolyn Jayne, CMT	

FIGURE 15.1
Sample handwritten chart note.

"error" above it and your initials. Do not scribble out the incorrect words. It is important to ensure that nothing appears to be covered up in the documentation, especially if legal action were ever threatened.

- If notes are is made in the wrong chart, cross out the entry using a single line, and write the word "error" above it.

- Use the accepted institutional terminology and abbreviations.

- Use the accepted charting style of the institution. In some facilities, a narrative style may be used; in others, the SOAP format may be the preferred way.

- Use terminology that will be understood by non-massage therapy care providers, such as nurses, physical therapists, social workers, and physicians.

- The use of sentence fragments is permissible.

- Enter the documentation in a timely manner, always before the end of the shift. If the entry is late, identify it as such: use the phrase "late entry" at the beginning of the entry. Be certain to list the time that the massage was given, not the time the documentation is entered into the chart.

Styles of documenting

There is no one way of documenting patient care and each institution establishes its own protocols. This text can only present some of the common methods of charting designed by massage therapy programs; it does not intend to make definitive policies. Many health care facilities have an employee or team that specializes in documentation. This person or team can assist massage therapy services as they create forms or establish charting protocols.

Chapter FIFTEEN

```
Date of Service: 9/17/2019
BEHP (if yes, visit number): {YESWILDCARD/NO:60}
Workers Comp (if yes, visit number): {YESWILDCAR/NO:60}

Chief Complaint:
No chief complaint on file.


SUBJECTIVE:
The patient complains of *** secondary to ***. ***
Goal for today's visit: ***
```

Time In	Treatment Start Time	Treatment End Time
***	***	***

	Pre-treatment	Post-treatment
Pain Scale:	{NUMBERS 0 - 10:11202} /10 {Anatomy; pain location list:11739} secondary to ***	{NUMBERS 0 - 10:11202} /10
Anxiety Scale:	{NUMBERS 0 - 10:11202} /10 secondary ***	{NUMBERS 0 - 10:11202} /10

```
OBJECTIVE:
***.  Hypertonicity noted in ***
ASSESSMENT:
Assessment:  ***. {AAINCREASE:12595} hypertonicity noted in  ***
PLAN:
***
```

```
X [] Sign at Close Encounter ∨
```

FIGURE 15.2
Screenshot of electronic intake form and SOAP note.

(Courtesy of Beaumont Hospital, Royal Oak, Michigan.)

Individual medical centers or health systems will have to make decisions about some of the following questions:

- Should massage therapists record in the medical record or document sessions on their own forms?
- Should massage therapists record in the medical record as well as maintain their own personal records?
- If massage therapists are to maintain their own charts, where should they be kept and for how long?
- What information may and may not be recorded to be compliant with local laws, such as HIPAA in the United States?

Session information is documented in a variety of ways. One of the most common methods is to record in the progress notes, or "notes" in the EHR. When the notations are made in the progress notes, a narrative style is usually used, although there is no reason the SOAP or other formats (examples of which are shared in the Appendix),

Therapist's journal 15.1
Writing careful notes is never a waste of time!

I received a phone call from the hospital's risk department about six months after I saw a fragile, elderly inpatient. They had gotten a complaint that the patient's arm was injured during the admission and were contacting everyone who was involved in their care. I only vaguely remembered the patient. I asked the investigator to read me back my note. I had written something like: "On intake, reported painful injury to right arm... Techniques used: Very gentle holds of the right arm." That refreshed my memory and I confirmed that my note was accurate and that I had done no manipulation or anything else that could have caused or exacerbated an injury. I never heard anything more about the incident. I figure that one note justified the thousands of notes I've written that I'm sure have never been read by anyone!

Lee Daniel Erman CMT

cannot be employed. This is true with electronic health records as well; however, templates or "smart phrases" are generally developed for ease and efficiency.

Narrative style

Include the following information when using the narrative style. Figures 15.3A&B illustrate the use of this recording style in the progress notes.

1. If nurses are allowed to give massage approval, enter a statement of authorization that includes the nurse's name. If approval is recorded in the chart by the physician, the statement of authorization is not necessary.

2. Date and time of session; length of session. Most medical centers will use military time and numbered dates. For example: 11/16/2020; 15:20. Do include year for accuracy.

3. Patient requests or complaints. This is often referred to as the presenting condition.

4. Action taken. Includes the parts of the body massaged. Always include a description of the amount

PROGRESS NOTES		Place patient label here
Instructions Date and time for each entry Describe the significant findings and actions taken Sign each entry in full		

Time	Date	Note significant findings and actions taken
14:30	4/6/20	Pt presented with frustration and back pain due to the hospital bed. Positioned Pt side lying for MFR x 30 mins. Released SI joint with Swedish and ROM. Pt was more at ease and comfortable. Pt stated "thank you" and would like me to come back again. Pt will be given priority for next shift. — Jen Poloski, CMT
(A)		

FIGURE 15.3A
Using the correct language is important when recording narrative style chart notes. Can you find the errors in these notes (**A**)? Compare with the notes shown (**B**).

of pressure used. Most often, words such as "light," "gentle," or "moderate" should be used to describe the amount of pressure. Whose lotion was used: the hospital's, the patient's, the therapist's? If any skin problems develop following the session, the lotion source will be on record in case follow-up is necessary.

5. Any unusual observations or findings about the patient. Document that the information was given to the patient's nurse.

6. Patient response. A verbatim or direct quote is most helpful.

7. Report. Identify nurse or method of report, as protocol indicates.

8. Signature of touch therapist.

Progress note examples

Compare the two examples of narrative style chart notes shown in Figures 15.3A&B. The first includes many

examples of inappropriate text. Can you identify the errors? The second example is more appropriate. Can you describe why?

Figure 15.3A demonstrates several common errors. To begin, it is inaccurate to state as a fact that the bed is the cause of the patient's low back pain. The touch practitioner cannot diagnose or define causes of pain; it is also possible that there are many contributing factors to the patient's pain. Secondly, abbreviations are not allowed except for the very few authorized by the organization. Examples of acceptable abbreviations include "Pt" for patient and "R" and "L" for right and left. "MFR" is a discipline-specific abbreviation and as such should not be used.

The phrase "was more at ease and comfortable" is not objective or measurable from the practitioner's simple observation and while likely true, should not be stated as

PROGRESS NOTES			Place patient label here

Instructions
    Date and time for each entry
    Describe the significant findings and actions taken
    Sign each entry in full			

Time	Date	Note significant findings and actions taken	
14:30	4/6/20	Pt presented with renal failure Hep C. Fragile skin Pt noted low back pain and frustration. Pt stated "I know its the bed." Positioned Pt side lying with pillows for support and comfort. Offered 30 min gentle myofascial release work, gentle Swedish with Range of motion intent to SI joint. Pt stated "better" and requested additional visits. Pt will be placed on list for next available shift. ——— Jen Polaski, cmt	

(B)

FIGURE 15.3B

fact. It is best to allow the patient to speak for themselves via a verbatim or direct quote. While gratitude can be noted, it does not indicate how the patient is physically feeling after the session. The use of the word "treatment" is also technically inaccurate from a narrow legal point of view and in medical settings should be avoided. Lastly, while it occasionally happens that a particular patient is specially requested to be seen on a particular date or time, all patients are "priority" and documentation should not suggest otherwise.

In Figure 15.3B, the language is more specific to the patient's report and opinion, which is relevant to their health care team. Quoting the patient's belief that the pain is being caused by the hospital bed may prompt the team to have the bed replaced, provide more pillows, or educate the patient on how to position properly and adjust settings on the bed. Next, by spelling out the modalities used, anyone on the team could research the method if curious or, in the case of an adverse event,[3] would have clear information to investigate if needed. For post-session verbatim reports, it is most helpful to find out how the patient is feeling. It is generally not required to record a pain scale number as such, but some level of comparison of pre- and post-session is best. Reporting the answer to the question: "How are you feeling now?" is the most frequently used method.

As an example from the Netherlands, Estelle Smits shares that she uses the same form for pre-session consultation and her post-session notes; these forms are kept as record of the work.[4] (See Appendix D for current form.)

Documenting in SOAP format

The SOAP format provides a common framework for record keeping. Because many therapists are taught this method of documentation in their training, it easily carries over to the hospital setting. In her book, *Hands Heal*, Diana Thompson describes the four components in the following way:

- Subjective: Data provided by the patient (symptoms and functional limitations).
- Objective: Data from the practitioner's perspective (movement tests, palpation findings, and visual observations, as well as treatment and the patient's immediate response to the treatment).
- Assessment: Functional goals and outcomes based on activities of daily living.
- Plan: Treatment recommendations and self-care education.[5]

However, when using the SOAP format in the hospital, it makes sense to slightly alter it from normal usage. Because the focus is generally on comfort rather than curative treatment, the "Assessment" component as normally used with healthy clients is less relevant. By replacing "Assessment" with "Action," the SOAP acronym can still be used. Also, since the average patient does not remain in the hospital long enough to be seen frequently by the massage therapist, the "Plan" component can be altered. Instead, "Progress" can be substituted. Thus, the four SOAP categories may be altered as follows:

- Subjective: Data provided by the patient.
- Objective: Practitioner findings.
- Action: Description of the massage session.
- Progress: Patient responses, including nonverbal ones.

Tip 15.2 Watch out for assumptions

When recording the session, be clear and concise, avoiding inferences and assumptions; document clear observations. It's important to write: "During the massage session, patient's heart rate decreased from 104 to 96", rather than: "Massage therapy resulted in an 8-point decrease in heart rate." It's impossible to know, in a single session with a single patient, if the touch therapy was what truly "caused" any changes observed. Similarly, when reporting observations, avoid such wording as: "Patient seemed calm." Instead, record something more objective, such as: "At the close of the session, patient's breathing was more regular than when the session began."[5]

Lauren "Cal" Cates and **Kerry Jordan**, Healwell

Subjective data

Information given by the patient, who is also referred to as the subject, is recorded in this section. Examples of common information reported by patients are:

- Physical complaints, such as back discomfort, sleeplessness, or pain.
- Emotional information such as anxiety, boredom, frustration, or feeling fragmented or stressed.

The subjective section is also the place to note goals the patient hopes to receive from the massage, such as relaxation or wholeness.

Objective data

Objective data is based on the factual observations of the therapist rather than opinion or guesses. Examples of objective statements are:

- Skin is well hydrated and intact.
- The right shoulder was tender to the touch.
- Skin coloring was pale.
- Patient spoke very little.

The following statements stray from the goal of making factual observations and should not appear in documentation unless they are direct comments from the patient:

- The patient appears very anxious about her upcoming procedure.
- Skin is dry from chemotherapy and insufficient water intake.
- Neck is sore from lengthy procedure this morning.

Action

In this section, the therapist records what was performed during the touch session or any suggestions offered to the patient. As when using the narrative style, the description should include:

- The physical parts addressed.
- The types of strokes, using easily understood terminology.
- The amount of pressure used. Most often, descriptive words such as "light," "gentle," or "moderate" are most appropriate.

Progress

The final section is reserved for patient responses, which will hopefully indicate some short-term progress that was made during the session. However, the massage therapist should also document patient complaints that remain unchanged or any new complaints reported.

Patient verbatim reports that express progress include: "I didn't know that would feel so good," "I feel whole again," or "I am going to sleep well tonight." These and others are often-heard reactions.

Objective changes include a drop on the pain-rating scale, report of being "relaxed" or "calm", slower breathing, or sleep.

Signature

It is required that each note be signed by the providing therapist. Name and credential should be legible. EHR entries will have an automatic signature based on the therapist's log in. Never share user ID and passwords to EHR programs. The therapist is legally responsible for the notes signed under their name.

Tip 15.3 Understanding adverse events, near misses, and errors[3]

According to the Patient Safety Network: "Adverse events refer to harm from medical care rather than an underlying disease. Important subcategories of adverse events include:

- Preventable adverse events: Those that occurred due to error or failure to apply an accepted strategy for prevention;
- Ameliorable adverse events: Events that, while not preventable, could have been less harmful if care had been different;
- Adverse events due to negligence: Those that occurred due to care that falls below the standards expected of clinicians in the community.

continued

Two other terms define hazards to patients that do not result in harm:

- Near miss: An unsafe situation that is indistinguishable from a preventable adverse event except for the outcome. A patient is exposed to a hazardous situation, but does not experience harm either through luck or early detection.
- Error: A broader term referring to any act of commission (doing something wrong) or omission (failing to do the right thing) that exposes patients to a potentially hazardous situation."[5]

Tip 15.4 Disposing of documents

Pieces of paper or notes containing patient information or names should be placed in the shredding bin before the therapist leaves the medical environment. There will be a multitude of these bins throughout the health care facility.

SOAP charting examples

Refer back to Figure 15.3B. It is written in narrative fashion, however, if it were documented in SOAP format, it would read as follows:

- S: Pt complained of low back pain and expressed frustration with hospital bed.
- O: Fragile skin; low back very tight; side-lying well tolerated.
- A: Offered gentle Swedish and myofascial release work, low back focus.
- P: Pain reported "relaxed" and additional sessions were requested.

Figure 15.4 illustrates a pre- and post-session intake form sample. The reader will notice it can be employed for both the intake assessment and post-session noting. After the form has been completed, the unit's protocol may require it to be placed in the back of the medical chart under a special section specifically for massage or integrative medicine therapies. If massage thera-

Inpatient Massage Therapy **Addressograph/medical records label**
Practitioner pre and post session intake

Before session

PT presenting condition(s) *Low back pain; frustration Primary Dx - renal failure*

☐ HOH ☐ Vision ☐ Speech ☐ Interpreter required. Language ______ ☐ Paralysis

Precautions

☒ Fall precautions ☐ Droplet ☐ Airborne ☐ Contact ☐ C. diff = contraindications

Position precautions

☐ Head↑ ☐ Flat ☐ No side-lying L/R ☐ Other ______

Site precautions

☐ Wound ☒ IV/PICC site *(R)* ☐ Skin *Fragile*

☐ Other ______

Platelet count ______ ☐ **Chemo, last** ______ ☐ **DVT, Loc** ______ ☐ **Febrile** ☐ **↓WBC**

Neuropathy? *X* **Location** *Feet*

Lymphedema? ______ **Present Hx** *(NA)* **Nodes removed, Tx? Where** ______

Current

Pain	0	1	2	3	4	5	(6)	7	8	9	10
Fatigue	0	1	(2)	3	4	5	6	7	8	9	10
Nausea	(0)	1	2	3	4	5	6	7	8	9	10
Anxiety	0	(1)	2	3	4	5	6	7	8	9	10

Goals and areas of MT session focus (List here) *Pain relief at low back, stress reduction*

Action taken *30 min gentle Swedish and Myofascial Release, low back focus. Lotion used*

continued

FIGURE 15.4
Sample intake form that includes a post-session pain scale and notation.

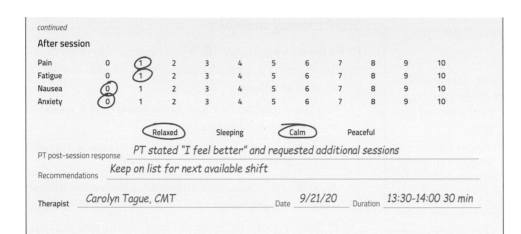

FIGURE 15.4 *continued*

pists are not allowed access to the chart, a consultation form is ideal for the massage therapy department to use when creating its own system of tracking patient care. If chart access is not allowed, the forms may be placed in a binder that is kept in the massage office or at the nurses' station. Most important is that the collection of documents is kept in a secured place away from public access.

Guidelines for charting in the medical record: Electronic health/medical record (EHR/EMR)

Guidelines for electronic health records are much the same as the previously described paper forms, therefore, it important that practitioners be familiar with all the material in this chapter. Whether using narrative or SOAP styles, electronic records have a number of advantages. For example, "smart phrases" are saved text that can be inserted into a note with a keystroke; generally, the text can be any length. Templates are another very efficient tool to help keep consistency in chart notes and allow for specific patient information to be entered without having to retype text that would otherwise be on a form (see Figure 15.5).

With simple instructions that will be provided by the medical center IT department, every user can create their own shortcuts. Some departments will have predeveloped templates and other tools that they will request massage therapists to use. With a little training or assistance, drop-down lists for selecting common text can be added to a note template: for example, the list might comprise common modalities that are offered: Swedish, craniosacral, myofascial, biofield therapy, other. Some EHR software programs allow for check boxes or radio buttons. Check boxes may be used for selecting a list of conditions commonly seen, for example: blood thinners, low platelets, fever, and types of precautions, such as Droplet or Contact. Radio buttons are typically either/or selections: a template may include "Lymphedema risk?" with a list – yes, no, current.

Additional guidelines for EHR progress notes (commonly referred to as "notes"), are as follows:

- **Keep it short.**
- Be consistent in placement of information (templates and smart phrases make this easy).
- Include verbatim reports in quotes.
- Know that everyone on the health care team has easy and quick access to your note. It is much more likely to be read than paper notes.

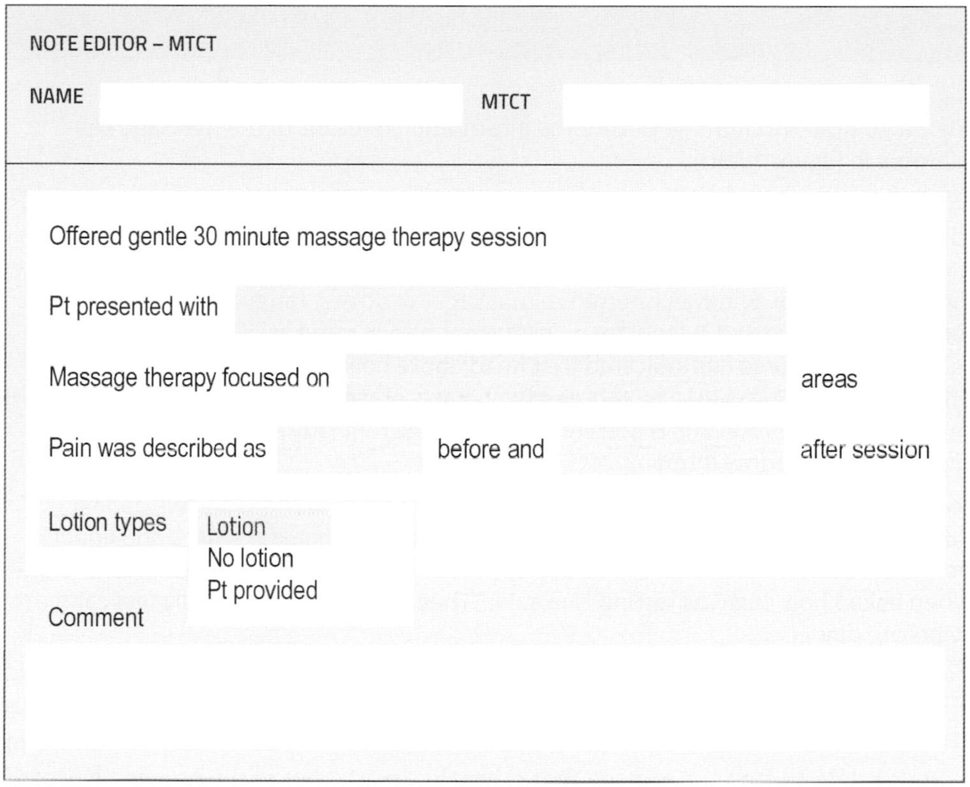

NOTE EDITOR – MTCT	
NAME	MTCT

Offered gentle 30 minute massage therapy session

Pt presented with

Massage therapy focused on   areas

Pain was described as   before and   after session

Lotion types   Lotion
           No lotion
           Pt provided
Comment

FIGURE 15.5
Simulated EHR chart note template. There will be a keystroke that moves the cursor from field to field to save time. Drop-down lists may be added to allow for quick access to common selections, such as lotion types shown here. In this example, the drop-down list could include: "Lotion", "No Lotion", "Pt provided."

Patient evaluations and feedback forms

In addition to recording post-session verbatim reports in progress notes, it is a highly recommended practice to implement a process for patients to give feedback about their massage therapy experience. Some medical centers use a simple hard copy form that is left with the patient after each session. Likert scale ratings of pain, fatigue, anxiety, nausea and others may be requested pre- and post-session. Open text lines for patients to write in are very helpful in sharing feedback about the service. Some centers will ask nurses or other staff to follow up and record satisfaction scores.

If research is a part of the medical center's goals, a third party may be involved to collect patient responses. Any opportunity for massage therapy practices to receive and collect data, especially direct quotes, is incredibly valuable. Number of patients seen, satisfaction scores, and handwritten expressions of positive outcomes can be presented to managers, administrators and donors. According to Diana Thomson: "The implementation of the Triple Aim has played a role in increasing awareness of and access to massage therapy because of patient surveys in hospitals and medical clinics: *patient satisfaction* is often linked to massage therapy in hospitals and clinics where it is provided."[5]

A routine feedback process also serves the important function of empowering the patient to share suggestions or report any discomfort. Overwhelmingly, evaluations are supportive and reinforce the dedication the touch practitioner has for this fulfilling work. See sample evaluation forms in Appendices E and F.

Chapter FIFTEEN

Case history 15.1	Exercise

Instructions: Use the case history below to practice charting. Record the information relevant to the massage session in narrative form (refer to the sample in Figure 15.3B).

Date: 8/23/19 Time: 13:10–13:50

Ms B is a 77-yo woman admitted to the hospital two days ago with a severe myocardial infarction and reports a few weeks of worsening headache. Ms B had emergency surgery to place a stent. The access point was through the L axilla. There is an IV line inserted in her R forearm. She was referred to massage for stress, fatigue and headache. Anti-nausea medications were given in the morning and Tylenol for pain. Current pain is rated as a 3/10. Pt notes her neck and shoulders feel unusually tight. The nurse has indicated that head above heart is best position for today. Prior to the heart attack Ms B was active and in good overall health. Her husband is present for the consultation but decides to go for a walk to get coffee during the session. Ms B does not get massage regularly so is happy to get the offer today. She is expected to be discharged tomorrow morning.

Because of positioning requirements, the patient was placed in a semi-reclining position without pillows behind her head for better access to shoulders and neck. Lotion was used for gentle massage to shoulders, neck and upper arms. Brief, gentle holds to head were offered. Provided foot reflexology and massage for half of the 30 minutes. Ms B rested well during the session. When asked how she was feeling, she said: "That was wonderful, I really feel calm. I think I am going to take a nap now before dinner."

Summary

Documentation is an integral part of the health care system. Everyone involved with patient care must record their actions and observations. The massage therapist who has previously found charting to be a difficult habit to establish will find it easier in this environment and will recognize its importance for excellence in patient care and building the service within the center. Creative writing is not required and is actually discouraged.

Each note should have a set of data fields or order of writing that takes the "work" out of the process. Recording patient outcomes and actual statements can serve to educate fellow providers on the efficacy of manual therapies. Collecting direct patient feedback will help to ensure patient satisfaction is consistently high and may prove to be helpful in securing and renewing funding for the service.

Please see the Appendix for more sample forms.

Test yourself

Complete the statements. Choose from: subjective; objective; electronic; narrative; template.

1. _____ information is that which the therapist observes.

2. _____ records were designed to share between clinics.

3. A _____ record is story-like.

4. _____ information is what the patient tells the therapist.

5. Electronic health records use _____ for ease of completing chart notes.

References

1. Walton T. Medical Conditions and Massage Therapy: A Decision Tree Approach. Baltimore: Wolters Kluwer Health, Lippincott Williams & Wilkins; 2011.

2. Health IT.gov. What is the electronic health record? Available from: https://www.healthit.gov/faq/what-electronic-health-record-ehr

3. Patient Safety Network. Adverse events, near misses and errors. Available from: https://psnet.ahrq.gov/primers/primer/34/Adverse-Events-Near-Misses-and-Errors

4. Smits E. Personal correspondence, 27 September 2019.

5. Thompson D. Hands Heal: Communication, Documentation, and Insurance Billing for Manual Therapists (5th edition). New York: Wolters Kluwer; 2019.

Additional resources

Chabner D. Medical Terminology: A Short Course (6th edition). St. Louis: Elsevier; 2012.

One thing that is unchanged since antiquity is that when you're seriously ill … you want someone to care for you – not just your family member but someone with scientific knowledge to also express care. [I am] hopeful that technology, such as artificial intelligence, can improve medical care, but only if it isn't done at the expense of human contact.

Abraham Verghese[1]

The beautiful cover image created for *Hands in Health Care* captures the timelessness of touch. It reminds us of human hands traced many thousands of years ago on dim cave walls, reaching out toward us. Glittering behind those hands is a starry firmament pulling us forward into a high-tech future. This text began with a look at the history of hospital massage, so it makes sense to end with some comments and speculation about the years ahead. Four topics are relevant to hospital massage as humanity progresses into the 21st century: technology, training of future hospital massage therapists, energy medicine, and the complications associated with aging and obesity – two conditions that will greatly impact health care over the next decades.

Technology

In 1982, John Naisbitt, in his book *Megatrends*, predicted ten new directions that would transform our lives. One of the ten directions he labelled "high-tech/ high-touch." Naisbett predicted that as computers came to predominate life, people would need more human touch. Once again, humanity is on the brink of profound technological innovations that will impact the way it lives, impelling people to adapt to these changes.

Every facet of our lives will be affected by changing technology. In health care this already includes increased use of video conferencing with patients, remote monitoring of symptoms and vital signs, the use of artificial intelligence, nanotechnology, robotic assists, and 3D-printing of synthetic tissues, to name just some. These capabilities will change the hospital, clinic and doctor's office of the future, though the exact nature of the impact remains to be seen. Will hospital stays become shorter and shorter? Will aging populations mean a need for more nursing facilities to care for those who can't remain at home? If technology-based care allows people to stay in their homes longer, how will community-based health care evolve? Given the likelihood that much of health care will be provided in a more remote way, how will humans respond? Will there be a paucity of human connection and, if so, how will that change outcomes?

Despite the growing sophistication of our knowledge, we still crave the comfort of human touch. We are still whole persons, and we bring our whole selves to the experience of illness and healing. Our fascination with the interrelationship between body and spirit is not likely to go away. Therapists wishing to work in health care settings or with medically complex patients would do well to seek training that prepares them to take their places in the changing landscape of health care. It may well turn out that massage therapists and other body workers will play an essential role in providing high-touch skills as a complement to high-tech care.

Training

Working in health care is a specialty that requires training rather than the "figure-it-out-as-you-go" approach that has been common since the 1990s. In addition to massage skills, this work requires an understanding of hospital dynamics, proficiency with terminology, basic knowledge of medical conditions and medications, competence in performing Standard Precautions, massaging around medical devices, the ability to cope with a high-intensity environment, and the chance to collaborate with other care providers. If massage therapists in the hospital setting are to be an essential part of the team, they need the same level of supervision and mentoring that nursing students and other practitioners in the health care setting receive. Massage training programs should form professional educational alliances with health care service providers that would allow

Chapter SIXTEEN

practicums and internships with supervised training in hospitals, clinics, nursing homes, rehab centers, and community-based care.

Training should center around competencies that specify key skills a practitioner needs in order to be prepared for work in health care settings. A list of competencies has been produced by the Hospital-Based Massage Therapy Task Force of the Academic Collaborative for Integrative Health (ACIH)[2]; The full competencies document is available on the ACIH website[2]; Info Box 16.1 contains a sample of the competencies listed for massage protocols in the hospital environment.

Info Box 16.1 ACIH Hospital-Based Competencies: Sample from Section 2

HBMT Competency 2 – Massage Protocols (MP)
General Competency Statement: Demonstrate understanding of massage protocols within a hospital environment.

- MP 1: Understand common medical conditions and symptoms and how they inform assessment and treatment plan of the massage session.
- MP2: Demonstrate ability to appropriately adjust massage techniques based on the patient's medical diagnosis and condition, including psycho/social condition. Treatment adjustments include pressure, positioning, site, pacing, duration and dosing.
- MP3: Understand indications, contraindications and precautions for massage therapy including infection control measures, health risk factors based on patient's presenting condition(s), and practitioner's safety needs.
- MP4: Demonstrate ability to provide massage therapy around hospital equipment such as hospital beds, wheelchairs, and infusion chairs.
- MP5: Recognize one's limitations in skills, knowledge, and abilities. [ACIH Competency: RR2]
- MP6: Demonstrate correct body mechanics for the hospital environment.[2]

All health care practitioners, such as nurses, doctors, respiratory therapists, physical and occupational therapists, phlebotomists, and social workers, receive the benefit of supervised field experience. Creation of this type of infrastructure is needed to fully integrate massage therapy as a service into medical and nursing settings. Without this, massage will remain a marginalized specialty, lacking the respect of more fully developed and standardized professions.

Another piece of the infrastructure needed for the future evolution of hospital massage is a professional organization around which therapists and institutions can coalesce. Hospital massage needs an association to help it become concrete and visible. Just as general massage, sports medicine, and oncology massage have associations, hospital massage must establish and monitor qualification standards for its practitioners. Continued professional development, a certification program, dedicated research efforts, and collegial support will move the profession forward in a cohesive way that garners respect from other health care professionals.

Energy medicine

Another sphere that heralds from the past but holds potential for the high-tech future in health care is energy medicine. A term commonly used in clinical settings and research instead of energy medicine is *biofield therapy*. The term was coined during the US National Institutes of Health Conference in 1992. It is defined as: "interacting fields of energy and information that surround living systems."[3] By whatever name, there are several well-established modalities within energy medicine that are regularly found in medical centers and whose use may surge in the future. These modalities can be delivered by direct touch, indirect touch off the body, or remotely.

As was discussed in Chapter 1, the history of health care has always shown a cross-pollination between cultures that evolved based on the needs of the times. The same can be seen in the use of energy medicine modalities. For example, Therapeutic Touch was developed by nurse Dolores Kreiger and Dora Kunz in the early 1970s, and was in part a response to the developers' belief that *anyone* can be taught to be a conduit for healing energy, not just a gifted few. This idea was radical at the time and is still often met with healthy skepticism.

Another widely recognized energy medicine modality is Reiki, which is said to have been rediscovered by Mikao Usui in Japan in the 1920s. Reiki is currently offered in many facilities as it is non-invasive and has some evidence of benefit for fatigue and anxiety, among other positive outcomes.[4]

Acupressure, which was the precursor in Traditional Chinese Medicine to acupuncture, should not be overlooked as an established energy medicine type of bodywork. The research presented in Chapter 2 is very supportive of its use. Patients and providers seek acupressure for pain, muscle tension, nausea, and the symptoms of labor and delivery.

Perhaps, over time, the clinical research of distance healing and non-touch modalities being done by Ann Baldwin PhD, Shamani Jain PhD and others will be more incorporated into health care settings. The Covid-19 pandemic of 2019-2020 is an unprecedented example of the need to be physically distant to those who need care the most. In the future, Reiki distance healing might be sought to help in situations like these. Other common circumstances might warrant the use of a non-touch modality, such as severely low platelets, surgery, or a lumbar puncture.

Aging and obesity

Two of the strongest influences on future global health will be aging and obesity. Both intersect with a long list of complications: diabetes, cancer, heart, liver, and kidney disease, joint problems, mental health issues, social life, mobility, and early mortality.

In 2016, according to the World Health Organization, 39% of adults were overweight and 13% were obese.[5] This accounts for more than half of all adults. It is estimated that if the trend continues at this rate, half of the adult population will be obese by 2030.[6] The social, medical, and economic burden of this phenomenon is staggering. One study suggests that the cost is comparable to that of smoking or armed conflict, war, and terrorism.[7] The United Nations notes that older people will outnumber children under the age of 10 by 2030 and that by 2050 they will outnumber youth ages 10–24. Globally the number of people over 80 will increase threefold between 2017 and 2050.[8] With an aging population, earlier detection of diseases, and better treatments, a growing number of people are living longer with a greater number of comorbidities and new medications to treat them. Patients of the future will be undoubtedly be more medically complex.

Are massage curricula geared up for these changing demographics? Are therapists sufficiently trained to adjust their treatment plans for more complicated scenarios? Are they given adequate supervised experience in school clinics and in health care settings? The massage curriculum of the future may need to be less about sports massage and more about addressing the needs of medically complex people.

Summary

Many bodywork disciplines are centered around elemental theory, which involves the archetypal energies of fire, earth, air, and water. Therapists who work in this realm help clients find balance and expression between the elements. Elemental theory can also be applied to the spirit of the times. The upcoming era will be one that emphasizes the air element – ideas, inventiveness, quick movement, and technology – all associated with the head. Finding ways to stay connected to the earth element will be vital. The body is one such way. Touch therapies can play an essential role in facilitating healing and balance.

Today's complementary practitioners bring comfort and help to manage symptoms, yet they have the potential to be so much more. Massage therapists can serve as a bridge between clinical practice and human needs, providing essential contact as health care is practiced at arm's length. This bridge, where technology and heart are joined, is the space where integration and healing take place.

Chapter SIXTEEN

When sick, we want someone to care for us, "someone with scientific knowledge" to express care. Enhanced, specialized training and experience will help touch therapists assume their places as respected clinical team members at the hospital bedside. Massage therapists need improved training, but they must also rise to the occasion of a future that requires unprecedented vision, ambition, and creativity. There is great opportunity for growth in this challenge, both professional and personal. The moment is ours for the making.

References

1. Harris R. As artificial intelligence moves into medicine, the human touch could be a casualty. 2019. Available from: https://www.npr.org/sections/health-shots/2019/04/30/718413798/as-artificial-intelligence-moves-into-medicine-the-human-touch-could-be-a-casual.

2. Academic Collaborative for Integrative Health. Hospital Based Massage Therapy: Competencies for Optimal Practice in Integrated Environments. 2017. Available from: https://static1.squarespace.com/static/55861f1ae4b01ea9a58583a7/t/5b365b-12352f537eda523d69/1530288918205/HBMT_Competencies_2018.pdf.

3. Jain S, Hammerschlag R, Mills P, Cohen L, Krieger R, Vieten C, Lutgendorf S. Clinical Studies of Biofield Therapies: Summary, Methodological Challenges, and Recommendations. 2015. Available from: https://www.ncbi.nlm.nih.gov/pmc/articles/PMC4654788/.

4. Baldwin A. Reiki in Clinical Practice: A Science-Based Guide. Edinburgh: Handspring Publishing; 2020.

5. WHO. Obesity and overweight. 2020. Available from: https://www.who.int/news-room/fact-sheets/detail/obesity-and-overweight.

6. Finklestein EA, Khavjou OA, Thompson H, Trogdon JG, Sherry B, Dietz W. Obesity and severe obesity forecasts through 2030. 2012. Available from: https://www.ajpmonline.org/article/S0749-3797(12)00146-8/fulltext.

7. Dobbs R, Swinburn B. Global obesity threat. McKinsey Global Institute. 2015. Available from: https://www.mckinsey.com/mgi/overview/in-the-news/the-global-obesity-threat.

8. United Nations. World Population Ageing 2017 Highlights. 2017. Available from: https://www.un.org/en/development/desa/population/publications/pdf/ageing/WPA2017_Highlights.pdf.

APPENDIX

Therapist Name _____   Date ___ / ___ / ___

Client Name _____   Age _____

Setting _____

Condition of Client
(current medical condition, areas of physical pain or discomfort, special needs, mental and emotional state, etc.)

_____

_____

_____

_____

Before session: _____ physical pain or discomfort (0 = none 10 = highest level)

_____ emotional pain or discomfort (0 = none 10 = highest level)

Action Taken
(massage techniques used, parts of body touched, position of client, length of session)

_____

_____

_____

Response of Client
(physiological changes noted during and after the session, i.e. breathing and changes in body tissues, nonverbal feedback, verbal feedback, etc.)

_____

_____

_____

After session: _____ physical pain or discomfort (0 = none 10 = highest level)

_____ emotional pain or discomfort (0 = none 10 = highest level)

Evaluation
(expectations or plan for next session, recommendations to client, suggestions to other caregivers, etc.)

_____

_____

_____

Appendix A Sample CARE notes. Copyright © 2019 Mary Kathleen Rose.

OB/GYN Massage Patient Data Form

Part A: (Nurse)

Patient name _Anna Kim_   DOB _11/20/95_

Unit _MBu_   Room _42_   Nurse _Kathy_   Today's date _01/05/21_

Dx _____   Dx procedure _____

Surgery _C-Section_   Surgery date _01/05/21_

Sensory impairment: ☐ Blind   ☐ HOH   ☐ Speech

Pressure restrictions: (Y) N

☐ DVT   ☐ Phlebitis   ☐ Varicose veins   ☐ Long-term bedrest   ☐ Easy bruising   ☒ Recent surgery

Site restrictions: (Y) N   **Position restrictions:** (Y) N

_____ Skin condition	_____ Epidural	☐ No walking ☐ Lie flat
Abd. Incision	_____ Diagnostic monitor	☒ No prone ☐ No side-lying
_____ Infection	_____ Labor stim points	_____ Elevate extremity or head
(L) wrist IV site	_____ Severe varicosity	

Gloving required: Y (N)

☐ Open wound (patient or LMT)   ☐ Skin condition   ☐ Presence of body fluids

Check if the patient has any of the following conditions:

☐ Hepatitis   ☐ Herpes   ☐ Other contagious disease   ☐ Allergy to lotion

Other: _On pain meds_

Part B: (Patient)

Has the patient ever received a professional massage?   Y (N)

What would the patient like from the massage session?

Subjective – _Relief from headache and fatigue, Relaxation._

Part C: SOAP Notes (Therapist)

Objective – _Flat facial expression, untalkative. Restricted movement in neck. Trapezius and levators tight on both sides._

Action – _Semi-reclining position : moderate pressure effleurage and petrissage to upper back, neck, & occiput. Effleurage and acupressure to face & scalp._

Progress – _Began smiling half way through. Pain rating dropped from 7 to 2._

Therapist's name – _Monica Southwell_   Length of session _30 min._

Appendix B Sample SOAP notes. Developed by Gayle MacDonald

Massage Therapy Session Note

You will need to type this into the open dialogue box EVERY TIME:
PAL CARE Massage Therapy Note

Time: _20:30_-20:50_ (this will be exact time your spent with your hands touching the patient)

Was patient receptive to massage? Explain briefly.
Patient was receptive, but tired and expressed that he may need to stop the session if he became too exhausted; also slightly nauseated

Was family present?

Yes, for whole session
Yes, for beginning of session
No
Other (explain briefly)

Patient's aunt came to visit in middle of session; patient was glad to see aunt

Briefly describe patient position and any changes made to position during session and reason for changes. Session supine

Please indicate areas of the body addressed, approximate amount of time spent on each, Walton Scale pressure and use of lotion

Head 5 minutes; pressure 2; no lotion

Neck 2 minutes; pressure 1; lotion

Shoulders 5 minutes; pressure 2; no lotion

Feet 10 minutes; pressure 3; lotion

Legs

Arms

Hands 10 minutes; pressure 3; lotion

Back 3 minutes; pressure 1; lotion

Please describe any adjustments to technique made as a result of medical appliances, patient comfort, side effects/complaints unrelated to massage, physiological concerns, etc.

Pt indicated that he was having pain in his L shoulder and would prefer not to lie on that side; pt also has active DVT in R gastroc, so did not work with R leg

Were there any interruptions (family/visitor arrival, nursing, etc)

Respiratory therapy arrived, but indicated that they would come back after the session was complete

How was patient dressed? Fully clothed? Hospital gown? Partially undressed to allow skin to skin contact?

Patient wore hospital gown

Please make any additional notes on the back of this page.

Appendix C Example EHR entry. Courtesy of Cal Cates, Healwell.

Intake Form: Oncology Massage in the Hospital			
Name of patient:		Room:	Date:
Name of MT:			
Date and reason for admission:			
Type of cancer + location:			
Metastases/location:			

Physical condition	Yes/no	Location	Remarks
Fever?			
Lymph nodes removed?			
Lymphedema?			
Neuropathy?			
DVT/thrombosis/pulmonary embolism?			
Surgery			
Radiotherapy			
Chemotherapy			
Immunotherapy			
Low blood counts?			
Pain?			
Pain medication?			
Delirium/confused/stress/mood?			
Infectious diseases/wounds?			
Isolation? If yes, what type?			
Other complaints/diseases			
Other remarks			

Appendix D Courtesy of Estelle Smits; English version. *Continued*

Report

- Contraindications:

- Adjustments:

- Pressure level/duration:

- Massage description:

- Reaction of patient:

- MT findings during/after massage:

- Notes for medical staff:

Appendix D Courtesy of Estelle Smits; English version.

UCSF Reflexology Foot Massage During Chemotherapy

Provided by UCSF Osher Center for Integrative Medicine
Evaluation Form

Date: _____

This is a pilot program and your feedback is greatly appreciated in helping us evaluate it. Please circle the number that best describes your answer.

Overall, how would you rate your experience?

Excellent	Good	Average	Poor	Very Poor
5	4	3	2	1

How did foot massage impact your chemotherapy session today, compared to previous chemotherapy sessions without foot massage?

Much Better	Slightly Better	About the Same	Slightly Worse	Much Worse
5	4	3	2	1

Would you recommend this foot massage to others receiving chemotherapy?

Definitely	Probably	Maybe/Not Sure	Probably Not	Definitely Not
5	4	3	2	1

Any additional comments? (Optional)

_____

_____

_____

_____

_____

This program is sponsored in part by: **UCSF** Health
Osher Center for
Integrative Medicine

Appendix E Courtesy of UCSF Osher Center for Integrative Medicine

BMT/SCT Inpatient Massage Therapy
Practitioner Pre and Post Session Intake

Please put patient label here

We would appreciate hearing about your experience with massage therapy as a patient at UCSF Medical Center.

Circle the number that represents how you are feeling after your massage therapy session.

Areas of massage therapy session focus (list here): _____

AFTER SESSION

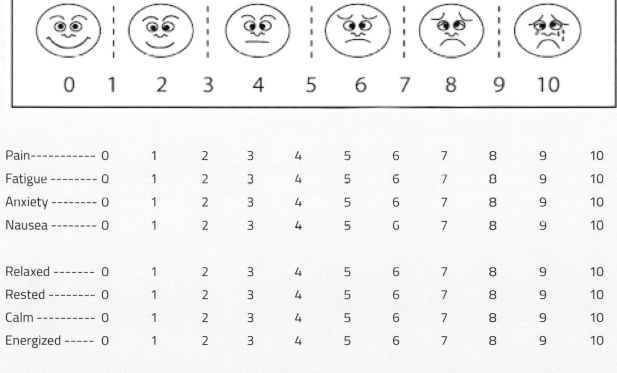

	0	1	2	3	4	5	6	7	8	9	10
Pain-----------	0	1	2	3	4	5	6	7	8	9	10
Fatigue ---------	0	1	2	3	4	5	6	7	8	9	10
Anxiety --------	0	1	2	3	4	5	6	7	8	9	10
Nausea --------	0	1	2	3	4	5	6	7	8	9	10
Relaxed -------	0	1	2	3	4	5	6	7	8	9	10
Rested --------	0	1	2	3	4	5	6	7	8	9	10
Calm -----------	0	1	2	3	4	5	6	7	8	9	10
Energized -----	0	1	2	3	4	5	6	7	8	9	10

On a scale of 0 to 10 (10 being best) - how satisfied were you with your massage? _____

Patient Comments: _____

_____

_____

_____

Appendix F Courtesy of UCSF Osher Center for Integrative Medicine

TEST ANSWERS

Chapter 2

1. F
2. F
3. T
4. T
5. F
6. F
7. T
8. F
9. T
10. F
11. T
12. T

Chapter 3

1. F
2. T
3. T
4. F
5. F

6. T
7. F
8. F
9. T
10. F
11. F
12. F

Chapter 5

Multiple choice:

1. B, C
2. B, C
3. B
4. A
5. A, D

True or False:

1. T
2. F
3. T
4. T
5. F

6. F
7. F
8. F
9. T
10. F
11. T
12. F

Chapter 6

1. A, B
2. A
3. A, B, C, D
4. B, C, D
5. A, B
6. A, B, D
7. A, B, D
8. A

Chapter 7

1. B
2. A, C, D

3. No correct answer.
4. D
5. A, B, C
6. A, B, C
7. A, B, C, D
8. A, B, D
9. A, B, C, D
10. B, C, D
11. C
12. B, C, D
13. A, B, C, D
14. B
15. C, D

Chapter 8

1. A, B, C
2. C, D
3. B, C, D
4. A, D
5. B, D
6. B

Test answers

7. C, D

8. B

9. A, B

10. A, B, D

11. A, B, C

12. B, D

13. A, B, C, D

Chapter 9

1. A, B, C

2. B

3. Matching: 1-D; 2-E; 3-B; 4-C; 5-A

Chapter 10

1. C

2. B

3. C

---

4. A

5. B

6. C

7. C

8. B

9. C

10. A

Chapter 12

1. T

2. T

3. F

4. F

5. T

6. F

7. T

---

8. T

9. T

10. F

Chapter 13

1. A

2. A, C

3. B

4. A, C, D

5. A, D

6. A, C

7. C

8. A

9. B, C, D

10. A, C, D

Chapter 14

1. B

2. C

3. D

4. B, C

5. D

6. B, C

7. A

8. A, B, C

Chapter 15

1. Objective

2. Electronic

3. Narrative

4. Subjective

5. Template

INDEX

Note: Boxes, figures, and tables are indicated by b, f, or t respectively following page numbers.

A

Academic Collaborative for Integrative Health (ACIH), 320
  hospital-based competencies, 320b
  Hospital-Based Massage Therapy Task Force of, 320
Accessories, in medical facilities, 46
Acetaminophen, and massage, 209b
ACIH. *See* Academic Collaborative for Integrative Health
Active dying, 300–301
  clinical considerations, 301
  mottling during, 300f
  offering massage during, 300
Activities of daily living (ADL), 117
Acupressure, 321
Addiction, 107–110
  drug and alcohol recovery, 108
  mood disorders, 109
  co-occurring conditions, 107, 110
  touch therapy, 107–108
  trauma, 108–109
Adornments, in medical facilities, 46
Agitation, at end of life, 290
Airborne isolation, 83
ALS. *See* Amyotrophic lateral sclerosis
Amyotrophic lateral sclerosis (ALS), 133–134
Analgesics, 207–209
  antipyretics, 208
  narcotics, 207–208
  non-narcotic, 208
  nonsteroidal anti-inflammatory drugs, 209
Aneurysm, 117
Angina, 115
Anorexia, at end of life, 287
Antenatal, 135
Anti-Alzheimer's drugs, 210
Antianxiety drugs, 210
Antibiotic-resistant organisms, 77b
Antibiotics, 210–211

Anticoagulants, 211
Anticonvulsants, 211–212
Antidepressants, 212
Antidiabetics, 212–213
Antiemetics, 213–214
Antifungals (systemic), 214
Antilipemics, 216–217
Antiplatelet medications, 217
Antipyretics, 208
Antispasmodics (skeletal muscle relaxants), 214–215
Antitumor (antineoplastic) drugs, 215–216
Antiviral and antiretroviral drugs, 216
Anxiety
  at end of life, 288–289
  research studies of massage in treatment of, 7
Apnea
  at end of life, 289–290
Armstrong, Karen, 239
Aromatherapy, 263–275
  aroma diffuser, 273, 273f
  aromapatch, 272
  aromatherapy service, setting up, 265–266
  blends, 270
    for malodor, 273b
    naming, 270
    nausea, 272b
  defining/understanding, 264–265
  essential oils. *See* Essential oils
  and health care, 264
  history of, 263–264
  nasal inhaler aromastick (NIAS), 271f, 272, 272f
  room spray or spritzer, 273, 273f
  tissues or cotton ball, 273, 273f
  treatment process in, 266–267, 267f
Arrhythmias, 115
Arteriosclerosis, 115
Arteriovenous fistula, 195, 196f
Arteriovenous malformation (AVM), 117

Arthroscope, 195
Ascites, 153–154
  clinical considerations, 154
  malignant, 153
Atherosclerosis, 115
Authentic communication, to build therapeutic relationships, 61–64
  holding space, 62
  motivational interviewing, 63–64
  patients under stress, understanding, 61–62
  practitioner vulnerability, 62–63
  therapeutic active listening, 62

B

Baldwin, Ann, 321
Bedside chart, 305
Benzodiazepines, 203
Beta-blockers, 217
Biopsy, 192
Blood poisoning, 123
Body mechanics, during massage session, 250–253, 251f, 252f, 253f
Bodyworkers, 45, 47
Brachytherapy, 113
Brain shunts, 186
Bruising and bleeding, 154–156
  applying lotion, 155
  clinical considerations, 156
  platelet count, 155
Buckle, Jane, 264

C

CABG. *See* Coronary artery bypass graft
Cachexia, at end of life, 287
Calvert, Robert, 1
Cancer, 110–114
  chemotherapy, 110, 111–112
  immunotherapy, 112
  metastasis, 110, 111

radiation therapy,   113
   surgery in,   114
   targeted drug therapies,   112
   vaccines,   112
Cardiac ablation,   192
Cardiac catheters and devices,   182–185
   clinical considerations,   182–183
   defibrillators,   183–184
   pacemakers,   183–184
   stents,   182–183
   Swan-Ganz catheter,   184–185
Cardiac glycosides,   217–218
Cardiac procedures,   192–194
   arrhythmia treatments,   192
   cardiac ablation,   192
   catheterization procedure,   192–193
   clinical considerations,   194
   open-heart surgery,   193
Cardiology patients
   massage research studies,   14, 15t–19t
Cardiovascular diseases (CVDs),   114–119
   anticoagulants in,   114
   arrhythmias,   115
   arteriosclerosis,   115
   atherosclerosis,   115
   congestive heart failure,   115–116
   major lifestyle changes in,   114
   myocardial infarction,   116
   stroke,   117–119
Cardiovascular drugs,   216–219
   antilipemics,   216–217
   antiplatelet medications,   217
   beta-blockers,   217
   cardiac glycosides,   217–218
   vasodilators,   218
Care/caring,   61–69
   authentic communication and,   61–64
   diversity, equity and inclusion,   67–68
   equality of,   52–53
   self-care practices,   68–69
   skillful compassion,   64–67
   spectrum of,   66t
   team,   47–50
Carrier oils,   269
Catheters,   178–182
central venous catheters,   180
   external urinary catheters,   179–180
   Foley catheter,   179, 179f

intravenous catheters,   180–182
peripherally inserted central catheter
   (PICC),   75, 180
   Swan-Ganz catheter,   184–185
Cellulitis,   123
Central venous catheters,   180
Chaplains,   49
Charts,   305–306
   bedside chart,   305
   electronic health record,   306
   kardex,   305
   medical chart,   306
Chemotherapy-induced peripheral
   neuropathy (CIPN),   170
Chronic obstructive pulmonary disease
   (COPD),   157–158
CIPN. *See* Chemotherapy-induced peripheral
   neuropathy
Cirrhosis,   128
Clever, Linda,   67
Clostridioides difficile (C. diff),   72, 231
Clothing, in medical facilities,   46
Collection devices,   178, 178f
Colostomy bags,   187
Colposcope,   195
Compression devices,   185, 185f
Computed tomography (CT),   199
Conflict of interest,   58
Confusion,   at end of life,   290
Congestive heart failure,   115–116
   drug combinations for,   219b
Constipation,   156–157
   acupressure points for,   157
   clinical considerations,   157
   at end of life,   291
   massaging abdomen,   157f
   research studies of massage in treatment
      of,   10–11
Contact isolation,   84
Contact Precautions sign,   82f
Continuous glucose monitors,   188–189
Continuous passive motion device,   189
COPD. *See* Chronic obstructive pulmonary
   disease
Coronary artery bypass graft (CABG),   193
Coronary artery bypass graft (CABG)
   surgery,   115
Corticosteroids,   219

Craniosacral Therapy,   92, 252f
Cystoscope,   195

D

Data Protection Act 1998,   53
Deep vein thrombosis (DVT),   172
Defibrillators,   183–184
Dementia,   132
Depression
   research studies of massage in
      treatment of,   11
Dermatitis,   163
Diabetes,   119–121
   clinical considerations,   121
   drug combinations for,   213b
   influences of,   120
   low blood sugar, signs and
      symptoms of,   121
   patients with uncontrolled,   120
Diuretics,   117, 219–220
Documentation,   305–317
   bedside chart,   305
   charts,   305–306
   disposing of documents,   313b
   electronic health record,   306
   kardex,   305
   medical chart,   306
   medical record, guidelines for
      charting in,   306–316
   narrative style,   309–310, 310f
   patient evaluations and feedback
      forms,   315
   progress note,   307f,
      310–312, 309f, 310f
   purpose of,   305
   SOAP format,   308f, 311–314
   styles of,   307–311
Drains,   185–187
Droplet isolation,   83–84
Drugs/medication. *See also* specific drug
   types
   common side effects of,   206b
   most prescribed, list of,   203b
   reference table for manual
      therapists,   204t–205t
Dunn, Tedi,   244
Dyspnea,   157–158

causes of, 158
chronic obstructive pulmonary
disease, 157–158
clinical considerations, 158
at end of life, 291–292
organ failure and, 158

E

Edema, 159
at end of life, 292
Edematous tissues, 159
Electrocardiograph (ECG) monitors, 188
Electronic health record (EHR),
227–228, 306
additional guidelines for, 314
guidelines for charting in, 314–316
orders, 229
simulated chart note template, 316f
Emesis bag, 178f
Emphysema, 158
EMR template, 239f
End of life
active dying, 300–301
adapting massage for, 285–286
anorexia and cachexia at, 287
anxiety at, 288–289
apnea at, 289–290
common symptoms at, 286–296
confusion, agitation and restlessness
at, 290
constipation at, 291
dying in hospital, 283–284
dyspnea at, 291–292
early decline, 297–298
edema at, 292
fatigue, 292–293
fractures and other injuries, 293
functional period, 297
late decline, 298–299
loss of communication, 293
loss of mobility, 294, 294f
pain during, 294–295
pre-active dying, 289–300, 289f, 301
self-care, 302
skin change during, 297
stages of dying, 296–302

Endoscopy, 194–195
Energy medicine, 320–321
Equality of care, 52–53
Escherichia coli (E. coli), 85
Essential oils (EOs), 264
approved, 266b
chemistry and safety of, 267–269
dilution ratio of carrier oil, 271t
dropping into carrier oil, 270f
extracted from different plant
parts, 280t–281t
fragrance notes in, 268b
in health care setting, ways to
use, 270–274
properties of, 267
Rose otto, 263b
storing, 268
synergistic effect, 270
therapeutic action of, 269–275
on tissue, 273, 273f
Etiquette
in health care settings, 58
toward patients, visitors, and
staff, 56–58, 56f
European Centre for Disease Prevention and
Control (ECDC), 72
Evidence-informed practice (EIP), 5, 5b
evidence, levels of, 5b
External beam radiation, 113
External urinary catheters, 179–180
Extubation, 190

F

Fatigue, 160–161
at end of life, 292–293
research studies of massage in
treatment of, 11
Fatty liver disease, 127–128
Fetal monitor, 188
Fever, 161–162
Fluid replacement, 220
Foley catheter, 179, 179f
Fowler's position, 99, 100f, 135, 154
Functional magnetic resonance imaging
(fMRI), 199

G

Gaia Principle, 3
Gastric residual volume (GSV), 22
Gastric stimulator, 195
Gattefosse, Rene-Maurice, 264
Geriatric patients
massage research studies, 19, 20f,
20t–22t
Geriatrics, 121–122
Global Health Security Agenda, 71
Gloves
for giving massage, 78
types of, 78
use in different situations, 78–79
Gloving, 77–79, 80f
doffing, 79, 80f
donning, 79
Gowns or aprons, 80–81, 81f
doffing, 81, 81f
donning, 81
Graft-versus-host disease (GVHD), 142
Grooming, in medical facilities, 46
Group treatment, 257
Grumpectomy, 52
GSV. *See* Gastric residual volume
GVHD. *See* Graft-versus-host disease

H

Hand cleaning, 74–77
antimicrobial soap and water
procedure, 75–76, 76f
use of handrubs, procedure for, 76–77
Hand hygiene, 75
Health care-acquired infections (HAIs), 71
Health care workers (HCWs), 77, 78
Health Insurance Portability and
Accountability Act (HIPAA), 53
HELLP syndrome, 154
Hematopoietic drugs, 220–221
Hematopoietic stem cell transplantation
(HSCT), 141–144
allogeneic, 142
autologous, 142
clinical considerations, 143
patient feedback, 143f

recipients admitted to hospital,   142
types of,   142
vs. stem cell therapies,   141–142
Hemiparesis,   117
Hemodialysis,   194–196
   clinical considerations,   196–197
   complications,   196
Hemodialysis patient, massage to,   9f
Hepatitis,   128
High-risk pregnancy,   135–136
High-tech medicine,   3
HIPAA. *See* Health Insurance Portability and
   Accountability Act
Hospital
   bodyworkers in,   45
   dynamics,   46–47
   learning to function in,   45
   policies about massage of
      thrombocytopenic patient,   155
   professional appearance in,   45–46
Hospital-Based Massage Therapy (HBMT)
   program,   49
Housekeepers,   49
HSCT. *See* Hematopoietic stem cell
   transplantation
Hydrocephalus,   186
Hydrosols (aromatic waters),   273
Hypercoagulability,   172
Hypnotics,   223
Hypothermia,   123

I

ICU patients
   massage research studies,   22, 23t
IFPA. *See* International Federation of
   Professional Aromatherapists
Ileostomy and urostomy bags,   187
Immunity
   research studies on effect of massage
      on,   11–12
Immunosuppressants,   221–222
Immunosuppression,   162–163
Immunotherapy, in cancer,   112
Inclusion criteria for research studies,   6
Infection control practices
   exposure to body fluids and,   85
   fingernail length,   85–86
   handling of work clothes,   85

infection control techniques,   74–82
kneeling on floor,   87
lotion, use of,   86
notebooks and other items from
   outside,   86–87
overview,   71
protective practices,   72–73
ring wearing,   86
Standard Precautions,   73–74
staying at home,   87
Transmission-Based Precautions,   82–86
Infection control techniques,   74–82
   gloving,   77–79, 80f
   gowning, masking, and gloving in
      combination,   82
   gowns or aprons,   us of, 80–81, 81f
   hand cleaning,   74–77
   masking,   79–80, 80f
Infections,   122–124
   cellulitis,   123
   clinical considerations,   124
   pneumonia,   122–123
   septicemia,   123
   urinary tract infections,   123–124
Inflammation,   163
Intake form, massage therapy,   233,
   315f–316f
   bilingual, section of,   241f
   completed,   238f
   pre and post session,   235f
Intensive care unit, massage therapy
   in,   124–126
   communication with patient,   125
   maintain physical contact with
      patient,   125
   safe massage in, requirements of,
      124–125
   session planning for massage in,   124
   skills required for,   124
International Federation of Professional
   Aromatherapists (IFPA),   268–269
Intravenous catheters,   180–182

J

Jacket defibrillator,   184
Jain, Shamani,   321
Jonas, Wayne,   67
J-pouch,   187

K

Kahn, Janet,   6
Kardex,   305
Kidney disease,   126–127
   acute, 126–127
   chronic,   126
   clinical considerations,   127
   end-stage,   127
   peritoneal dialysis in,   127

L

Laparoscope,   195
Laxatives,   222
Leukopenia,   162
Lewis, Rhiannon,   272
Lewy body dementia,   129
Liability,   55
Linen handling,   84–85
Liver disease,   127–129
   cirrhosis,   128
   clinical considerations,   128–129
   end stage,   128
   fatty liver disease,   127–128
   hepatitis,   128
Loss of mobility, at end of life, 294, 294f
Lotion
   for bruising and bleeding,   155
   for infection control,   86
   massage,   249
Lou Gehrig's disease,   132
Lovelock, James,   3
Lumbar puncture,   197–198
Lymphedema,   163–167
   clinical considerations,   166–167
   lymphatic basics,   164–165
   massage adjustments,   165–166
   massaging person with,   167f

M

Magnetic resonance imaging (MRI),   199
Manual therapists, medications reference
   table for,   204t–205t
Masking,   79–80, 80f
Massage
   history of,   1–4
   during Middle Ages,   1–2

and nursing, 2–3
Massage research studies, 5–40
    patient populations in, 13–39
        cardiology patients, 14, 15t–19t
        geriatric patients, 19, 20f, 20t–22t
        ICU patients, 22, 23t
        maternity patients, 23–24, 24t–27t
        oncology patients, 27–28, 28t–33t
        procedural interventions, 34, 34t–37t
        surgery patients, 37, 37t–39t
    variables in, 6–13
    anxiety, 7
        constipation, 10–11
        depression, 11
        fatigue, 11
        immune-related, 11–12, 27
        length of stay, 12
        lesser-studied variables, 12–13
        nausea, 10
        pain, 7–8
        pain medication and potential cost
            savings, use of, 12
        sleep, 9–10
        vital signs, 8–9
Massage session
    body mechanics during, 250–253, 251f,
        252f, 253f
    closing/ending of, 247–249
    components of, 244–250
    draping, 250
    length of, 255–256
    massage lotion, 249
    overview, 243
    patient safety during, 257–258
    skillful communication during start
        of, 247
    starting, 246–247, 246f
    tasks after, 258–259
    tasks before, 243–244
    touch modalities for medically complex
        patient, 253–255
    touch session, suggestions for, 256–257
Massage sessions for staff, 50
Massage therapy intake form, 233
Matched unrelated donor (MUD), 142
Maternity patients
massage research studies, 23–24, 24t–27t
Maury, Marguerite, 264

McIntosh, Nina, 50
Measure Yourself Concerns and Wellbeing
        (MYCaW), 267
Measure Yourself Medical Outcome Profile
        (MYMOP), 267
Medical chart, 306
Medical devices, 177, 178t
    brain shunts, 186
    cardiac catheters and devices, 182–185
    catheters, 178–182
    collection devices, 178
    colostomy bags, 187, 187f
    compression devices, 185, 185f
    drains, 185–187
    emesis bag, 178f
    ileostomy and urostomy bags, 187
    monitors, 188–189
    orthopedic devices and equipment,
        189–190
    oxygen delivery devices, 190–191
    pain management devices, 191
    resections and collection bags, 187–188
    shunts, 186–187
    tubes, 186–187
Mennell, James, 92
Methicillin-resistant *Staphylococcus aureus*
        (MRSA), 72, 75
Micra pacemakers, 183
Military Massage Corps, 2
MND. *See* Motor neurone disease
Monitors, 188–189
Motivational interviewing, 63–64
Motor neurone disease (MND), 133–134
Multiple gated acquisition (MUGA)
        scan, 200
Multiple sclerosis, 132
MYCaW. *See* Measure Yourself Concerns and
        Wellbeing
MYMOP. *See* Measure Yourself Medical
        Outcome Profile
Myoclonus, 300–301

N

NAFLD. *See* Nonalcoholic fatty liver disease
Naisbitt, John, 4, 319
Narcotics, 156, 207–208
Nasal cannula, 190

NASH. *See* Nonalcoholic steatohepatitis
Nasogastric (NG) tube, 186
Nausea and vomiting, 167–168
    acupressure points for, 168
    clinical considerations, 168
    controlling, 168
    research studies of massage in treatment
        of, 10
Networking, within medical setting, 49
Neurological disorders, 129–134
    amyotrophic lateral sclerosis, 133–134
    dementia, 132
    multiple sclerosis, 132
    Parkinson's disease, 132–133
    spinal cord injury, 129–130
    traumatic brain injury, 129
NHS Care Record Guarantee, 53
Nightingale, Florence, 74
Nociceptive pain, 295
Nonalcoholic fatty liver disease
        (NAFLD), 127–128
Nonalcoholic steatohepatitis (NASH), 128
Nonsteroidal anti-inflammatory drugs
        (NSAIDs), 209
Nursing
    massage and, 2–3
    staff, interacting with, 48
Nursing assistant/medical assistant, role
        of, 49

O

Obstetrics (OB), 134–138
    antenatal, 135
    clinical considerations, 137–138
    C-sections, overuse of, 135
    high-risk pregnancy, 135–136
    labor and delivery, 136–137
    postnatal, 137
    pregnant patient in left side-lying
        position, 135f
Oncology patients
    massage research studies, 27–28,
        28t–33t
Opioid, crisis in America, 207b
Opioid analgesics, 207–208
Orders, 228–230
    combination of methods, 229–230

electronic health record, 229
initiating, via text, 229
note in medical chart, 229
obtaining, 228–229
signed, 229
standing, 229
verbal, 230
Organ transplantation, 138–140
clinical considerations, 139–140
drug combinations for, 221b–222b
post-transplant, 139
pre-transplant, 138
Orogastric tube, 186
Orthopedic devices and equipment, 189–190
clinical considerations, 190
traction devices, 189
Orthopedic patients, 140–141
clinical considerations, 141
positioning of, 140
Oxygen delivery devices, 190–191

P

Pacemakers, 183–184
Pain, 168–170
applying heat for, 295
approach of cultures to, 169
clinical considerations, 170
during end of life, 294–295
explaining, 169b
medication, 12
nociceptive, 295
non-pharmacologic treatment modalities, Joint Commission reviews of, 9b
research studies of massage in treatment of, 7–8
Pain management devices, 191
Parkinson's disease, 132–133
Pathogenic substances, potential, 73b
Patient-controlled analgesia (PCA), 191
Patient data, collection of, 230–240
contractors or third-party massage therapy providers, 240
intake information from nurse, 232–239
intake taken directly with patient, 239–240
medical health record, consulting, 231

medical health record vs. nurse, consulting, 231–232
skillful interviewing for, 234–239
Patient evaluation and feedback forms, 315
Patient privacy and confidentiality, 53–55
Patients under stress, understanding, 61–62
Patient–therapist boundaries, 50–52
Pericardial effusion, 183
Peripheral artery disease, 115
Peripherally inserted central catheter (PICC), 75, 180
Peripheral neuropathy, 170–171
Persad, Randall, 120
Personal hygiene, in medical facilities, 46
Personal protection equipment (PPE), 73
Petechiae, 96
Phlebitis, 172
Pneumonia, 122–123
Polarity Therapy, 155
Portacath, 180
Positioning adjustments, 98–104
align patient hips with fold in bed, 99b
basic positions for receiving massage, 99, 100f
draw sheet, use of, 102–103, 103f–104f
indications for, 99b
propping, 101, 101f–102f
Positron emission tomography (PET), 199–200
Practitioner vulnerability, 62–63
Pre-active dying, 299–300, 299f
clinical considerations, 301
offering massage during, 300
Pregnancy-related drugs, 222
Pressure modifications, 92–96
Pressure scale for patients, in health care settings, 93t–94t
Preterm labor, 135
Private practitioner, 230
Procedures (medical), 191–192
Professional appearance, in hospital, 45–46
Progress note, 307f, 310–312, 310f, 311f
Propping, 101, 101f–102f
Protected information, of patient, 53b
Protective practices, 72–73

Pulmonary embolism (PE), 158, 172–173
Pulse ox, 188, 189f

Q

Qualitative studies, 5
Quantitative data, 6
Quasi-experimental design, 6

R

Randomized controlled trial (RCT), 5, 6
Referrals, 227–228
getting new, 230
Reiki, 6, 11, 97, 145, 159, 286, 321
above body, 110
for medically complex patient, 253
practitioners, 74
in thrombocytopenic patients, 111
Resections and collection bags, 187–188
Restlessness, at end of life, 290
Reverse/protective isolation, 84
Rose otto, 263b

S

Scans, 198–200
computed tomography, 199
functional magnetic resonance imaging (fMRI), 199
magnetic resonance imaging (MRI), 199
multiple gated acquisition (MUGA), 200
nuclear imaging, 199, 200
positron emission tomography (PET), 199–200
ultrasound, 200
X-rays, 198–200
Scope of practice, for massage therapists, 55–56
Sedatives, 223
Self-care practices, 68–69
Semmelweis, Ignaz, 74
Sepsis, 123
Septicemia, 123
Shunts, 186–187
Signed orders, 229
Site considerations, 96–97, 97b

Skillful compassion, to build therapeutic relationships, 64–67
  compassion, 65
  empathy, 65
  in patient–practitioner conversation, examples of, 67
  sympathy, 65
Skin conditions, of hospital patient, 171–172
Sleep
  research studies of massage in treatment of, 9–10
SOAP format, documentation in, 308f, 311–314
  action, 312
  categories, 311
  charting examples, 313–314, 313–314f
  objective data, 312
  progress, 312
  signature, 312
  subjective data, 312
Social media awareness, 54b
Social workers, 49
Spasticity, 117
Spinal cord injury (SCI), 129–130
Staff (hospital)
  educating, 50
  etiquette toward, 56–58, 56f
  massage sessions for, 50
  medical, engagement with, 48
  nursing, interacting with, 48
  working with, 47–50
Standard Precautions, 72, 73–74
Standing orders, 229
Statins, 115
Stem cell transplantation, 141–144
  matched unrelated donor, 142
Stenosis, 115
Sternotomy, 193
Stroke, 117–119
  clinical considerations, 119
  hemiparesis, 117
  ischemic, 117
  positioning in caring of stroke survivors, 118

  spasticity and, 117, 118
Superficial lymph drainage patterns, 164f
Surgery patients, 144–145
  massage research studies, 37, 37t–39t
Swan-Ganz catheter, 184–185
Swedish massage, in edema, 159

T

Targeted drug therapies, in cancer, 112
Team care, 47–50
  chaplains, 49
  educating staff, 50
  engagement with medical staff, 48
  housekeepers, 49
  interacting with nursing staff, 48
  massage sessions for staff, 50
  networking within the medical setting, 49
  nursing assistant/medical assistant, role of, 49
  social workers, 49
  unit secretaries, 49
Technology, 3–4, 6, 319
TENS. *See* Transcutaneous electrical nerve stimulation
Therapeutic active listening, 62
Therapeutic relationships
  authentic communication for, 61–64
  definition of, 61
  habits for successful, 68
  skillful compassion for, 64–67
Thromboemboli, 172
Thrombolytics, 223
Thrombophlebitis, 172
Thrombosis, 172–173
Total parenteral nutrition (TPN), 13
Touch modalities, for medically complex patient, 253–255
Touch session, suggestions for, 256–257
Touch therapy session workflow, 243f
Tracheotomy tube, 190
Traction devices, 189
Training, 319–320
  competencies and, 320

  in hands-on modalities, 3
Transcutaneous electrical nerve stimulation (TENS), 191
Transient ischemic attacks (TIAs), 117
Transmission-Based Precautions, 72, 82–86
  airborne isolation, 83
  contact isolation, 84
  droplet isolation, 83–84
  linen handling, 84–85
  reverse/protective isolation, 84
Traumatic brain injury (TBI), 129
Tubes, 186–187

U

Ultrasound, 201
Unit secretaries, 49
Urinary tract infection (UTI), 123–124

V

VAD. *See* Ventricular assist device
Valnet, Jean, 264
Vancomycin-resistant *Enterococcus* (VRE) species, 75, 77b, 85
Vasodilators, 218
Ventricular assist device (VAD), 138
Verbal orders, 230
Vital signs
  research studies of massage in treatment of, 8–9

W

Walton, Tracy, 40
Werner, Ruth, 94
Whole systems research (WSR), 5
Wounds, incision and drainage of, 197
WSR. *See* Whole systems research

Z

Zuther, Joachim, 165